Principles of Clinical Research

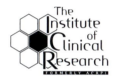

Principles of Clinical Research

edited by

Ignazio Di Giovanna
Director, CCA2000 Ltd, East Horsley, Surrey, UK

Gareth Hayes
Executive Liaison Officer, The Institute of Clinical Research,
Maidenhead, Berkshire, UK

WRIGHTSON BIOMEDICAL PUBLISHING LTD
Petersfield, UK and Philadelphia, USA

The Institute of Clinical Research is an organisation for all clinical development professionals; it is respected as a key decision-maker and body of expertise with regard to the scientific, ethical and practical conduct of clinical research. Its aims are to increase the standing of its members and of clinical research in general.

PO Box 1208, Maidenhead
Berkshire SL6 3GD, UK
Telephone: 44 (0)1628 829900
E-mail: info@instituteofclinicalresearch.org
Website: http://www.instituteofclinicalresearch.org

Published by:

Wrightson Biomedical Publishing Ltd
Ash Barn House, Winchester Road, Stroud,
Petersfield, Hampshire GU32 3PN, UK
Telephone: 44 (0)1730 265647
Fax: 44 (0)1730 260368

British Library Cataloguing in Publication Data
Principles of clinical research
    1. Clinical medicine – Research
    I. Di Giovanna, Ignazio   II. Hayes, Gareth   III. Institute of
    Clinical Research
    610.7'2

Library of Congress Cataloging in Publication Data
A catalog record for this book is available from the Library of Congress

ISBN 1 871816 45 9

Composition by Scribe Design, Gillingham, Kent, UK
Printed in Great Britain by Biddles Ltd, Guildford

Contents

Foreword

This is a significant period in the history of The Institute of Clinical Research and I am proud to be Chairman of our esteemed organisation at this exciting time. Over the last year, a dedicated group of Institute members from a variety of disciplines have devoted a great deal of time and energy, over and above their already considerable workload, to contribute chapters on their individual areas of expertise. The second edition of the *Handbook of Clinical Research*, published in 1994 and reprinted in 1997, was highly valued by all those working within the clinical research arena. However, the intervening years have witnessed enormous changes in clinical research, and it was felt that it would no longer be sufficient merely to revise the *Handbook* again. To reflect this period of change and to more accurately describe the scope and focus of the contributed chapters, the book has also been given a new title – *Principles of Clinical Research*.

I have no doubt that *Principles of Clinical Research* will prove to be even more valuable than its predecessors and that it will provide an appropriate complement to other Institute publications and to the Institute's educational programmes. *Principles of Clinical Research* will not only be useful as a textbook for those new to clinical research, it will also prove a sound source of reference for those with greater experience.

PENNY MAGUIRE
Chairman, The Institute of Clinical Research

Preface

Clinical research is a multidisciplinary, multibillion, multinational industry, governed by many complex and interrelated regulations and guidelines. Changes in working practices, company mergers, technological developments, and other factors have led to changes in personnel and management structures, affecting sponsor organisations, as well as CRO companies and study sites. The clinical researcher needs to be multidisciplined and to work alongside like-minded colleagues who complement and support the development of health care products across international borders. It is therefore vitally important that each person involved in clinical research has an understanding of other activities in order to grasp the 'big picture' and further develop the way they work. Hence, each chapter in this book is relevant to us all, not only in the pharmaceutical industry but also in academic research, as more and more 'pure' research comes under the same scrutiny as industry-sponsored research programmes.

This book builds on the success of its predecessor, the *Handbook of Clinical Research*. The reader will find that many of the chapters carried over have been simplified in a conscious effort to highlight the general principles governing each subject, hence our title: *Principles of Clinical Research*. We make no apology for omitting certain specialist topics because the scope of this book does not extend to such detail, and many chapters provide extensive bibliographies and/or suggestions for further reading for those who wish to delve deeper. Although most of the contributors are UK-based, this book has been written with an international readership in mind. It is our hope that by concentrating on principles, the book will be useful and relevant to clinical researchers wherever clinical research is conducted, despite the fact that the day of total international regulatory and ideological integration is still some way off, due to persisting differences between individual countries' requirements.

The book includes many chapters dealing with new or emerging issues: outsourcing has become commonplace in all companies to some degree; fraud and malpractice are, unfortunately, issues over which we must all be constantly vigilant; the requirement to archive the ever-increasing volume of clinical data is becoming a challenge for all companies; the development of medical devices increasingly parallels the development of pharmaceutical products; the trial master file is key to successful document management; and finally, ever-increasing competition and regulatory demands have ensured that health economics and outcomes research are among the fastest growing disciplines in clinical research.

Clinical research is a continually evolving discipline; almost by definition, change is part of its make-up and could be described as its only constant. The Declaration of Helsinki, the ICH GCP Guideline, the European Clinical Trials Directive and the Human Rights Act have all been revised/amended and/or released in the six months prior to this book going to press. Indeed, the Edinburgh revision of the Declaration of Helsinki was only issued in October 2000, and we have been able to make reference to the most relevant revisions and possible implications. The Human Rights Act came into force in the UK in October 2000, and it is too early to assess its impact on clinical research. The European Clinical Trials Directive, coming up for its second reading, will most probably come into force during the lifetime of this book, and is likely to affect early phase more than later phase clinical studies. In regard to clinical research conduct, any study that complies with ICH will undoubtedly also comply with the standards to be set by the European Directive. All these regulatory documents are underpinned by good clinical practice (GCP), which bases its human values on patient welfare and ethics control, and its scientific values on transparency of conduct and reproducibility of data.

The Institute of Clinical Research will continue to provide publications and educational programmes to support the immediate and future issues within clinical research such as gene regulation and 'e-trials'. There is no doubt, however, that this book is as up to date as it could possibly be.

This book will be of primary interest to new and recent recruits to clinical research, wherever they are based: in a pharmaceutical company, CRO, investigative site or academic institution. However, we believe it will also serve as a ready source of information and reference publications for the more experienced members in our industry. The content of each of these chapters represents the personal views of the individual authors, and not necessarily those of The Institute of Clinical Research. We are indebted to the authors for putting so much time and effort into preparing their texts; their work has been outstanding and they have our thanks. The efforts of Angie Major in providing administrative support and David Beattie in providing superb editorial services have been well beyond the call of duty. They have our utmost gratitude. It is also a pleasure to acknowledge our publisher, Judy Wrightson, and to thank her for her diligence and expert advice in bringing this book to press.

IGNAZIO DI GIOVANNA
GARETH HAYES

Contributors

Elizabeth Allen, *Guy's Drug Research Unit, 6 Newcomen Street, London SE1 1YR, UK*

Pippa Anderson, *Fourth Hurdle Consulting Ltd, 2 Fisher Street, Holborn, London WC1R 4QA, UK*

Roger Ashby, *Syne qua non Ltd, Navire House, Mere Street, Diss, Norfolk IP22 4AG, UK*

Pamela Charnley Nickols, *Charnley Nickols Associates Ltd, 6 Dove Lane, Long Eaton, Nottingham NG10 4LP, UK*

Angus Donald, *Stiefel Laboratories, Whitebrook Park, 68 Lower Cookham Road, Maidenhead, Berkshire SL6 8XY, UK*

Nina Downes, *Allergan Ltd, Coronation Road, High Wycombe, Buckinghamshire HP12 3SH, UK*

Brian D. Edwards, *Senior Director of Worldwide Pharmacovigilance, Parexel International Ltd, River Court, 50 Oxford Road, Denham, Uxbridge, Middlesex UB9 4DL, UK*

Helen Glenny, *9 Oak Piece, Welwyn, Hertfordshire AL6 0XE, UK*

Nicola Goodwin, *Millhaven, 98 Langley Road, Watford WD17 4PJ, UK*

Karen Grover, *Syne qua non Ltd, Navire House, Mere Street, Diss, Norfolk IP22 4AG, UK*

Linda Hakes, *Vice President, Preclinical Development, Schwarz Pharma AG, Alfred-Nobel-Strasse 10, D-40789 Monheim, Germany*

John Hall, *Vice President, Clinical Operations, Covalent Group Ltd, The Technology Centre, 40 Occam Road, Surrey Research Park, Guildford, Surrey GU2 5YG, UK*

Elizabeth Hooper, *Phlex Ltd, Dairy House, Churchfield Road, Chalfont St Peter, Buckinghamshire SL9 9EW, UK*

Bryan C. Hurst, *AstraZeneca plc, Mereside, Alderley Park, Macclesfield, Cheshire SK10 4TG, UK*

John Illingworth, *Clinical Development & Support Services (CDSS) Ltd, The Old Chapel, Hollin Lane, Higher Sutton, Macclesfield, Cheshire SK11 0NN, UK*

Richard Kay, *Parexel International Ltd, The Straddle, Victoria Quays, Sheffield S2 5SY, UK*

Hervé Laurent, *Président-Directeur Général, Parexel-Biostat, 15 Avenue des Droits de l'Homme, 45058 Orléans cedex 1, France*

Adam Lloyd, *Fourth Hurdle Consulting Ltd, 2 Fisher Street, Holborn, London WC1R 4QA, UK*

Julia Lloyd-Parks, *75 Springfield Park, Twyford, Berkshire RG10 9JG, UK*

Tim Mant, *Guy's Drug Research Unit, 6 Newcomen Street, London SE1 1YR, UK*

Brenda Mullinger, *Wordpower Projects, Larches, Green Road, Shipbourne, Tonbridge, Kent TN11 9PL, UK*

Paul O'Connor, *Clinical Trial Services, 9 Charlestown Road, Seagoe Industrial Estate, Craigavon BT63 5PW, Northern Ireland*

Gill Pearce, *GlaxoSmithKline, Greenford Road, Greenford, Middlesex UB6 0HE, UK*

Pauline Pentelow, *Syne qua non Ltd, Navire House, Mere Street, Diss, Norfolk IP22 4AG, UK*

Joan Perou, *16 Conway Drive, Ashford Common, Middlesex TW15 1RQ, UK*

Wolfgang Schaub, *CRO Contracts, Luisenstraße 13, D-65779 Kelkheim, Germany*

David Talbot, *Senior Clinical Project Manager, Leo Pharmaceuticals, Longwick Road, Princes Risborough, Buckinghamshire HP27 9RR, UK*

John C.C. Talbot, *Director, Global Drug Safety, AstraZeneca R & D Charnwood, Bakewell Road, Loughborough, Leicestershire LE11 5RH, UK*

Frank Wells, *MedicoLegal Investigations Ltd, Old Hadleigh, London Road, Capel St Mary, Ipswich, Suffolk IP9 2JJ, UK*

Shirley Wildey, *Quintiles (UK) Ltd, Ringside, 79 High Street, Bracknell, Berkshire RG12 1DZ, UK*

Andrew Willis, *Omnicare Clinical Research, Wessex Business Centre, Bumpers Way, Bumpers Farm, Chippenham, Wiltshire SN14 6NQ, UK*

Graham Wylie, *Medical Director, Parexel International Ltd, River Court, 50 Oxford Road, Denham, Uxbridge, Middlesex UB9 4DL, UK*

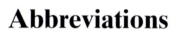

Abbreviations

ABPI	Association of the British Pharmaceutical Industry
ACE	angiotensin converting enzyme
ADR	adverse drug reaction
ADROIT	Adverse Drug Reaction On-line Information Tracking (UK)
AICRC	Association of Independent Clinical Research Contractors (UK)
AIM	active ingredient manufacturer
ALT	alanine aminotransferase (also SGPT)
ANDA	Abbreviated New Drug Application
ASPP	anonymised single patient print
AST	aspartate aminotransferase (also SGOT)
AUC	area under the curve
BMA	British Medical Association
BSE	bovine spongiform encephalopathy
BSI	British Standards Institution
CBA	cost–benefit analysis
CCOHTA	Canadian Co-ordinating Office for Health Technology Assessment
CCPPRB	Comité Consultatif de Protection des Personnes dans la Recherche Biomédicale
CDER	Center for Drug Evaluation and Research (FDA)
CD-ROM	compact disc – read-only memory
CE	conformité européenne
CEA	cost-effectiveness analysis
CFR	Code of Federal Regulations (USA)
CHF	congestive heart failure
CMA	cost-minimisation analysis
CMS	Concerned Member State
CNS	central nervous system
CPMP	Committee for Proprietary Medicinal Products
CQA	clinical quality assurance
CRA	clinical research associate = (study) monitor
CRF	case record (or report) form
CRO	contract research organisation
CSM	Committee on Safety of Medicines (UK)
CSR	clinical study report
CT	computed tomography
CTD	Common Technical Document
CTA	clinical trial administrator
CTX	Clinical Trial Exemption scheme
CUA	cost–utility analysis
CV	curriculum vitae (plural form: curricula vitae)
DCF	data clarification form
DMF	drug master file
DSMB	data safety monitoring board
DSRU	Drug Safety Research Unit (Southampton, UK)
DVD	digital versatile disc
ECG	electrocardiogram/ electrocardiography
e-CRF	electronic case record (or report) form
EEG	electroencephalogram/ electroencephalography
EMEA	European Agency for the Evaluation of Medicinal Products
EPAR	European Public Assessment Report
ESR	erythrocyte sedimentation rate

EU	European Union	MedDRA	Medical Dictionary for Regulatory Activities
EWG	Expert Working Group (ICH)		
FDA	Food and Drug Administration	MHW	Ministry of Health and Welfare (Japan)
GBP	pound sterling	MLI	MedicoLegal Investigations Limited
GCP	good clinical practice		
GLP	good laboratory practice	MREC	multicentre research ethics committee
GMC	General Medical Council		
GMM	genetically modified micro-organism	MRFG	Mutual Recognition Facilitation Group
GMO	genetically modified organism	MRI	magnetic resonance imaging
GMP	good manufacturing practice	MRP	mutual recognition procedure
GP	general practitioner	MS	Member State
GPRD	General Practice Research Database (UK)	NCE	new chemical entity
		NCR	no-carbon-required
HIV	human immunodeficiency virus	NDA	New Drug Application
		NHS	National Health Service
HMO	health maintenance organisation (US)	NICE	National Institute for Clinical Excellence
HRQoL	health-related quality of life	NSAID	non-steroidal anti-inflammatory drug
HTA	health technology assessment		
IB	investigator's brochure	NTA	Notice to Applicants
ICDP	international clinical development plan	ORI	Office of Research Integrity
		OTC	over-the-counter
ICDT	international clinical development team	PAP	product analysis print
		PASS	post-authorisation safety study
ICH	International Conference on Harmonisation of Technical Requirements for Registration of Pharmaceuticals for Human Use	PBAC	Pharmaceutical Benefits Advisory Committee (Australia)
		PCC	Professional Conduct Committee (of GMC)
IEC	independent ethics committee	PD	pharmacodynamic(s)
IND	investigational new drug	PE	pharmacoeconomics
IRB	institutional review board	PEM	prescription event monitoring
ISO	International Organization for Standardization	PFC	Professional Fees Committee (of BMA)
ISS	integrated safety summary	PIL	patient information leaflet
IT	information technology	PK	pharmacokinetic(s)
IVRS	interactive voice response system	PMS	post-marketing surveillance
		POM	prescription-only medicine
LCD	liquid crystal display	QA	quality assurance
LoI	letter of intent	QALY	quality-adjusted life year
LREC	local research ethics committee	QC	quality control
		QoL	quality of life
MAA	marketing authorisation application	RCGP	Royal College of General Practitioners (UK)
MAUI	multi-attribute utility instrument	RCT	randomised controlled trial
		R&D	research and development
MCA	Medicines Control Agency (UK)	RCP	Royal College of Physicians
		REC	research ethics committee
MDD	Medical Devices Directive	RFP	request for proposal
MDI	metered-dose inhaler	RMS	Reference Member State

SAE	serious adverse event	SMO	site management organisation
SAG	Scientific Archivists Group	SPC	summary of product
SAMM	safety assessment of marketed		characteristics
	medicines	SOP	standard operating procedure
SDV	source data verification	TMF	trial master file
SF-36	Short Form 36 (Health	USAN	United States approved name
	Survey)	USD	United States dollar
SGOT	serum glutamic-oxaloacetic	VAS	visual analogue scale
	transaminases (also AST)	WHO	World Health Organization
SGPT	serum glutamate pyruvate	WMA	World Medical Association
	transaminases (also ALT)	WTP	willingness to pay

1

The drug development process

John Hall

INTRODUCTION

This chapter will provide an overview of the lengthy and complex process of drug development. It will review the economic and legal frameworks in which the pharmaceutical industry operates worldwide and will provide a route map through the various stages of the drug development process, from discovery to the marketing of medicines. Much of the material covered briefly here will be addressed in greater depth by subject experts in later chapters.

HISTORICAL OVERVIEW

The pharmaceutical industry as such did not come into being until the start of the nineteenth century. Prior to that, providers of drugs and medicines had served society for thousands of years, but their products were based on the ancient art of pharmacy. The mid-nineteenth century saw increased demands for painkillers and antiseptics, principally as a result of military conflicts such as the American Civil War. The growth of the dyestuffs industry in Europe also had the spin-off effect of fostering the development of pharmaceuticals in the modern sense. Over the ensuing 100 years the pharmaceutical industry has grown steadily but the proper clinical testing of new medicines only became an established process as late as the 1950s. Since that time, the randomised, controlled clinical trial has become the definitive arbiter of safety and efficacy, and pharmaceutical legislation has grown exponentially, often in response to specific events, such as the thalidomide disaster in the early 1960s. The process of the clinical testing of drugs continues to evolve as a result of many factors, including attempts at global harmonisation. In the 1990s the outsourcing of clinical trials has led to the growth of contract research organisations (CROs) and there has been a corresponding shift away from permanent, in-house clinical research staff to an environment in which temporary staff are contracted in or studies or whole development projects are contracted out. Clinical trials have moved on from the time (only 50 years ago) when a mere 20 or 30 patients were treated before the launch of a new medicine.

THE ECONOMIC ENVIRONMENT

The introduction of modern pharmaceuticals has had a significant impact on clinical practice. Many more people can now be treated as outpatients, and diseases can be controlled, often with life-saving consequences. The pharmaceutical industry has enabled governments to save considerable sums of money by shortening hospital stay times, and has also made a significant contribution to the overall balance of payments in countries where medicines are produced for export. Pharmacoeconomics (PE), the quantification of savings made and of improvements in quality of life (QoL) for patients, has emerged as a science in its own right in the last two decades. Unfortunately in some respects, PE has become a necessary part of the drug development process, in order to justify the introduction of new medicines. Several countries around the world now demand PE data prior to launch, in addition to the 'usual' demands of proven quality, safety and efficacy. In the UK, the introduction of the National Institute for Clinical Excellence (NICE) in April 1999 has created a further hurdle for both new and existing medicines. This requires PE studies or modelling to demonstrate the cost-effectiveness of a medicine, and hence its 'value' to the National Health Service (NHS).

There is no doubt that governments are extremely concerned about the overall cost for the provision of health care, and justifiably so. The principal reason for escalating costs is the increasing number of elderly people in the population. These patients are the greatest consumers of health care resources, and their numbers will continue to grow in developed countries over the next few decades. Additionally, the introduction of high-technology procedures in medicine, e.g. magnetic resonance imaging (MRI), more complex surgical techniques, the continuing AIDS epidemic and, of course, the introduction of new expensive medicines have all placed increasing strain on limited financial resources. The natural reaction of governments is to look for ways either of increasing revenue or of minimising costs. These objectives can be achieved by a number of methods, but usually result in attempts to regulate the pharmaceutical industry by way of price control, profit control or reimbursement lists. The 'drugs bill' is a visible and easily identified expenditure and therefore a target for regulation. Because consumers do not generally regard the pharmaceutical industry in a positive light (medicines are expensive and have unpleasant side-effects, and pharmaceutical companies get rich on the proceeds of illness), there is no outcry when the industry is targeted. It is within this environment of cost control that the modern pharmaceutical industry operates.

RISK AND REWARD

The drug development process is a lengthy and risky business. It is highly regulated and although estimates vary, it costs approximately USD 350 million to develop a new drug from concept to market. The rewards for producing a 'blockbuster' can be huge, however, with the best-selling drugs returning revenues of more than USD 3 billion per year to their manufacturers. This appears to be a wonderful return on investment, and indeed it is – for the few drugs that ever attain such status. However, these statistics represent the tip of a pyramid of uncertainty: for every 10 000 chemicals screened, only 1000 have biological activity. Of those 1000, only 10 will ever advance so far as to be administered to humans, and only one will reach the market place.

Reaching the market place is in itself no guarantee of success, and the costs of marketing and advertising will add many millions more to the overall investment in the medicine. Moreover, those drugs that do reach market have to fund the development of all of those that never see the light of day. Furthermore, the patent life for any compound begins to tick away from the day the molecule is registered. By the time a drug is launched, only 5 to 10 years of patent life may remain to maximise the return on investment. After that time, one or several generic copies of the drug may appear at a lower price (generics companies generally have minimal research and development (R&D) activity and lower manufacturing costs). Generic copies are licensed as 'essentially similar' to the originator drug, and will be prescribed in preference to the original by cost-conscious doctors (i.e. the majority). In the UK, for example, the government has set a target for 75% of all prescriptions to be written generically rather than by brand name. This means that the pharmacist receiving the prescription can dispense the cheapest available version. In this environment it is increasingly important for companies to focus their R&D efforts not only on achieving registration, but also on future marketing to an increasingly critical group of buyers. It is possible in the UK, for instance, that an accolade from NICE may turn out to be the best route to high sales in the future.

Against this background of cost constraint and control by the purchasers, and cost-consciousness amongst prescribers, the costs of R&D have escalated. The reasons for this increase are manifold and include the need for highly sophisticated laboratory conditions and new high-tech equipment, increasing demands from the regulatory authorities, and the costs of implementing outcomes from the International Conference on Harmonisation of Technical Requirements for Registration of Pharmaceuticals for Human Use (referred to more conveniently as ICH).

The pharmaceutical industry's response to this hostile series of events has been to retrench to some extent. All R&D directors have had their budgets scrutinised in depth, and they have redoubled their efforts to bring medicines to the market even faster, thus effectively gaining a longer patent life. CROs have made claims that they can generate data faster, although probably not more economically, and there has been consolidation amongst the main pharmaceutical companies.

The pharmaceutical industry is very fragmented on a global scale. Even the largest companies have single-digit shares of the total market, and there are very many small companies, some of which are speculative biotechnology or gene therapy groups. Amongst the largest players, billion dollar mergers have been concluded in an attempt to gain economies of scale. This has changed the industry landscape by producing GlaxoSmithKline, AstraZeneca, Aventis, Novartis, an enlarged Pfizer (which also includes Warner Lambert), and several other 'new' companies. Alongside full-blown mergers and acquisitions, there is an emerging trend towards co-operation amongst companies, both in terms of co-marketing and in collaborative research. Companies with a somewhat thin pipeline of drugs in the later stages of development have forged collaborative agreements with other companies that perhaps have an embarrassment of riches. Sharing the costs and resources required to complete the drug development process ultimately earns a share of the royalties that are potentially forthcoming after marketing. Many of the small innovative groups engaged in discovery research on a 'shoestring budget' have been acquired or funded by multinational companies in the hope of rich rewards for the large company in the future. It remains to be seen whether or not this merger and acquisition frenzy will bear fruit. 'Good' mergers are those that are likely to yield synergies in development activity while achieving economies of effort and scale in the process. Some recent mergers may have had a more short-term goal, namely of appearing to increase immediate profitability (by adding sales and reducing head-counts), thus pleasing the financial markets. Where that is the case, more mergers will inevitably follow because R&D pipelines will not be any more promising after the merger than they were before.

RULES AND REGULATIONS

The pharmaceutical industry is one of the most highly regulated of all. It is constrained, for example, by local country laws, by European Directives (in the EU), by the Declaration of Helsinki, by regulatory authorities, by ICH guidelines, and by local country good clinical practice (GCP) guidelines.

The Declaration of Helsinki defines biomedical research, and as a statement of principles about the ethics of research in humans, it applies to all biomedical research activities in patients. As a succinct set of principles, it should be read and understood by everyone working in clinical research. Regulatory authorities exist in all the major countries, the most important in terms of future sales potential being those in the USA, Europe and Japan. Despite being a relatively smaller proportion of the world population, these areas account for more than 85% of all drug sales. The European regulatory scene changed dramatically in 1995 with the setting up of the European Agency for the Evaluation of Medicinal Products (EMEA). The agency is located in London but provides an alternative route for pan-European registration. It is now possible to apply directly to the EMEA in a centralised application; if successful, this will result in a positive approval for all EU countries. Alternatively, it is possible to obtain approval in one member state, and then to apply for mutual recognition in some or all of the other member states. The EU has introduced many other directives, for example, relating to clinical trial design, policies and procedures, and special patient populations, as well as marketing and advertising.

The Food and Drug Administration (FDA) controls the licensing of new medicines in the USA. The requirements for the approval of new medicines are generally similar to those in Europe, although the process is rather different, and certainly more interactive. The licensing process in Japan is different again, although since the advent of ICH, the data requirements are now very similar to those in Europe and the USA.

ICH began as an attempt to reduce unnecessary duplication of research, to harmonise requirements between the USA, Europe and Japan, and to apply best practice from the formerly quite different approaches adopted in each of those major regions. The process of harmonisation has been largely successful and has led to improvements in many areas. Among others, harmonised guidelines have been produced on tests in geriatric patients, on requirements for population exposure, and on requirements for drugs involving chronic therapy. ICH has also produced a synthesis of the best aspects from the various GCP guidelines that existed previously.

The ICH GCP guideline sets out the obligations of sponsors, investigators, and monitors, and also demands the application of properly constituted standard operating procedures (SOPs). All pharmaceutical companies and CROs will have their own SOP versions, with some being exhaustive in every detail, while others state guiding principles only. GCP has undoubtedly brought great improvements to the clinical research process, and has resulted in far greater acceptance and credibility of the data generated in clinical trials. It has improved confidence in the industry, and has helped to ensure the safety of trial subjects. Furthermore, it has done much to eradicate fraudulent practice in clinical trials, although this does still raise its head from time to time. It is now much easier to follow a document trail to assess the validity of data, and this necessarily brings an increased level of confidence. However, these laudable and essential changes have also increased the resources, both human and financial, now required in order to conduct clinical trials. This is undoubtedly one of the drivers of the increasing cost of drug development. Nevertheless, GCP in its various guises has been a vital factor contributing to successful drug registration.

DRUG DISCOVERY

Although there is still the occasional example of serendipity providing a company with a multi-million dollar product (exemplified most recently by Viagra (sildenafil), which started out as a treatment for a medical indication rather different from male erectile dysfunction), most drug development is by rational drug design. The last 25 years or so have seen biology evolve from the random evaluation of large numbers of molecules, to their selective screening in models of the putative disease process. There has been enormous growth in enabling technologies, such as molecular biology. This has allowed the development of new concepts in therapy, including gene therapy and antisense drugs, but has also led to a deeper understanding of the underlying pathologies as a precursor to new drug design by the medicinal chemist. It is now possible to go through a process of rational screening, the objective being to design a molecule that will act, for example, as an agonist or antagonist, or that will mimic the actions of a chemical target. The chemist and biologist work together to identify several lead candidates, from which the eventual drug candidate will be derived. A prototype structure with an appropriate level of biological activity is defined, and the pharmacodynamic profile based on predetermined biological criteria to produce drug candidates will then be quantified. Random screening of vast libraries of chemical compounds is still used, although nowadays the process resulting in the generation of lead compounds is generally rapid. These lead compounds then need to be optimised in order to produce the lead candidate, which becomes the potential new drug.

During the initial evolution of a drug, the medicinal chemist and the pharmacologist interact to develop a molecule designed to elicit a maximal response from a specific target receptor in *in-vitro* tests. Further tests will determine the selectivity of the putative drug for its proposed action in the body. Invariably, the potential drug has to be formulated eventually into a variety of medicinal products that can be easily handled and administered in a number of pharmaceutical forms. These may be injections, oral formulations, patches, creams or products for inhalation. All these formulations will contain drug plus a variety of excipients, the purpose of which is to enhance product performance. During this process, the drug must retain its promising pharmacological activity, and must provide a predictable response in patients. It will have to be stable, packaged and available for administration. It must be capable of manufacture in an economical way on a large scale, without danger to those working in the manufacturing plant. The process will have to comply with all the regulatory requirements of the countries in question, and must be in accordance with good manufacturing practice (GMP). Given all these requirements, pharmaceutical development will be an integral part of the early process. Before any development studies can be performed, fundamental physicochemical information on the new drug must be obtained. The initial formulation of a new drug is likely to be an injectable form for basic pharmacological, pharmacokinetic or toxicological studies in animals or man. The final drug may exist in a number of different formulations, depending upon whether or not it is needed for local or systemic action, and depending upon the characteristics of the compound itself. Formulation changes at a late stage can be very costly, and may necessitate re-testing in clinical trials using the new formulation. In tandem with pharmaceutical development, there is an initial priority to develop an analytical method to detect the compound, any intermediate compounds and degradation products as a basis for future investigations.

The basic physicochemical properties of the drug will be determined to provide essential information for interpreting future studies. Its chiral properties will be assessed, with a view to separating out enantiomers with different pharmacological properties, or indeed with no activity in man. Successful formulation then depends upon the selection of appropriate excipients that do not react with the drug or with each other. Prior to launch, the manufacturing process will have to be scaled up from relatively small amounts of drug to much larger quantities. Pre-registration Phase II and Phase III studies will themselves potentially require large volumes of drug supplies, probably with matching placebo to preserve the double-blind conduct of the studies, thus eliminating any potential bias that may be introduced into the results. The blinding of clinical trial supplies is a complex and vital part of any development process, and can be extremely costly if not performed accurately, as this may potentially nullify the results of a multi-million dollar study.

PRE-CLINICAL TESTING

Pre-clinical studies are carried out primarily to assess safety and biological activity, in an attempt to understand the therapeutic ratio of the compound. Various types of study exist, ranging from *in-vitro* models to *in-vivo* animal studies. A minimum set of toxicology requirements has been defined, both for a compound to enter clinical trials for the first time, and ultimately to achieve registration. ICH has specified the duration of repeated-dose animal studies required to justify administration of single doses to humans, with further defined requirements for administration to humans lasting up to 2 weeks, 1 month, 3 months and 6 months. For registration purposes, however, a much broader battery of tests is specified, covering genotoxicity, acute, sub-acute and chronic toxicity, oncogenicity, and fertility and reproduction.

Genotoxicity

Genotoxicity refers to the potentially harmful effects of the compound upon genetic material occurring directly as a result of mutations in the amount or structure of the DNA within cells. This may happen as a result of gene mutation (changes in nucleotide sequence), chromosomal mutation (changes in the gross structure of chromosomes), or genomic mutation (changes in the number of chromosomes in a genome). Mutagenic properties may represent a potential hazard in terms of the subsequent carcinogenic potential of the compound. The studies in question look for gene mutation in bacterial cells, assays are conducted for chromosomal aberrations (in cell line cultures), mammalian cells (cell lines) are tested for gene mutation, and rodent bone marrow is investigated for chromosome damage (mouse micronucleus test). Tests are also conducted to detect unscheduled DNA synthesis (*ex-vivo* assay in rodent liver). The tests are usually performed in step-wise fashion, depending upon the outcome of the *in-vitro* tests in the first instance. Drugs intended for topical use are also tested for irritation and sensitisation potential to the skin.

Toxicity

Toxicity studies are performed to enable the toxicologist to advise the clinician of the possible risks of exposing humans to the compound. Safety in humans can only be proven from extensive and detailed human data. There is a biological basis for the view that toxic effects caused by drugs in animals are often predictive of adverse reactions in humans. It is assumed that increasing the dose and prolonging the duration of exposure will somehow improve the sensitivity and predictive power of the tests. The guidelines for toxicity testing prior to human exposure are predicated on this principle. A six-month study at high doses is presumed to give a more accurate answer than a one-month study at low doses. Toxicologists debate this point, however, with many believing that a properly conducted short-term study is equally useful.

According to the ICH guidelines, the toxicology programme and the clinical programme may run in parallel. Preclinical safety pharmacology aims to establish whether potential drugs have side-effects that might preclude or limit their therapeutic use. It also provides an indication of potential safety margins. Tests would normally include the determination of overt pharmacodynamic effects in conscious animals, the determination of cardiovascular and respiratory effects and, possibly, tests for abuse potential.

Single-dose studies are usually performed in two animal species, using two routes of administration. Preliminary studies provide an indication of the maximum non-lethal dose. These are followed by definitive studies conducted for up to 14 days with subsequent autopsy to provide tissue samples for macroscopic and microscopic examination. They provide information about potential target organ toxicity, and offer some indication of the consequences of massive overdose in patients.

Repeated-dose studies are usually performed in a rodent species, and probably also in dogs. The longer the proposed duration of therapy in humans, the longer the required duration of the repeated-dose toxicity studies. Doses are usually based upon preliminary dose-escalation studies. Maximum repeatable dose studies are often the first to be carried out, for each species and by each route of administration. The aim is to provide a profile of toxic effects, including target organ toxicity, that can then be related back to systemic exposure and give an indication of the relationship between dose and effect. Subsequent assessment of safety margins can be useful in helping to define the appropriate dose in man.

Studies lasting one, three, six and 12 months will follow, in an attempt to characterise any target organ toxicity identified in earlier studies. These studies will look for any new target organs, check whether the previously identified kinetics change after repeated daily administration, and establish whether any drug-related effects are readily reversible on cessation of treatment.

Oncogenicity

Oncogenicity studies are lifetime bioassays in animals to detect whether or not a compound has the potential to cause neoplastic changes in a tissue or tissues. These studies are required when the drug is intended to be used continuously for long periods, where its chemical structure suggests oncogenic potential, or where there is other cause for concern, e.g. arising from the genotoxicity studies. In view of their size and duration, oncogenicity studies are usually conducted towards the end of the development of a compound, when clinical efficacy has been established and the majority of toxicity studies have been completed. The route of administration should be similar to the intended clinical route, with oral administration being used most frequently. Meticulous records are essential, as a vast corpus of data will be generated and a detailed autopsy will be required on every animal.

Reproductive toxicology

Reproductive toxicology studies assess new pharmaceutical products for their effects on the complex mammalian process of reproduction that includes gametogenesis, fertilisation, implantation, embryogenesis, foetal growth, parturition, postnatal adaptation, development and ageing. The lengthy and carefully documented studies for general reproductive effects examine the possibility that agents may affect male or female fertility. Developmental effects are investigated in order to detect abnormalities in the developing offspring: the studies are difficult to design because of variable inter-species response, and because of the spontaneous emergence of abnormalities. Reproductive toxicology studies have three basic strands: segment I examines fertility and general reproductive performance; segment II is the teratogenicity study; and segment III is the perinatal and postnatal study.

Ideally, toxicology studies should be as faithful a representation as possible of exposure in humans. The route of administration should therefore mimic the intended clinical route. Special studies may be needed to examine topical irritancy, absorption, and systemic toxicity, e.g. following inhalation or intranasal application. Such studies would be used throughout where these are the planned routes of administration in man.

Toxicity studies are costly in terms of animal and financial resources. It is incumbent upon the industry to minimise the excessive use of animals, and great efforts have been made in this regard over the last decade. Most of the studies conducted now are the result of regulatory requirements, and it is indeed inconceivable that drugs would be administered with man as the first 'whole body system'.

CLINICAL DEVELOPMENT

Phase I

Drug development in human subjects usually begins with the investigation of tolerability, pharmacokinetics and pharmacodynamics in healthy volunteers. This is not always the case, however, because initial dose-escalation studies for some drugs are conducted in patient volunteers. Whatever the scenario, these early clinical development studies help to achieve a number of objectives. They assist decision-making about the future of the putative drug, particularly in terms of establishing the dose–response relationship in small numbers of people, and they define to some extent the tolerability of the drug, and its pharmacokinetics, in humans. This stage is often referred to as Phase I, although studies in healthy volunteers may also be performed at different stages throughout the drug development programme. For example, drug interaction studies and pharmacokinetic studies of new formulations are frequently conducted shortly before submission of the product licence application, and clinical pharmacology studies to support line extensions may be conducted years after the original product licence has been granted.

To avoid the confounding influence of other diseases, other medications and age, the first administration in humans usually occurs in young healthy volunteers. It may well be necessary, however, to involve other populations later, e.g. people with hepatic or renal impairment, or the elderly. There are many specialist clinical pharmacology units with panels of volunteers available for such studies. The volunteers are all carefully screened to avoid exposing them to any major risk as far as possible. Although volunteers are paid for their participation, the sums are not excessive in order to avoid the impression that 'danger money' is being offered.

Administration to humans entails many more responsibilities and much greater costs than hitherto in the drug development programme. The decision to enter Phase I will not have been taken lightly, and will be based on the careful characterisation of dose/concentration–response relationships *in vitro* and *in vivo*. Furthermore, the available toxicology results will have been reviewed very carefully. The Phase I studies will provide information on the tolerability of a range of doses, the pharmacokinetics of the drug, and early dose–response relationship findings. Data will also be generated on plasma concentrations and on pharmacodynamic activity, broadening understanding of the bioavailability of the drug, its clearance mechanisms, metabolites and other important issues relating to its behaviour in humans (*see Chapter 6*).

A successful outcome to these initial studies will engender confidence to proceed with the full development programme, usually involving a series of international studies to achieve marketing authorisation in all the major countries. Good trial design in the early stages will allow the company to design subsequent trials using dosage regimens that are rational and justifiable. The full clinical development programme must take account not only of all the requirements of the regulatory authorities, but also increasingly of the needs of future purchasers. The commercial prospects for the drug must be exhaustively reviewed prior to embarking on what will be the most expensive part of the development process thus far. Assuming that the decision is taken to proceed, important information needs to be collected in the ensuing clinical trial programme. Licences are granted on the basis of efficacy, safety and quality. Sufficient data must be generated in all these areas to enable the submission dossier to pass speedily through the regulatory agency. The studies will all be conducted to GCP standards and must be carefully designed to maximise the ability of the reviewer to understand the key features and benefits of the new drug.

Phase II

The first trials in patients with the disease to be treated, diagnosed or prevented will be relatively short: Phase II is usually the first time that patients rather than volunteers will be exposed to the drug. Phase II studies are conducted in units with specialist investigators, and will require prior regulatory approval as well as ethics committee approval. It is likely that surrogate end-points will be measured, particularly in diseases of chronic duration. In other words, markers of the disease may be measured (e.g. by blood tests, scans or other means) rather than conducting studies for the long period of time that would be necessary to measure the disease outcomes themselves.

As the drug moves forward through these initial studies in patients, identification of the optimum dose becomes very important. These studies will attempt to identify the dose that produces efficacy with a minimum of side-effects. The design of the studies will allow for relatively short-term exposure to the drug, will usually include a placebo control, and will often use specialist investigators to measure surrogate end-points. At the end of Phase II, the company must have a clear idea of the small range of doses to carry forward into the largest and most expensive studies of the entire development programme, the pivotal Phase III studies.

Phase III

In Phase III, the company should be seeking to assess real outcomes in a variety of patients approximating to the 'real-life' population of patients who will receive the drug once it has been launched. Regulatory and ethics committee approval is mandatory for Phase III, and ethics committee approval in particular may be the rate-limiting step when the company is eager to start the study. Unless the drug is ultimately intended for use in specialist centres only, it is important now to move to a more general range of investigators. Even at this final stage of development, the clinical study protocol will still exclude many 'real-world' patients, e.g. those with other serious medical conditions, those receiving a range of other medications, and women of child-bearing age unless using accepted contraceptive precautions. It is debatable whether or not these studies provide a true test for the new drug, compared with what will happen on the first day of launch. When that time comes, prescribing doctors will probably give the drug to their most difficult patients, i.e. those fitting many of the categories specifically excluded from the clinical trial programme. Despite these reservations, the precautions needed in Phase III are relevant and necessary to protect patients who have essentially volunteered to be a part of the drug development programme. The use of placebo comparators in Phase III studies is a subject in itself, and the decision taken will depend on the therapeutic area concerned and the specific disease and drug category being investigated. The regulatory authorities must be convinced of the efficacy of the drug and sometimes this can only be achieved satisfactorily using a placebo control.

Clinical trial design methodology will be addressed elsewhere (*see Chapter 5*), but it may suffice here to emphasise that innovation is important, rather than simply following the protocol and case record form (CRF) template used earlier in the programme. The current climate of having to satisfy requirements other than those of the regulators underlines how vital it is to think carefully about the best design to achieve a defined end-point.

Safety data will have been collected throughout the development programme. In the early stages reliance is placed upon understanding the class effect where other drugs belonging to the same class already exist. As the programme progresses through pre-clinical and clinical studies, specific safety data collection becomes vital. Knowledge of the effects of the compound itself upon target organ systems, and predictions concerning potential side-effects in man, will accumulate on an ongoing basis. The specific studies in the toxicology and pharmacology programmes will provide much evidence for the physicians to review. Many of the events that will be seen in man can be predicted from a knowledge of the pharmacology of the drug. Other events are not predictable, and these are potentially the most serious, both to patients and to the continued success of the drug. Examples abound of unpredictable side-effects that have led to tragic consequences for patients, and ultimately to the withdrawal of the drug in question. Vigilance at all stages is the only way to recognise signals as they arise. If the company takes action promptly, there is some chance that patients will be protected through warnings introduced into the summary of product characteristics (SPC) and the drug may be saved from withdrawal. It must be remembered that the regulatory agencies are all interested in weighing the risk–benefit ratio for the drug. The risk to patients must never exceed the potential benefit. This judgement of balance will change, depending on the severity of the disease and the availability of other compounds to treat it, but it is fundamental to the licensing of drugs, emphasising the paramount importance of collecting good quality safety data.

Phase IIIb

Studies which start pre-launch, but which are not intended to form part of the regulatory dossier, are conventionally referred to as Phase IIIb studies. These are conducted predominantly for marketing purposes, and are sometimes intended as the main support for the required cost/value arguments. Phase IIIb studies typically use the market leader as a comparator, the hope being to achieve a benefit over and above that of the existing drug, thus enabling the marketing and sales groups to maximise performance after launch. This may or may not be possible, but at the very least the Phase IIIb studies provide further data to support the safety and efficacy of the drug. At the time of the dossier submission, only a few thousand patients will have been treated with the drug, and all within the confines imposed by clinical trial programmes and their protocols. Further data are important, and will bolster the confidence of future prescribers.

Pharmacoeconomics

PE has come to play an increasingly important role in the drug development process. Many companies already include QoL scales in their pivotal studies in an attempt to quantify other benefits of their drug for the patient, apart from simple efficacy in the disease process. Furthermore, there has been rapid growth in identifying outcomes in clinical research beyond the straightforward measurement of empirical end-points. For example, does lowering of blood pressure matter *per se*, or should one also measure the effect of lowering blood pressure on mortality due to stroke and heart disease? This kind of question is ultimately more important to the patient as well as to those responsible for making decisions about the funding of therapy.

The measurement of QoL is important as part of the overall assessment of the benefit of a drug. It may be necessary to measure direct utility scales to permit later calculation of quality-adjusted life years (QALYs) as well as disease-specific scales to permit judgements of efficacy. Specific QoL scales have been designed and validated for many major diseases and these should be used wherever possible. If such a scale does not exist, it may be necessary for a company to work with health psychologists and others to devise and validate a scale that will be useful later. The calculation of QALYs or, more importantly, cost per QALY is an exercise beloved of health economists. The satisfactory calculation of these variables demands that QoL be measured using the available highly specific utility scales that have been validated.

There are four main forms of PE evaluation: cost-minimisation, cost-effectiveness, cost–utility and cost–benefit (*see Chapter 14*). All these analyses measure cost as one side of the equation, but they differ in terms of the other measurements required. *Cost-minimisation* is probably the most straightforward of the analyses in that it assumes that the outcomes from compared treatments are identical, and measures cost alone. *Cost-effectiveness* attempts to measure the outcomes of treatment in terms of therapeutic effectiveness. The results are usually expressed in terms of the cost of successfully treating a patient using each of the interventions. *Cost–benefit*, on the other hand, measures everything in terms of money, and outcome may be expressed in terms of the savings made by using one intervention rather than another. This analysis may be appropriate, for example, when comparing drug treatment with surgery for a particular disease. Even though surgery may be a 'one-off' event, there may well be expensive sequelae that need to be taken into account. *Cost–utility* analysis seeks to assign a quality weighting to a patient's health status at a particular point in time. This is compared with health status after treatment, and with the theoretical outcome without treatment. In this way a QALY statistic can be assigned to the 'health gain' achieved. The point of such an analysis is usually to allow comparison with QALYs in other interventions in other disease states. Only thus can those bodies charged with public health responsibilities make decisions on how to spend their cash-limited budget in order to bring health gain to the maximum number of patients. The sad but true fact is that not all diseases or conditions will qualify for routine funding.

Post-launch studies

The drug development programme should not cease after the drug has been launched. Instead, the pharmaceutical company should have elaborated a well-formulated strategy to develop new formulations, to expand the patient population, to seek new indications, and to work with prescribers to identify optimum patient profiles. Patent expiry will often mean that at least half the revenue from a drug will potentially be lost. This trend can be countered by fragmenting the market, thus making it more likely that revenue will be preserved. These and other strategies should be evolving immediately the drug is launched. It may also be that a specific safety study is required after launch. Separate rules exist for safety assessment of marketed medicines (SAMM) studies, an idea that originated in the UK and is now used in other countries too. Discussions should take place with the regulatory authority as to optimum study design: however, these studies are not clinical research in the true sense because data are usually collected in the form of case-control studies or classical post-marketing surveillance (PMS) studies.

CONCLUSION

Drug development is a lengthy and expensive process that is fraught with risks. It also brings people together from many disparate backgrounds and professional disciplines to form cohesive teams, all striving for the same goal. That goal is a drug that will benefit patients, satisfy prescribers and bring some profit back to the company to enable the whole process to start over again. Drug development is not always successful, but when it does lead to a new drug being made available to patients and doctors, it is extremely satisfying for all concerned.

FURTHER READING

Applied Clinical Trials (various issues).
Bäumler, E (1984). *Paul Ehrlich – Scientist for Life*, Holmes and Meier, New York.
Clinical Research Focus (various issues).
Day, S (1999). *Dictionary for Clinical Trials*, John Wiley, Chichester.
Hutchinson, DR (1997). *How Drugs Are Developed*, Brookwood Medical Publications, Richmond.
ICH Guideline (1996). *Topic E6: Good Clinical Practice – Consolidated Guideline*, International Federation of Pharmaceutical Manufacturers Associations, Geneva (Issued as CPMP/ICH/135/95).
Jadad, A (1998). *Randomised Controlled Trials*, BMJ Publishing Group, London.
Kremers, E and Urdang, G (1976). *The History of Pharmacy (4th edn)*, Lippincott, Philadelphia.
Poynter, FNL (1965). *The Evolution of Pharmacy*, Pitman Medical, London.
Raven, A (1997). *Consider it Pure Joy. An Introduction to Clinical Trials (3rd edn)*, Cambridge Healthcare Research, Cambridge.
Sneader, W (1985). *Drug Discovery: The Evolution of Modern Medicines*, John Wiley, Chichester.
Spilker, B (1991). *Guide to Clinical Trials*, Raven Press, New York.
Trease, GL (1964). *Pharmacy in History*, Baillière, Tindall and Cox, London.
Walker, SR (1991). *Creating the Right Environment for Drug Discovery*, Quay Publishing, Lancaster.

Winslade, J (1997). *Dictionary of Drug Development*, ACiX SCiENTiFiC Publications, Aldershot.
Winslade, J and Hutchinson, DR (1993). *Dictionary of Clinical Research*, Brookwood Medical Publications, Richmond.

2

Medicinal product regulations in the 21st century

Andrew Willis

INTRODUCTION

This chapter is intended to provide an overview of the regulatory systems currently in operation in the European Union (EU), and to provide insight into the rationale for those systems. Starting with a concise history of medicinal product regulations, it will guide the reader through regulatory aspects of the clinical development programme and ultimately describe the marketing authorisation procedures applicable in Europe. In addition, brief summaries are provided with respect to the US regulatory environment and the future of regulations for the pharmaceutical industry.

HISTORY AND BACKGROUND TO REGULATIONS OF MEDICINES

Regulations of medicines were originally concerned not with the efficacy or safety of the drug substance and product, but with its quality. The quality of the drug substance was established primarily by determining its identity and its purity. The earliest written code for quality control in Britain was the Ordinances of the Guild of Pepperers of Soper Lane in 1316. These ordinances also applied to apothecaries and prohibited the mixing of ingredients of different quality and price, detailed standards for the weighing of goods, and prevented the falsifying of weight by wetting.

The evolution of medicinal product regulation over the ensuing two or three centuries is somewhat confused. However, the direction of drug regulation became clearer with the emergence of the first medicinal product formulation scientists, and their subsequent division into those who ultimately became general medical practitioners and those who became chemists and druggists.

This led to the formation of the Pharmaceutical Society, whose members are now referred to as pharmacists. It was not until 1607 that King James I recognised the apothecaries. Ten years later, in 1617, James granted the apothecaries a charter as 'The Worshipful Society of the Art and Mystery of Apothecaries', to separate and distinguish them from the Grocers.

In 1540, the College of Physicians passed one of the earliest British statutes on the control of drugs, empowering physicians to appoint inspectors of 'Apothecary Wares, Drugs and Stuffs'. This gave physicians the right to search apothecaries' shops. If any search showed that drugs were not pure or not suitable to be administered as medicines, the material was destroyed. These powers were modified in 1553 in order to strengthen the search capabilities and systems.

Throughout Europe, the quality control of drug substances and their corresponding products was furthered by the development and issue of pharmacopoeias (Greek *pharmakon*, a drug + *poiein*, to make). The first official modern pharmacopoeia in Europe was published in 1498 in Florence. Other cities followed with the publication of such formularies, notably Barcelona in 1535 (*Concordia Pharmacolorum Barcinonesium*) and Nuremberg in 1546 (*Dispensatorium Valerii Cordis*). Similar compilations were also issued in Mantua (1559), Augsburg (1564), Cologne (1565), Bologna (1574), Bergamo (1580) and Rome (1583).

In Britain, the first 'official' edition of the *Pharmacopoeia Londinensis* was not published until 1618. However, King James I issued a proclamation, laying down the expectations placed on apothecaries and binding them to use the pharmacopoeia: 'Apothecaries within this our Realm of England or the dominions thereof do not compound or make any medicine, or medicinable receipt of prescription by any other books or Dispensatories whatsoever but after the only manner and form that hereby is, or shall be directed, prescribed and set down by the said book and according to the weights and measures that are or shall be therein limited and not otherwise upon pain of our high displeasure, and to incur such penalties and punishment as may be inflicted upon offenders herein for their contempt or neglect of this our royal commandment.'

In 1650 the second *London Pharmacopoeia* was issued and further pharmacopoeias appeared at intervals until the tenth was published in 1851. In Britain, pharmacopoeias were also issued in Edinburgh and Dublin.

With its creation in 1858, the General Medical Council (GMC) was given the task of compiling a single pharmacopoeia for the whole of the United Kingdom. The *British Pharmacopoeia* then became recognised as a source of both drug and drug product information throughout the world, a position it has held to the present day. It is now harmonised with the *European Pharmacopoeia*, a work that is regarded as the gold standard throughout the EU.

It is approximately 30 years since the Convention on which the work of the *European Pharmacopoeia* was based, following the signing of an agreement between the original eight Member States. The *European Pharmacopoeia* is based on the European Treaty Series No. 50, as amended by the protocol to the Convention (European Treaty Series No. 134), and is signed by the governments of Austria, Belgium, Bosnia-Herzegovina, Croatia, Cyprus, Denmark, Finland, France, Germany, Greece, Iceland, Ireland, Italy, Luxembourg, Netherlands, Norway, Portugal, Slovakia, Slovenia, Spain, Sweden, Switzerland, the Former Yugoslav Republic of Macedonia, Turkey, UK and the European Community.

The purposes of the *European Pharmacopoeia* are to:

- develop a harmonised European approach to quality;
- facilitate the free movement of medicinal products in Europe; and to
- ensure the quality of medicinal products exported from Europe.

The monographs contained in the *European Pharmacopoeia* are detailed summaries of the testing criteria and limits of acceptance applied to drug substances and are accepted by all European Member States. However, particular care should be taken over the suitability of the monograph to ensure adequate control and quality of the drug substance or medicinal product.

There have been extensive efforts to achieve global harmonisation in terms of the policies, standards, monograph specifications, analytical methods and acceptance criteria of all these pharmacopoeias. These activities have led to greater mutual recognition between the USA, Europe and Japan concerning the specific requirements and testing procedures for drugs, drug products and excipients. The emergence of further mutual recognition agreements with other regions across the world has also ensured greater co-operation.

Following on from the original emphasis placed on the quality of the drug substance, medicines regulation has broadened to encompass clinical use, particularly with regard to safety and efficacy. At present, medicinal product regulations have progressed significantly, and include detailed directives and guidelines for the control of drug development. This control extends not only to those issues concerning quality and purity of formulations but also to the data supporting routine use in patients, thus ensuring that the efficacy and safety of the medicinal product are well understood and documented.

Within Europe the current regulations are an integral part of every aspect of the discovery, development, manufacture, presentation, marketing, distribution and use of medicines. The Member States of the European Union all have country-specific mechanisms for approving medicinal products. The first steps towards harmonising these different regulatory frameworks were taken in 1965. Directive 65/65/EEC is the fundamental regulation governing the sale and supply of medicinal products and ensures that each Member State authorises a medicinal product before it is placed on its national market. It also sets out a common framework for the manner in which this should occur and also indicates the data package necessary to obtain approval.

Regulation of medicines in Europe has evolved from Directive 65/65/EEC into a comprehensive system of directives, regulations and guidelines that define the contents of a marketing authorisation application (MAA). These regulations and directives are enshrined in the national law of each Member State, forming a Europe-wide system for the regulation of medicinal products. This framework of regulations governs the largest pharmaceutical market in the world, dictates how patients gain access to innovative medicines and determines benchmarks for quality, safety and effectiveness of medicines in use.

THE LEGAL BASIS OF CONTROL BY REGULATORY AUTHORITIES

The regulatory infrastructure in the EU consists of directives and guidelines adopted by the European Parliament, with the former subsequently endorsed into the national legislation of each Member State. This infrastructure is primarily concerned with public health and the need to assure quality and establish the safety of products.

A series of directives and regulations has been designed in order to take into consideration the differences between Member States and to create the conditions that will allow a single market. However, innovation and the need to develop new medicinal products have not been forgotten and guidelines have been published to facilitate these aspects.

The publication of Directive 65/65/EEC ensured that marketing authorisation (often referred to as a product licence) was required before a new medicinal product could be placed on the market. This Directive also laid down the basis for the evaluation of new medicinal products, ensuring that the critical points of safety, quality and efficacy were fully addressed, and outlined the concept of the summary of product characteristics (SPC).

Subsequently, a series of additional directives has been created. These include Directive 75/320/EEC, which created the Pharmaceutical Committee, and Directive 75/319/EEC, which defined the overall framework for the operation of the single market. This Directive also established the Committee for Proprietary Medicinal Products (CPMP) and the multistate application procedure. Over the past three decades, further directives have been issued in order to clarify, extend and amend the original directives. These include Directive 83/570/EEC relating to data requirements and CPMP procedures, Directive 89/341/EEC extending the scope to cover all medicinal products, Directive 89/342/EEC relating to immunological products, Directive 89/343/EEC relating to radiopharmaceuticals, Directive 89/381/EEC relating to blood products, and Directive 87/21/EEC which addressed the issue of protection for the first applicant.

Data requirements for marketing authorisations have primarily been defined in Directive 75/318/EEC (further amended with directives 83/570/EEC, 91/207/EEC, 83/571/EEC and 87/18/EEC).

Table 1. Medicines regulation in the EC – key elements.

Directive	Comments
65/65/EEC	Sets out scope and definitions. Requires Member States to grant marketing authorisations for new medicines on the grounds of safety, quality and efficacy. Elaborates the summary of product characteristics (SPC).
75/318/EEC	Data requirements for physicochemical, pharmaceutical, pharmacotoxicological and clinical testing.
75/319/EEC	Further definition of the general framework, particularly with regard to manufacturing. Establishes the CPMP, and the multistate procedure (first phase). (Revised by 78/420/EEC, which was subsequently repealed).
75/320/EEC, 78/25/EEC, 83/570/EEC	Council decision to establish the Pharmaceutical Committee. Permitted colourings for medicines (amended by 81/464/EEC). Amends 65/65/EEC, 75/318/EEC, with regard to data requirements, and 75/319/EEC with regard to CPMP procedure (introducing second phase).
83/571/EEC	Council recommendation introducing guidelines for safety and efficacy testing.
87/19/EEC	Amends 75/318/EEC and introduces the regulatory committee procedure to enable rapid update of guidelines and data requirements to take technical progress into account.
87/21/EEC	Amends 65/65/EEC with regard to protection against the second applicant for biotechnology products (concertation procedure), and high technology products.
87/22/EEC	Concertation procedure for biotechnology and high technology products.
87/176/EEC	Council recommendation with further guidelines.
89/341/EEC	Amends 65/65/EEC, 75/318/EEC, and 75/319/EEC to extend the scope to cover all medicinal products and other technical changes, including requirements for patient information, and export certification.
89/342/343 and 381/EEC	Three directives introducing special provisions for biological (vaccines, sera and allergens), radiopharmaceuticals, and blood/plasma products.
91/507/EEC	Updates the Annex to 75/318/EEC (as amended by 83/570/EEC).
2309/93	Centralised procedure from 1 January 1995. Decentralised (mutual recognition) procedure from 1 January 1995.
93/39/EEC	Repeals concertation procedure from 1 January 1995.
Transparency	
89/105/EEC	Regulates the way in which Member States control pricing and reimbursement of medicines.
Intellectual property	
1768/92	Introduces the supplementary protection certificate.

The critical step in the evolution and completion of the harmonisation process was the development of the European Marketing Authorisation System. Council Regulation 2309/93 set up the centralised procedure and created the European Agency for the Evaluation of Medicinal Products (EMEA). In addition, this directive put in place a new pharmacovigilance system. Directives 93/39/EEC and 93/40/EEC established the decentralised procedure, commonly referred to as the mutual recognition procedure (MRP). The implementation of the centralised and mutual recognition procedures with effect from 1 January 1998 has led to the present harmonised approach to the authorisation and maintenance of proprietary medicinal products throughout Europe.

The key elements of the European directives and regulations providing the framework for the present European system for controlling the approval of medicines for marketing are detailed in Table 1.

REGULATORY ASPECTS OF THE CLINICAL DEVELOPMENT PROGRAMME

The safety and efficacy of a new medicinal product have to be demonstrated before it can be introduced into clinical practice. In determining the level of evidence necessary to obtain a product licence, those engaged in clinical trial design must understand how regulatory aspects impinge upon the clinical development programme. The design of clinical trials initially focused on randomisation to reduce bias by confounding factors and to reduce observer bias. Fundamentally, a new medicine must be thoroughly assessed in patients with the illness that it is intended to treat before it is licensed for use.

The team designing a clinical study, whether it is an individual trial or part of a series, must possess a comprehensive understanding not only of the medical considerations but also of any regulatory limitations. The team should be fully aware of the context in which the trial is to be conducted, and be able to anticipate consequential action, depending on outcome. In addition, the study design chosen will be that which is best suited to achieving the desired objective. At this level, the involvement of the regulatory affairs group is fundamental to the principles of good project management. The pharmaceutical market place is now global and the medicines developed by the industry must be marketable throughout the world. Only such a strategy will ensure maximum reward from the extremely costly process of drug development. Knowledge of global regulations is therefore crucial for the clinical development of a potentially global product.

In the context of obtaining marketing authorisation for a medicinal product, the SPC occupies a central position. This document is a distillation of the research results from all non-clinical, early phase, pharmacokinetic and pharmacodynamic studies through to the pivotal efficacy and safety studies required to satisfy the regulations for any medicinal product to be placed on the market. It is therefore reasonable to postulate that the development studies should be designed in order to reflect the intended SPC. As such, a draft SPC should be created early in the clinical development programme. This draft can be treated as the product wish list; however, it must equally be recognised that this draft SPC will develop and grow as new data and greater understanding emerge during the clinical development of the medicinal product.

The design of clinical studies must take account of country-specific requirements, medical practice in the countries where the trial is being conducted, and common global standards now in place thanks to the efforts of the International Conference on Harmonisation (ICH). A well-designed study will also make allowances for nuances of regulatory and medical practice in the countries where the product is to be marketed.

A design philosophy such as this will ensure that individual clinical studies and the overall investigational plan for a new medicinal product are based on the data requirements stipulated by regulatory bodies throughout the world. Instead of being equated merely with the timely completion of the individual processes of a clinical study, success then comes to be defined as delivery of the end product, i.e. the granting of marketing authorisation. Moreover, the clinical study report will meet regulatory requirements in terms of compliance and sound statistical analysis, and will ultimately support the proposed product labelling.

At the present time in Europe, the principal document underpinning all clinical trials is the ICH Harmonised Tripartite Guideline for Good Clinical Practice (GCP). GCP originated from a series of requirements imposed by the US Food and Drug Administration (FDA) during the 1970s. These requirements made it progressively more difficult for clinical data generated in countries other than the USA to be accepted for New Drug Applications (NDAs). In Europe a series of rules and guidelines was developed in conjunction with ICH, many of which pertained to clinical research. This common standard has allowed the globalisation of the pharmaceutical industry to progress significantly over the past two decades.

Accordingly, clinical research conducted in the EU should comply with the ICH Tripartite Guideline for GCP; the requisite data protection laws; any specific national additions above and beyond ICH requirements for GCP; and any specific regulatory requirements and ethics committee requirements.

In addition to GCP, the design of any clinical study should also take into account a wide range of guidelines, some of which refer to general principles that apply to all clinical studies, while other, more specific guidelines address the critical points of certain disease areas. The guidelines detailed in Table 2 refer to the general guidance provided by the CPMP.

Obtaining approvals for clinical trials is now a significant part of the successful management of a study. As outlined above, the approach should address the

Table 2. Clinical guidelines – adopted guidelines published in the *Rules Governing Medicinal Products in the European Union. Volume 3C* (EudraLex, 1998).

Title	Date of item (date of effect)	Reference documents
Good Clinical Practice. *(ICH Topic E6 (including E6A and E6B) Step 4 adopted May 1996).*	July 1996 (January 1997)	CPMP/ICH/135/95 (including III/5085/94) (Updated the Volume III Addendum (1990) guideline: III/3976/88 which updated the Volume III (1989) guideline: III/411/871)
Explanatory note and comments to ICH Topic E6.	September 1997	
Structure and Content of Clinical Study Reports. *(ICH Topic E3. Step 4 adopted November 1995).*	December 1995 (July 1996)	CPMP/ICH/137/95
Pharmacokinetic Studies in Man.	February 1987 (October 1988)	Volume III (1989)[a]
Dose-Response Information to Support Product Authorisation. *(ICH Topic E4. Step 4 adopted in March 1994)*	May 1994[b] (November 1994)	Volume III Addendum 3 (1995) (CPMP/ICH/378/95) (III/3376/93)
The Extent of Population Exposure to Assess Clinical Safety for Medicines intended for Long-term Treatment of Non-life threatening Conditions. *(ICH Topic E1. Step 4 adopted October 1994).*	November 1994 (June 1995)	Volume III Addendum 3 (1995) (CPMP/ICH/375/95) (III/5084/94)
Clinical Investigation of Medicinal Products for Long-term Use.	February 1987 (August 1987)	Volume III (1989)[a]
Biostatistical Methodology in Clinical Trials.	December 1994 (July 1995)[c]	Volume III Addendum 3 (1995) (III/3630/92)

Subject	Date	Reference
Clinical Investigation of Medicinal Products in Children.	September 1988 (March 1989)	Volume III (1989) (III/535/86)
Clinical Investigation of Medicinal Products in Geriatrics. *(ICH Topic E7. Step 4 adopted June 1993)*	September 1993 (March 1994)	Volume III Addendum 3 (1995) (CPMP/ICH/379/95) (III/3388/93) (Updated Volume III (1989) guideline: III/536/86)
Fixed-Combination Medicinal Products.	April 1996 (October 1996)	CPMP/EWP/240/95 (III/5773/94) Updated the Volume III (1989) guideline[d]
Clinical Testing of Prolonged Action Forms with Special Reference to Extended Release Forms.	July 1990 (January 1991)	Volume III Addendum (1990) (III/1962/87)
Clinical Requirements for Locally Applied, Locally Acting Products containing known Constituents.	November 1995 (June 1996)	CPMP/239/95 (III/3664/92)
Clinical Safety Data Management: Definitions and Standards for Expedited Reporting. *(ICH Topic E2A. Step 4 adopted October 1994). See also Table 8.*	November 1994 (June 1995)	Volume III Addendum 3 (1995) (CPMP/ICH/377/95) (III/3375/93)
Clinical Safety Data Management: Periodic Safety Update Reports for Marketed Products. *(ICH Topic E2C. Step 4 adopted November 1996). See also Table 8.*	December 1996 (June 1997)	CPMP/ICH/288/95 (III/3175/93)
Investigation of Bioavailability and Bioequivalence.	December 1991 (May 1992)	Volume III Addendum 2 (1992) (III/54/89) (Updated Volume III (1989) guideline[a])

[a] These guidelines were originally published in Recommendation 87/176/EEC.
[b] The guideline in Volume 3C has a date of May 1993. It appears to be essentially the same as the May 1994 CPMP guideline adopted by ICH in March 1994.
[c] The guideline in Volume 3C has a date of May 1993. It appears to be essentially the same as the guideline adopted by the CPMP in December 1994.
[d] These guidelines were originally published in Recommendation 83/571/EEC.

data requirements of all participating countries, ensuring compliance with the regulatory requirements of all countries in which the study is to be conducted.

The majority of countries within Europe require that an application be submitted in order to start a clinical trial. Such a submission should contain a number of key documents:

- application forms;
- protocol or summary of the protocol;
- investigator's brochure; and
- supporting data.

Data requirements

Supporting scientific data is possibly the only section that is not fully defined and requires greater clarification. While these data differ in degree between countries, it is prudent with such requirements to operate to the highest common denominator. The supporting data should provide a description of the rationale for the product, its relationship to other dosage forms of the same drug substance, and any information on the product relevant to other countries, including reasons for refusal or revocation of a product licence in such countries, if applicable.

Pharmaceutical section

The pharmaceutical section should include data on:

- Composition
- Method of preparation
- Control of starting materials
- Control tests on intermediate products
- Control tests on the finished product
- Stability
- Other information.

If the product to be used in clinical trials is covered in all respects by a marketing authorisation and a statement is provided to this effect, no data need be provided in the pharmaceutical section.

Non-clinical pharmacology and toxicology studies

Data may be required under some or all of the following headings:

- *New dosage level:* toxicity data may be necessary if the dosage is raised significantly.
- *New route of administration:* relevant sections on toxicity, irritancy and metabolism may be required, although this will depend both on the new route and the route already licensed.

- *New mixtures:* information may be required on the toxicity of the new combination of substances, although if two substances are commonly used together in clinical practice, this may not be necessary.
- *Little known substances:* these are substances that are not widely used and are poorly documented in the literature. Information may be required in this section.

Data are not normally required for the following:

- Well established pharmacopoeial substances to be used by the normal route in standard dosage.
- If the health authority has already approved the drug substance in question, it is possible to cross-refer to these data and not repeat the data in this section.

Studies in humans

There are no requirements that studies in humans should be completed before clinical trial approval is granted. However, if any studies have been undertaken, they must be reported. These should include any studies in healthy volunteers or in patients.

Labelling

Labelling is another key issue complicating the smooth operation of clinical trials within Europe. However, the GCP guidance documents state that good manufacturing practice (GMP) should be followed. The subject of the labelling of clinical trial supplies is discussed in *Chapter 10*.

Once all the data requirements are known, the difficulty shifts to the specific regulatory requirements of the individual countries in which a study is to be conducted. The present situation within Europe is highly complex and procedures differ from country to country. Currently, EU countries have different regulatory requirements with regard to type of application, period for approval, and documentation required both for ethics committees and for regulatory bodies. This situation is further complicated by the regulations relating to different clinical study phases within the same country. The current situation will change dramatically with the implementation of the European Clinical Trials Directive. For the present, however, it is more appropriate to identify the differences between the countries of Europe and to provide overviews of the timings and data requirements within the specific countries.

Table 3 demonstrates the complexity of regulatory approvals for clinical trials within the EU. As stated previously, the emergence of the global market is widening the range of countries where such studies are being performed. Central and Eastern Europe is now an emerging geographical zone for clinical development, and Table 4 again illustrates the difficulties

Table 3. Health authority requirements for clinical trials within the EU.

Type of application	Clinical phase		
	I	II and III	IV
Authorisation	Austria, Denmark, Spain, Greece, Ireland, Italy, Sweden	Denmark, Spain, Greece, Ireland, Italy, UK, Sweden	Denmark, Spain, Greece, Ireland, Italy, UK, Sweden
Notification	Germany, Belgium, Finland, France, Netherlands, Portugal	Austria, Germany, Belgium, Finland, France, Netherlands, Portugal	Austria, Germany, Belgium, Finland, France, Portugal
No health authority requirement	UK		Netherlands

Table 4. Health authority requirements for clinical trials in Central and Eastern Europe.

Type of application	Clinical phase		
	I	II and III	IV
Authorisation	Bulgaria, Estonia, Hungary, Poland, Czech Republic, Romania, Russia, Slovak Republic, Slovenia	Bulgaria, Estonia, Hungary, Poland, Czech Republic, Romania, Russia, Slovak Republic, Slovenia	Bulgaria, Poland, Russia, Slovenia
Notification			Estonia, Hungary, Czech Republic, Romania
No health authority requirement			Slovak Republic

facing the clinical research team in ensuring that all requirements and official national procedures are adhered to.

The conduct of multinational clinical studies is further complicated by inter-country differences in approval times. These differences in health authority and ethics committee approval times are an obstacle to the accurate planning of clinical programmes, resulting in protracted studies if all such nuances are not taken into account (Table 5).

Finally, the clinical research professional must consider precisely which documentation is required by the review bodies of the countries where the study is to be conducted. Table 6 identifies the document requirements

Table 5. Health authority and ethics committee timings for clinical trials in the EU.

Country	Health authority	Ethics committee
Austria	Ethics review prior to ethics committee vote: 4–8 months Notification in parallel with ethics committee: 4 weeks	Approval required: 2–3 months
Belgium	Notification after ethics committee	Approval required: 1–3 months
Denmark	In parallel with ethics committee: 2–4 months + data protection: 4 weeks	Approval required: 6–10 weeks
Finland	After half ethics committee vote: 60 days	Approval required: 5 weeks
France	After ethics committee vote: max. 8 weeks	Approval required: 5 weeks
Germany	After ethics committee vote (ethics committee responsible for *Leiter der Klinischen Prüfung*)	Approval required: 1–2 months
Greece	After ethics committee vote: 1–3 months	Approval required: 1–2 months
Ireland	Approval required: 6–12 weeks in parallel with ethics committee	Approval required: 6–12 weeks
Italy	NCE: before ethics committee: 1–2 years Non-NCE: ethics committee submission only	Approval required: 1–3 months Approval required: 3 months
Netherlands	Notification by Import Licence: 2–9 weeks	Approval required: 1–4 months
Portugal	Notification after ethics committee: 2–3 weeks	Approval required: approx. 3 months
Spain	PEI: 3 months[a] RA after ethics committee vote: 60 days[a]	Approval required: approx. 2 months
Sweden	After or parallel with ethics committee: 6–10 weeks	Approval required: 1–2 months
UK	CTX: 35 days CTC: 6 months	MREC: approx. 5 weeks LREC with MREC: 6–8 weeks LREC only: 4 weeks

[a]PEI, productos en investigación; RA, regulatory approval.

Table 6. Document requirements for health authorities (HA) and ethics committees (EC) in the EU.

Document type	Austria		Belgium		Denmark		Finland		France		Germany		Greece	
	HA	EC	HA	EC	HA	EC	HA	EC	HA	EC	HA	EC	HA	EC
Covering letter	✓	✓	✓	✓	✓	✓	✓	✓	✓	✓	✓	✓	✓	✓
Application forms	✓	✓	–	–	✓	✓	✓	–	✓	–	✓	✓	✓	–
Protocol	✓	✓	✓	✓	✓	✓	✓	✓	✓	✓	✓	✓	✓	✓
Protocol summary	✓	✓	–	–	–	–	–	–	✓	✓	–	–	–	–
Protocol amendments	✓	✓	–	✓	✓	✓	✓	✓	✓	✓	✓	✓	✓	✓
Patient information leaflet	✓	✓	–	✓	✓	✓	✓	✓	✓	✓	✓	✓	✓	✓
Informed consent form	✓	✓	–	✓	✓	✓	✓	–	✓	✓	✓	✓	✓	✓
Investigator's brochure	✓	✓	–	–	✓	✓	✓	–	✓	✓	✓	✓	✓	✓
Labelling	–	✓	–	–	✓	–	✓	✓	✓	–	–	–	–	–
CRF	–	✓	–	✓	✓	✓	–	✓	✓	✓	✓	✓	✓	✓
Summary of non-clinical data	✓	–	–	✓	✓	–	–	–	–	–	✓	–	✓	–
Summary of previous human experience	✓	–	–	–	✓	–	–	✓	–	–	–	–	✓	–
Chemistry, manufacture and control data	–	–	–	–	–	–	✓	–	–	–	–	–	–	–
GMP certification	✓	–	–	–	✓	–	–	–	–	–	–	–	–	–
Expert opinion	✓	–	–	–	–	–	–	–	–	–	–	–	–	–
Investigator CV	✓	✓	–	–	–	–	–	–	–	✓	✓	–	–	–
List of investigators	–	✓	✓	–	–	✓	✓	–	✓	✓	–	✓	–	–
Insurance certificate	–	✓	–	✓	–	–	–	–	✓	✓	–	✓	–	✓

Table 6. *Continued.*

Document type	Ireland HA	Ireland EC	Italy HA	Italy EC	Netherlands HA	Netherlands EC	Portugal HA	Portugal EC	Spain HA	Spain EC	Sweden HA	Sweden EC	UK HA	UK EC
Covering letter	√	√	√	√	√	√	√	√	√	√	√	√	√	√
Application forms	√	√	√	–	–	√	–	–	√	√	√	√	√	√
Protocol	√	√	–	√	√	–	√	–	√	–	√	√	–	√
Protocol summary	–	√	–	√	–	√	–	√	–	√	–	–	√	√
Protocol amendments	√	√	–	√	√	–	√	√	√	√	√	√	–	√
Patient information leaflet	√	√	–	√	–	√	√	√	√	√	√	√	√	√
Informed consent form	√	√	–	√	–	√	√	–	√	√	√	√	√	√
Investigator's brochure	–	√	√	–	√	√	–	√	√	–	–	√	√	√
Labelling	–	–	–	√	–	√	–	√	–	–	√	–	–	–
CRF	–	–	–	√	–	–	–	–	√	–	√	–	–	–
Summary of non-clinical data	√	–	√	–	–	–	√	–	√	–	√	–	√	–
Summary of previous human experience	√	–	√	–	–	–	√	–	√	–	√	–	√	–
Chemistry, manufacture and control data	√	√	–	–	–	–	√	–	√	–	√	–	√	–
GMP certification	–	–	–	*a*	–	√	–	–	–	–	–	–	–	–
Expert opinion	–	–	–	–	–	–	–	–	√	–	–	–	–	–
Investigator CV	–	–	√	√	–	–	√	–	–	–	√	–	–	–
List of investigators	√	–	–	√	*b*	–	√	√	–	–	√	–	–	–
Insurance certificate	–	√	–	√	√	√	√	√	√	–	–	√	–	√

a Sometimes required.
b Investigative sites rather than investigators required.

throughout the EU, both for health authorities and ethics committees. While highlighting the overlap between document requirements for health authorities and ethics committees within countries, it also emphasises the differing degrees of documentation required between countries.

As if the above challenges were not enough, one further complication must be considered: language. Documentation must be submitted to the health authority and/or ethics committee in the correct language(s). However, this may not apply to all documents, since many EU Member States accept English versions. This aspect needs to be organised and planned when scheduling a clinical trial in several countries across Europe. Careful consideration should be given to the validity of the translations, and the translation activity should be viewed as an integral part of clinical trial management. Appropriate standard operating procedures (SOPs) should be available for the conduct of such work, in accordance with the basic principles of GCP.

While the current regulatory procedures for conducting clinical trials in Europe are diverse and complex, a successful outcome is possible with careful planning based on comprehensive information. The major differences between countries include the type of approval required (authorisation/notification), the time for such approvals to be granted, and the diversity of documentation required. The European Clinical Trials Directive will inevitably encourage a more harmonised approach to clinical trials in Europe. This will go hand in hand with further mutual recognition agreements as the 'march of globalisation' leads to common technical packages and a total sharing of information between countries.

MARKETING APPLICATIONS

Directive 65/65/EEC requires that each European Member State should authorise medicines before they are placed on the national market and sets out the common framework within which this should occur. The primary purpose of the rules, as set out in Directive 65/65/EEC concerning the production and distribution of proprietary medicinal products, is to safeguard public health. The current European directives define the content of a marketing authorisation. These rules lay down the principles of the dossier format and content and identify the different types of application that can be made.

Application types

A number of different types of application may be submitted, including:

- Abridged applications: *informed consent* from a Marketing Authorisation Holder (Article 4.6 (a)(i) of Directive 65/65/EEC); *essentially similar products* (Article 4.6 (a)(iii) of Directive 65/65/EEC); *others* – line extensions, including hybrids.

● Full applications (new chemical entities/NCEs).
● Bibliographical applications (Article 4.6 (a)(ii) of Directive 65/65/EEC).

Three main categories of abridged applications may be considered. Such applications take account of the cross-referral to reference products, thus minimising the volume of information required, usually with regard to the non-clinical and clinical data.

Applications may be abridged when:

1. The product is essentially similar to the marketed, already approved product and where the original marketing authorisation holder has granted permission for the new applicant to refer to the original authorisation.
2. The product is a generic or is essentially similar (i.e. pharmaceutically equivalent and bioequivalent) to an already approved product which has been authorised within the European Community for at least 6 years (10 years in some Member States). In such cases full chemistry and pharmacy data, bioequivalence data and appropriate labelling would be required. The expert reports would need to appropriately assess the available data (all expert reports being required) and justify the route of submission.
3. The product meets the requirements to be considered in respect of other types of abridged applications. These requirements may include:

   ● new salt or ester;
   ● new or different indication;
   ● new route of administration;
   ● new dosing schedule;
   ● new strength;
   ● supra-bioavailable product; or
   ● new combination of active ingredients.

Full applications apply to all products where the exemptions granted to applications of abridged authorisations do not apply. In such cases, full supporting data on pharmaceutical quality, and on non-clinical and clinical development will need to be supplied.

Bibliographical applications may be made when the product is well established and already has established efficacy and safety. A full justification will be needed for such an application and it is not uncommon for these applications to be supplemented with new clinical and non-clinical data. The full pharmaceutical data requirements would still apply.

The dossier

As stated above, Directive 65/65/EEC specifies the content of the dossier for a marketing authorisation within the European Community. The European dossier is divided into four main sections:

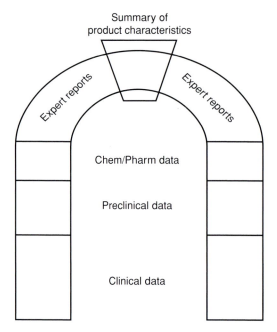

Figure 1. The dossier.

- Part I – Administrative (including SPC and expert reports)
- Part II – Chemistry and pharmacy
- Part III – Non-clinical/preclinical data
- Part IV – Clinical data

Figure 1 demonstrates the building blocks comprising a dossier for marketing approval. It can be clearly seen that the SPC is the element that locks the structure together.

The dossier itself will be defined more fully by reviewing the respective sections below.

Part I

The submission needs to comply with the Notice to Applicants (NTA) and completion of the appropriate European or national application form is required. This section of the dossier is in itself subdivided into three sections: Part IA (Administration), Part IB (Labelling) and Part IC (Expert reports).

Part IA contains the application forms (now in a European standard format), details of the structure and contents of the dossier and, usually, the appendices detailing a series of documents that an applicant is required to provide. These additional documents may include:

- letter of access to the drug master file (DMF) of the active ingredient manufacturer (AIM), if appropriate. The DMF contains information pertinent to the synthesis, control and structure of the drug substance;
- notarised version of the manufacturer's licence and contract manufacturer's licence, if applicable;
- declaration of commitment to current GMP;
- certificate of use of bovine spongiform encephalopathy (BSE)-free excipients/active ingredients.

Part IB refers to the proposed labelling and is a key section within the dossier, incorporating the SPC. The SPC details the specific indications, contra-indications and special warnings in all European countries. Specific formats should be followed for the completion of the SPC and details must be provided under the following headings:

- TRADE NAME OF THE MEDICINAL PRODUCT
- QUALITATIVE AND QUANTITATIVE COMPOSITION
- PHARMACEUTICAL FORM
- CLINICAL PARTICULARS
    Therapeutic indications
    Posology and method of administration
    Contra-indications
    Special warnings and special precautions for use
    Interaction with other medicaments and other forms of interaction
    Pregnancy and lactation
    Effects on ability to drive and use machines
    Undesirable effects
    Overdose
- PHARMACOLOGICAL PROPERTIES
    Pharmacodynamic properties
    Pharmacokinetic properties
    Preclinical safety data
- PHARMACEUTICAL PARTICULARS
    List of excipients
    Incompatibilities
    Shelf-life
    Special precautions for storage
    Nature and contents of container
    Instructions for use/handling
- MARKETING AUTHORISATION HOLDER
- MARKETING AUTHORISATION NUMBER
- DATE OF FIRST AUTHORISATION/RENEWAL OF AUTHORISATION
- DATE OF (PARTIAL) REVISION OF THE TEXT

In addition, a proposed patient information leaflet (PIL) should be provided, together with full-colour mock-ups of the labels, and these need to comply with current guidelines.

Part IC includes the expert reports, of which there are three: the Pharmaceutical, Chemical and Biological Expert Report; the Non-clinical Expert Report; and the Clinical Expert Report. Many applications, particularly for new active substances, also include a written summary. Because the European approval process places heavy reliance on these expert reports, it is important to understand the detail and format of their structure.

The expert reports are critical assessments of the methodology, results and conclusions of all studies conducted with the medicinal product. Written summaries and tabular formats may supplement the expert reports, which form a critical section of the dossier, allowing the competent assessing authority to perform its evaluation in a rapid, structured manner. The expert reports summarise the relevant data or specific studies contained within the dossier; based on these the expert will draw conclusions and provide an overall critical assessment. It is important to emphasise that the expert should be fully convinced that the product as developed is both safe and efficacious. As such, the expert should adopt a defined position on the product, taking current scientific knowledge into consideration. The following guidance is generally given concerning the length of expert reports:

● Pharmaceutical, Chemical and Biological – up to 10 pages;
● Non-clinical – up to 25 pages; and
● Clinical – up to 25 pages.

The nature and content of the expert report may differ, depending on the type of application. Abridged applications (essentially similar products, line extensions and hybrids) and bibliographical applications may concentrate more specifically on certain points, e.g. an essentially similar product may concentrate on pharmaceutical aspects and bioequivalence.

Technical documentation

Parts II, III, and IV of the application dossier consist of the chemical, pharmaceutical and biological documentation; the toxicological and pharmacological documentation; and the clinical documentation, respectively.

Part II of the dossier provides data to the health authority on the quality control and pharmaceutical aspects of the new medicinal product. It is divided into sections and follows a standard format.

Part IIA – Composition: includes data relating to the composition, containers, clinical trial formulations and development pharmaceutics.

Part IIB – Method of manufacture: summarises the overall manufacturing process, supplies a flow diagram illustrating the process, and provides details of the site of manufacturing.

Part IIC – Control of starting materials: provides detailed information on the active ingredient, excipients used and packaging components. Data on the active ingredient should be consistent with those stipulated in the DMF. Excipients and packaging components should be tested to European pharmacopoeial standards, where available. Certificates of analysis should be provided to show compliance with the *European Pharmacopoeia.*

Part IID – Intermediate products: supplies data on any intermediates created in the manufacturing process, giving details of specifications and testing procedures.

Part IIE – Control tests on the finished product: gives the full product specification, together with details of test procedures and appropriate validation data for such tests. The validation reports will be required for all assay test procedures employed and should comply with ICH criteria. In addition, certificates of analysis must be supplied for three finished-product batches.

Part IIF – Stability of the active and finished product: provides stability data on the active component; these data should be presented in tables and comply with ICH stability criteria. A re-test period should be provided, with appropriate justification, together with details of packaging and storage conditions for the active ingredient. This section also includes a stability study on the finished product, compliant with current ICH guidelines. The stability data should be presented in tables, together with a detailed commentary of results. The release and end of shelf-life specifications should be given, with appropriate justification for any deviations.

Parts IIG, H and Q: refer to data on the bioavailability/bioequivalence, environmental risk, and other information, respectively.

Part III: provides information on the safety and toxicity of the product and active drug substance. The data are provided in a set format in accordance with a specific itemised list:

● Toxicity
    Single-dose studies ?
    Repeated-dose studies
● Reproductive toxicity
● Embryo-foetal and perinatal toxicity

- Mutagenic potential
  - *In-vivo*
  - *In-vitro*
- Carcinogenic potential
- Pharmacodynamics
  - Pharmacodynamic effects relating to proposed indication
  - General pharmacodynamics
- Pharmacokinetics
  - After single dose
  - After repeated doses
  - Distribution
  - Biotransformation
- Local tolerance
- Other information
- Environmental risk assessment/ecotoxicity

Part IV: like Part III, Part IV of the dossier follows an agreed format, and conveys the data obtained from the clinical trials performed and/or bibliographical information available. Directive 91/507/EEC ensures that any trials reported should have been conducted in accordance with GCP. Therefore, the raw data (clinical trial reports) should be presented in accordance with the guidance provided by the Committee for Proprietary Medicinal Products (CPMP) and with GCP. The structure of Part IV is as follows:

- Pharmacodynamics
  - Summary
  - Results
  - Conclusions
  - Bibliography
- Pharmacokinetics
  - Results in healthy volunteers
  - Results in patients
  - Results in special populations
  - Conclusions
- Clinical experience
  - Clinical trials: for each trial, there should be a summary, detailed description, results, discussion and conclusion
- Post-marketing experience
- Published and unpublished experience
- Other information

Application procedures

The current European rules for the approval of medicines for marketing have been in place since 1 January 1995, with a transitional phase until 1998. The procedures fall into two categories: the centralised procedure; and the decentralised (or mutual recognition) procedure.

In order to utilise the MRP, a pharmaceutical company must first obtain a national licence. Strictly speaking, therefore, there are three procedures. The stand-alone, national procedure must be followed by MRP if further approvals in the EU are to be sought. However, there are certain exceptions to this rule, e.g. bibliographical applications.

Before reviewing the two main procedures, it will be helpful first to clarify which products can be processed by the respective procedures. The centralised procedure applies to biotechnological products (Part A) and new active substances (Part B), whereas the MRP applies to abridged applications and NCEs, but does not apply to biotechnological products. (Part A and Part B of the Annex to Council Regulation no. 2309/93 are explained below.)

Because the centralised procedure and the MRP each have advantages and disadvantages for the applicant, a detailed understanding of the two procedures is required, and a strategic regulatory plan should be in place before any application is made.

Centralised procedure

The centralised procedure has been in full use since 1 January 1998 and was created by Council Regulation 2309/93. These regulations created the EMEA and, by default, the CPMP which advises on the scientific control and review of medicinal products. The key point of the centralised procedure is that it allows the granting of a marketing authorisation that is valid for the entire EU market. The technical sections of the dossier for a centralised application are as described earlier; however, the administrative procedure is comprehensive and must be adhered to punctiliously.

As stated previously, the types of products for which the centralised procedure is appropriate include those that meet the criteria for Part A, for Part B or for abridged applications where the reference product was granted under the centralised procedure.

Part A products are medicinal products that have been developed by one of the following biotechnological processes:

- recombinant DNA technology;
- controlled expression of genes coding for biologically active proteins in prokaryotes and eukaryotes, including transformed mammalian cells;
- hybridoma and monoclonal antibody methods.

For medicinal products falling under the scope of Part B of the Annex, applicants have the option of using the centralised procedure. Part B products include:

- medicinal products developed by other biotechnological processes which constitute a significant innovation;
- medicinal products administered by means of new delivery systems which constitute a significant innovation;
- medicinal products presented for an entirely new indication which are of significant therapeutic interest;
- medicinal products based on radioisotopes which are of significant therapeutic interest;
- new medicinal products derived from human blood or human plasma;
- medicinal products, the manufacture of which employs processes which demonstrate a significant technical advance, e.g. two-dimensional electrophoresis under micro-gravity;
- medicinal products intended for administration to human beings and containing a new active substance which, on the date of entry into force of Council Regulation (EEC) no. 2309/93, as amended, was not authorised by any Member State for use in a medicinal product intended for human use.

Assuming that a product satisfies the criteria for either Part A or Part B, the process by which the application is made will now be examined. However, the overall procedure commences well in advance of the actual submission. Figure 2 is a flow chart illustrating the centralised procedure, from submission notification through to the final issue of the European Public Assessment Report (EPAR). The different stages in the procedure are explained below.

Stage 1: Pre-submission administration: Approximately 4–6 months before submission of the dossier, the applicant must notify the EMEA of its intention to submit the application. The EMEA emphasises the importance of pre-submission meetings with the applicant. These meetings provide an opportunity for applicants to obtain procedural, regulatory and legal advice from the EMEA. When notifying its intention to submit the application, the applicant must supply the EMEA with the following documentation:

- Draft SPC
- Justification for eligibility under Part A or Part B. (If the intended product falls under the scope of Part B, the applicant should notify and submit evidence that the medicinal product can be classified under such criteria. Any such request, together with relevant supporting documentation, should be submitted at least 15 working days before the following CPMP meeting. The outcome of the CPMP discussions will be forwarded to the applicant directly after the CPMP meeting.)
- Type of application
- Details of scientific advice received. (Scientific advice may be obtained from the EMEA (CPMP) if necessary, and a set procedure exists for this. It should be noted that any such advice given is not binding on the EMEA.)

- Classification of the product
- DMF submission intent, if relevant
- Rapporteur and co-rapporteur choice
- Commitment to genetically modified organism (GMO) release regulations, if relevant
- Manufacturer's location details
- Any request for waivers
- Details of any regulatory issues already identified.

Stage 2: Pre-submission (appointment of rapporteurs). On acceptance that an application falls within the scope of Part A or Part B, the EMEA will notify the applicant, approximately 3 months prior to the actual submission date, of the name of the rapporteur and co-rapporteur and provide information on the applicable fees and dossier requirements of the different CPMP members.

Stage 3: Submission. Following agreement between the applicant and the EMEA, the dossier will be submitted in parallel to the EMEA, the rapporteur and the co-rapporteur. In addition, the applicant will pay the requisite fee. The dossier will consist of one full copy, including the applicant's part of the DMF, and two copies of Part I, including a copy in each of the 11 official EU languages of Part IB.

Stage 4: Validation. Following acknowledgement of receipt of the dossier by the EMEA, validation will take place over the next 10 days. Assuming a positive validation, the EMEA project manager will notify the applicant accordingly and advise on which volumes/parts of the dossier are to be sent to different CPMP members. Subsequently, the EMEA project manager will enter details of the application on to the EMEA tracking system. Simultaneously, the rapporteur and co-rapporteur, having acknowledged receipt of the full application, will notify the Secretariat to start the procedure, effectively setting Day 0 in the flow chart (see Figure 2).

Stage 5: Review procedure. The review process follows a structured, well-defined timetable. Once the procedure has started, the rapporteur and co-rapporteur review the dossier. Following this initial review, an assessment report is generated by the rapporteurs and sent to the CPMP members. By Day 100 of the process, all CPMP members will have returned any comments to the rapporteur and co-rapporteur. This list of comments, together with the original assessment at Day 70, will be compiled into a comprehensive draft list of questions and circulated to the other CPMP members. The agreed list of questions, together with the overall conclusions and overview of the scientific data, are sent to the applicant by Day 120. At that point the timetable is stopped (referred to as a 'clock stop') to allow the applicant to assess the comments and provide suitable and full responses to any of the questions

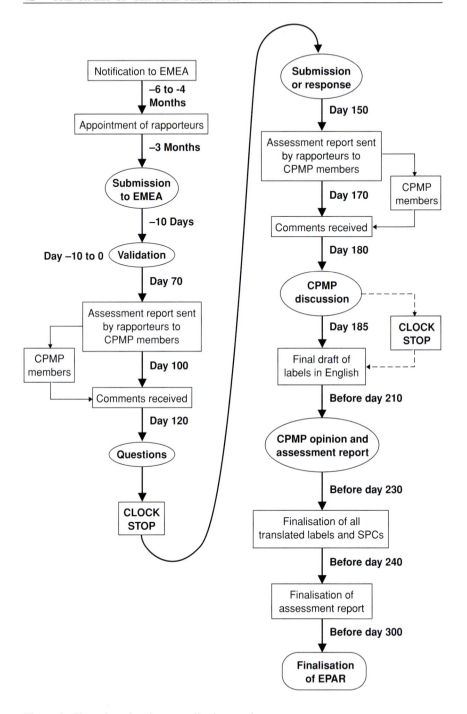

Figure 2. Flow chart for the centralised procedure.

raised. It is clearly in the best interests of the applicant to minimise the response time by being prepared for possible queries that have been identified previously.

Following the submission of responses by the applicant, the timetable is re-started, i.e. at Day 121. However, it should be noted that there are 11 official re-start dates per year. By Day 150 of the procedure, a common assessment report is generated by the rapporteurs and distributed to the CPMP members and the EMEA. Comments from CPMP members are then returned to the rapporteurs by Day 170. The full CPMP meeting to discuss the application is carried out by Day 180 and any need for oral explanations is reviewed. An additional 'clock stop' is possible at this stage to allow the applicant to prepare suitable oral explanations for any remaining issues. Following this and, if necessary, any oral explanation, the final draft of the labelling (including the SPC) is provided by the applicant to the rapporteur, and a CPMP opinion, with draft assessment report, is generated.

Stage 6: CPMP opinion. The CPMP opinion is achieved by Day 210 of the procedure, and takes into consideration all the data presented thus far, including any oral presentations made by the applicant. The opinion is usually achieved by consensus. However, in cases where no overall consensus is obtainable, a majority opinion will be adopted. Assuming that the opinion is positive, the follow-up and issue of the licence then begins.

Stage 7: Follow-up to CPMP opinion. Within 5 days of the opinion (i.e. by Day 215 of the procedure), appropriate translations of the SPC, labels and patient information leaflet (PIL) are provided by the applicant for review by the EMEA and CPMP members. Fifteen days later, the applicant provides the CPMP members with the final translations in accordance with any feedback received. The EMEA receives the final versions of the SPC, labels and PIL, in all 11 official languages, by Day 230 (i.e. 20 days following the opinion).

By Day 240 of the procedure (30 days after CPMP opinion), the final CPMP assessment report and opinion are transmitted by the EMEA to the Commission, Member States and the applicant. By Day 300 of the procedure, the finalisation of the European Public Assessment Report (EPAR) is generated and issued.

It should be noted that the opinion of the EMEA (governed by the scientific review of the rapporteurs and other CPMP members) may be negative. In such cases, the applicant has the right to appeal against the decision using a structured appeal process.

Mutual recognition procedure

The MRP or decentralised procedure has been available since 1995, and has been in full, compulsory operation since January 1998. The legal basis for the procedure is found within Directives 65/65/EEC and 75/319/EEC. The purpose of the MRP is to allow access to a single market, providing an environment of co-operation between Member States. As such, an applicant may obtain approval in a single Member State (first approving state, referred to as the Reference Member State or RMS), and have the application mutually recognised by other Member States (referred to as Concerned Member States or CMSs). This leads to greater understanding between the competent authorities and, most importantly, to the harmonisation of medical practice for specific products (i.e. a harmonised European SPC).

Recommendation by the RMS that a licence should be granted will allow an applicant to proceed with the MRP. The dossiers and an assessment report, generated by the RMS, are updated to include any new information sent in response to questions during the national procedure. This updated version of the dossier and the updated assessment report are then sent to each of the other Member States (the CMSs) selected by the applicant. Mutual recognition of the original marketing authorisation should then occur within 90 days. The individual stages in the MRP are described below.

1: Application to the first Member State or RMS. Each Member State has its own competent licensing authority. A company wishing to license a product in just one Member State must submit an application for marketing authorisation to that national authority. The dossier is assessed, summarised and reviewed by an expert assessor or group of assessors. Usually, the authority will send a list of questions, points for clarification or request for more data to the applicant after approximately 150 days. From the moment the questions are sent until the time when a response is received, the 'clock' is stopped. When all the questions have been answered, the competent authority will either recommend that a licence is granted, request further data, or reject the application. The entire process is usually completed within 210 days (plus the 'clock stop' time to allow responses to queries). The flow diagram in Figure 3 illustrates the overall national procedure, with some 'typical' time periods incorporated.

2: Update of the dossier and request for mutual recognition. Prior to entering the MRP, the application must undergo an updating process (Figure 4). The extent and manner of updating is dependent upon when the initial authorisation was obtained from the RMS, i.e. recently approved applications or older applications.

For recently approved applications, it is likely that no variations to the application will have taken place; as such, the updating of the dossier should be consistent with the questions and responses raised during the national review process. This may include updates to the expert reports and various technical data sections of the dossier. A typical example in this context may be updates to the finished product specification in line with the health authority comments.

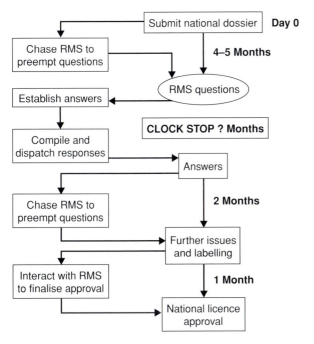

Figure 3. Flow chart for the national procedure.

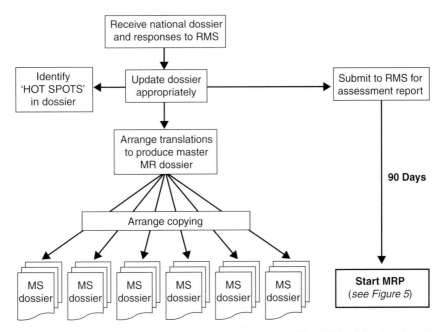

Figure 4. Update of national submission for mutual recognition (MS = Member State).

For older products, the updating process may be somewhat more complex and have to take account of any variations, new data and pharmacopoeial changes that have occurred during the life of the product.

Once the updating process has been completed, the dossier is re-submitted to the RMS with the request to produce an updated assessment report for the purposes of the MRP. The RMS has 90 days in which to generate this updated assessment report; this will be supplied to the applicant's desired CMSs, and the applicant will simultaneously provide the dossier to the same countries. During this stage the applicant simultaneously arranges appropriate translations and copying of the dossier in readiness for submission to the desired CMSs.

3: Validation and submission to CMSs. After being updated, the dossier (including translations of the SPC, PIL and label) is supplied in appropriate format to the applicant's chosen CMSs. The applicant will arrange for fees to be paid to the respective health authorities. Simultaneously, the RMS will supply the updated assessment report to the same CMSs. The validation period, scheduled to last for 10 days, commences on submission. Following validation, Day 0 of the mutual recognition process will be set by the RMS, usually in accordance with a schedule to allow Day 75 of the process to coincide with one of the year's pre-set Mutual Recognition Facilitation Group (MRFG) meetings.

If any country has issues with the data submitted, the validation of the dossier by the CMSs can take longer than the designated 10 days. Equally, however, this part of the process should not focus on inadequacies in the actual technical data except where these relate to concerns over public health.

4: Mutual recognition to the other selected Member States. After Day 0 has been set by the RMS, the mutual recognition process proper will begin. This part of the procedure has a set timetable that lasts for a total of 90 days. Figure 5 presents an overview of MRP from initial updating of the dossier and submission through to final licence issue by the respective CMSs. The procedure focuses on the pivotal 90-day period after Day 0 has been set. A number of critical dates fall within this period:

- All questions (concerns over public health) should be raised by CMSs and relayed to the applicant by Day 55 of the procedure.
- All responses to queries raised should be returned to CMSs by Day 65 of the procedure. (It should be noted that all responses to all queries are relayed to all CMSs involved.)
- Day 75 sees the MRFG meeting during which final resolution of queries and SPC issues can be addressed. The aim of the MRFG is to ensure agreement of a harmonised SPC.
- Day 85 sees finalisation of the SPC.
- Day 90 marks the end of the procedure and the mutual recognition of the original RMS approval.

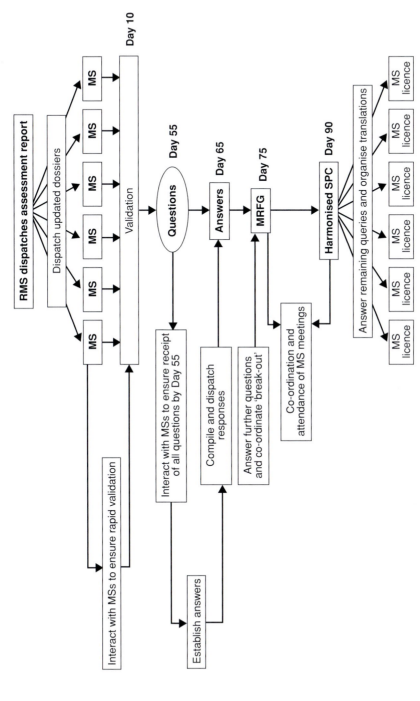

Figure 5. Overview of MRP (MS = Member State).

It is possible to withdraw the application from all or any individual Member States during the process if there are insurmountable but genuine public health concerns. Because the process is still very political, the applicant may view withdrawal as preferable to arbitration.

5: Issue of national licences. Following Day 90 and the recognition of the first national approval by the respective CMSs, the applicant must re-submit to all the CMSs the appropriate updated translations of the SPC, PIL and labels, in accordance with agreed changes following the MRP. The applicant should provide these updated translations of the documents to the CMSs within 14 days following Day 90. Accordingly, the CMSs then have a period of 30 days in which to issue the product licences. This time frame assumes that there are no country-specific issues with the national language versions of these key documents; it is not unusual for this period to be significantly longer than the designated 30 days.

In addition to the above, the applicant must also arrange/apply for required reimbursement status in certain European countries.

Summary. Both the centralised procedure and the MRP are comprehensively described in documentation issued by the EMEA and both can be regarded as successful methods for obtaining harmonised marketing authorisations throughout Europe. Under the current legislation, however, the applicant is faced with a significant dilemma during drug development: which procedure is more appropriate? Table 7 summarises the features of the two systems.

Table 7. Features of the mutual recognition procedure v. centralised procedure.

Mutual recognition procedure	Centralised procedure
<ul><li>210 days + 90 assessment report + 90 mutual recognition</li><li>+ 30 (issue licence)</li><li>Early market access in Reference Member State</li><li>Flexibility</li><li>Difficulties in time to authorisation in some Concerned Member States</li><li>Flexibility for co-marketing/licensing arrangements</li><li>Facilitates regional marketing strategy</li><li>Withdrawal route offers access to majority markets</li><li>Failure during arbitration prevents access to all</li><li>Labelling approved after evaluation</li></ul>	<ul><li>210 days + 110 (decision-making process) + clock stop</li><li>Lengthy process</li><li>Predictable timelines</li><li>Pan-European authorisation/Commission decision-making process</li><li>Multiple applications overseen by Commission</li><li>All or nothing</li><li>Labelling approved in parallel with evaluation</li></ul>

THE FUTURE SYSTEM OF MEDICINAL PRODUCT REGULATION

Any survey of key areas in which global advances are being made towards improved harmonisation will highlight the following achievements:

- The ICH Steering Committee and its technical Expert Working Groups (EWG) are still making significant progress on the Common Technical Document (CTD) and on the electronic version of the CTD, specifically under the aegis of the EWG on Electronic Standards for Transfer of Regulatory Information (ESTRI).
- ICH is involved in a number of other important initiatives. Progress is being made on safety pharmacology and on the topic of GMP for active pharmaceutical ingredients. Furthermore, harmonisation work on pharmacopoeias has progressed well and further advances are anticipated.
- The ICH Steering Committee plans to further develop the concept of harmonisation in gene therapy.
- The FDA has significantly advanced the use of the Medical Dictionary for Regulatory Activities (MedDRA), and the Coding Working Party of ICH has developed points to consider on MedDRA™ Term Selection.

While numerous advances are being made in terms of global harmonisation, led by ICH, it is felt that the major advances for Europe will focus on the development of an agreed clinical trial administration procedure and on improvements in the marketing authorisation process. This summary of future developments relating to the regulation of medicinal products will concentrate on two principal areas: the European Clinical Trials Directive and the CTD.

The European Clinical Trials Directive

In April 1999 the Commission adopted its amended proposal for a European Parliament and Council Directive on the approximation of the laws, regulations and administrative provisions of the Member States relating to the implementation of good clinical practice in the conduct of clinical trials on medicinal products for human use. The amended proposal takes into account the first reading by the European Parliament, the opinion of the Economic and Social Committee, as well as discussions with Council representatives. In order to ensure more efficient implementation of the Directive, the Commission has introduced a number of amendments aimed either at clarifying and strengthening some of the initial provisions or at adding new provisions to bring the proposal more closely into line with existing Community legislation on medicinal products.

The principal purpose of the European Clinical Trials Directive is to ensure that the ICH Tripartite Guideline for GCP is implemented into European law. In addition, it is envisaged that the Directive will allow the harmonisation of regulatory requirements and country-specific nuances to be addressed, thus permitting a standardised approach to clinical trials to be adopted throughout Europe.

In summary, in addition to incorporating the ICH Tripartite Guideline for GCP into European law, the Directive will:

- allow implementation of an audit procedure;
- impose specific requirements on sponsors to inform health authorities of the start of any clinical study, effectively forming a standard approach to regulatory approval of trials;
- create the basis for an exchange of information on clinical trials in the EU;
- enforce GMP;
- standardise labelling requirements; and
- standardise pharmacovigilance in clinical trials.

The European Clinical Trials Directive will compel all ethics committees to operate within a detailed framework, thus providing a consolidated central approach to the ethical review of clinical trials. This in turn should lead to the better acceptability of EU clinical data by the FDA, a major factor given the global nature of the pharmaceutical research industry today. It is currently envisaged that the Directive will be implemented into EU law, and subsequently into respective Member States' national laws, during 2001 and 2002.

The Common Technical Document

Under the terms of ICH, views concerning a common standard for clinical reports have been firmly understood for a number of years. The format of clinical study reports has been agreed and a single format for reporting the core clinical studies comprising the clinical section of a registration dossier has been established.

It therefore seems sensible to move towards harmonisation of the marketing application in terms of the CTD. The harmonisation process is intended first to address the technical content of those sections of the data where significant differences have been identified between regulatory requirements. One aim of the CTD is to remove redundancy and duplication in the development and review process. As ICH is approaching this target of a single data format for a new product, the development of the CTD for reporting these data to the regulatory authorities has become increasingly important.

In principle, the proposed structure of the CTD follows a defined system consisting of five modules, as described below.

- *Module I:* Regional administrative information (e.g. application form with signatures, declaration of fees, table of contents, proposals for packaging text, labelling and package leaflet).

- *Module IIA:* Executive summaries:
    Quality
    Non-clinical
    Clinical
- *Module IIB:* Non-clinical summaries:
    Written summary
    Tabulated summary
- *Module IIC:* Clinical summaries:
    Written summary
    Tabulated summary
- *Module III:* Quality
- *Module IV:* Non-clinical data study reports
- *Module V:* Clinical data study reports

One major implication of the CTD, especially with respect to the US FDA system, is that the raw data from each of the individual studies are not part of the CTD. This has been overcome by ensuring that such data are available upon request.

The format of CTD modules III, IV and V will now be examined in greater depth. Module III (Quality) will consist of the following sections:

- Description of manufacturing process controls for:
    new chemical entities
    biotechnology products
- Control of materials for biotechnology
- Process validation or evaluation
- Container closure system
- Pharmaceutical development report
- Description of manufacturing process and process controls
- Container closure system
- Description of biotechnology facilities and equipment
- Viral safety evaluation

However, some obstacles still need to be overcome with regard to the data supplied in Module III. One of these concerns the fact that in the USA, the quality of drug substances, excipients, or containers manufactured by a third party may be documented by the supplier in a DMF and filed with the FDA separately. The manufacturer of the drug product may then simply refer in the application to DMFs. This procedure is restricted to active ingredients in the EU, and does not exist at all in Japan. Another challenge for the Quality module of the CTD is the difference in specifications: in the USA and Japan, drug substance and drug product specifications set limits that are valid until the re-test date of the substance or throughout the shelf-life of the product. In the EU, in addition, a release specification valid at the time of batch release after manufacturing has to be supplied to the authorities as part of the registration documentation.

Module IV (Non-clinical) of the CTD follows a logical order that reflects the sequential pathway of drug development:

- Table of contents
- Study reports
- Pharmacology
    Primary pharmacodynamics
    Secondary pharmacodynamics
    Safety pharmacology
    Pharmacodynamic drug interactions
- Pharmacokinetics
    Analytical methods and validation reports (if separate reports are available)
    Kinetics (including studies of absorption and excretion)
    Tissue distribution
    Metabolism
    Pharmacokinetic drug interactions (non-clinical)
    Other pharmacokinetic studies
- Toxicology
    Single-dose toxicity
    Repeated-dose toxicity
    Genotoxicity
    Carcinogenicity
    Reproduction toxicity
    Fertility and early embryonic development
    Embryo-foetal development
    Pre-natal and post-natal development, including maternal function
    Local tolerance
    Other toxicity studies (if available)
    Antigenicity
    Immunotoxicity
    Mechanistic studies (if not included elsewhere)
    Dependence
    Metabolites
    Impurities
    Other
- Key literature references

Module V (Clinical data) of the CTD will be organised as follows; among other documents, it will contain the individual clinical study report:

- Table of contents
- Tabular listing of all human studies
- Human study reports

- Bioavailability and bioequivalence studies
    Bioavailability
    Bioequivalence
    In-vitro/in-vivo comparison
    Bioanalytical and analytical methods
- Studies using human biomaterials pertinent to absorption or disposition
    Plasma protein binding
    Hepatic metabolism and interaction studies
    Studies using other human biomaterials
- Human pharmacokinetics (PK) studies
    Healthy subject PK and initial tolerability
    Patient PK and initial tolerability
    Intrinsic factor PK
    Extrinsic factor PK
    Population PK study
- Human pharmacodynamics (PD) studies
    Healthy subject PD and PK/PD
    Patient PD and PK/PD
- Efficacy and safety studies
    Controlled clinical studies pertinent to the claimed indication
    Uncontrolled clinical studies
    Analyses of data from more than one study
    Other study reports
- Post-marketing experience
- Case report forms and individual patient listings

The proposed CTD will have to be discussed with authorities in countries outside the ICH territory, including Australia, New Zealand, South Africa, and other members of the World Health Organization (WHO). Canada and Switzerland have always participated in ICH discussions, and Norway and Iceland as well as countries in Central and Eastern Europe usually adopt ICH and EU guidelines. Further points still to be addressed include extending the CTD to pharmaceutical products containing drug substances other than just new active substances.

THE REGULATORY ENVIRONMENT IN THE USA

The FDA ensures that food, cosmetics, medicines, medical devices and radiation-emitting consumer products (e.g. microwaves) are safe and effective. Of particular relevance to the pharmaceutical industry, the FDA oversees regulations for medicinal products and devices, with respect to both the clinical development and ultimately the marketing of such products.

Authorised by the US Congress to enforce the Federal Food, Drug and Cosmetic Act and several other public health laws, the FDA monitors the manufacture, import, transport, storage, and sale of USD 1 trillion worth of goods annually. The FDA employs over 9000 people in 157 US cities, among whom are 2100 scientists, including 900 chemists and 300 microbiologists, who work in 40 laboratories across the country. In addition, the FDA employs 1100 investigators and inspectors.

The section of the FDA involved in control of human medicines is the Center for Drug Evaluation and Research (CDER). Its function is to evaluate new drugs before they can be sold. The CDER ensures that safe and effective drugs are available to improve the health of consumers, and that prescription and over-the-counter drugs, both brand name and generic, work correctly and that their health benefits outweigh the known risks.

The clinical development of a new drug is covered by FDA regulations and an investigational new drug (IND) application needs to be made when clinical studies in humans are to be carried out. An IND application is a request for the FDA to authorise the new drug to be given to humans. Such an authorisation must be secured before administration of any new drug. The IND regulations are contained in Title 21, Code of Federal Regulations (CFR), Part 312.

The rules laid down in CFR 21 require that a drug be the subject of an approved marketing application before it is transported or distributed across state lines. Because a sponsor will probably wish to transport investigational drug to study sites throughout the USA, an exemption from that requirement must be sought. The IND allows the sponsor to by-pass these transporting rules.

During a new drug's early non-clinical development, the sponsor's primary goal is to determine whether the product is reasonably safe for use in humans and whether the compound exhibits any pharmacological activity. Once a suitable product has been identified, the focus then shifts to collecting the data and information necessary to establish that the product will not expose humans to unreasonable risks when used in limited, early-phase clinical studies.

The role of the FDA in the development of a new drug begins when the sponsor company wishes to test the drug's diagnostic or therapeutic potential in humans. At that point, the legal status of the molecule changes under the Federal Food, Drug, and Cosmetic Act and it becomes a new drug subject to specific requirements of the drug regulatory system.

In addition to the standard IND, there are three further types of IND:

- An Investigator IND is submitted by a physician who both initiates and conducts an investigation, and under whose immediate direction the investigational drug is administered or dispensed. A physician might submit an Investigator IND to propose the study of an unapproved drug, or of an approved product for a new indication or in a new patient population.

- Emergency use IND allows the FDA to authorise the use of an experimental drug in an emergency situation where there is insufficient time to submit an IND. It is also used for patients who do not meet the criteria of an existing study protocol, or in cases where an approved study protocol does not exist.
- A Treatment IND is submitted for experimental drugs that show promise in clinical testing for serious or immediately life-threatening conditions while the final clinical work is conducted and the FDA review takes place.

The IND application must contain information in three broad areas:

- Animal pharmacology and toxicology studies: preclinical data to permit an assessment as to whether the product is reasonably safe for initial testing in humans. Also included here is any previous experience with the drug in humans, e.g. from use in other countries.
- Manufacturing information: information pertaining to the composition, manufacture, stability, and controls used for manufacturing the drug substance and the drug product. This information is assessed to ensure that the company can adequately produce and supply consistent batches of the drug.
- Clinical protocols and investigator information: detailed protocols for proposed clinical studies to assess whether the early phase trials will expose subjects to unnecessary risks. Information is also provided on the qualifications of clinical investigators – professionals (generally physicians) who oversee the administration of the experimental compound – to assess whether they are qualified to fulfil their clinical trial duties. Finally, commitments are given to obtain informed consent from the research subjects, to obtain review of the study by an institutional review board (IRB), and to adhere to the IND regulations.

Once the IND has been submitted, the sponsor must wait 30 calendar days before initiating any clinical trials. During this period, the FDA has an opportunity to review the IND for safety to ensure that research subjects will not be subjected to unreasonable risk.

Following successful implementation of a development programme, the sponsor may wish to apply for a marketing authorisation. As with the situation in Europe, the FDA has specific application procedures and dossier requirements for both New Drug Applications (NDAs) and Abbreviated New Drug Applications (ANDAs).

The NDA is the process that allows sponsors to apply to the FDA to approve a new pharmaceutical for sale and marketing in the USA. The data gathered during the animal studies and human clinical trials of an IND become an integral part of the NDA. Sufficient information should be provided in the NDA to allow the FDA reviewer to reach a decision on the drug's safety, effectiveness, quality and labelling suitability. The documentation required in an NDA should convey the complete picture of the development of the drug,

Table 8. Sections of US NDA compared with those of a European marketing application (MA).

NDA	MA
1. Index	Part I
2. Labeling	Part I
3. Application summary	
A. *Annotated package insert*	Part I.B. Summary of product characteristics
B. *Pharmacologic class* Scientific rationale Intended use Potential clinical benefits	Incorporated in clinical expert report
C. *Foreign marketing history*	Not required
D. *Chemical manufacturing controls summary*	Part I.C.1. Pharmaceutical expert report
E. *Non-clinical pharmacology and toxicology summary* 1. Pharmacology 2. Toxicology 3. ADME	Part I.C.2. Pharmaco-toxicological expert report
F. *Human pharmacokinetics and bioavailabilty summary*	Part I.C. Clinical expert report
G. *Clinical data summary and results of statistical analysis*	Part I.C. Clinical expert report
H. *Benefit/risk, proposed postmarketing studies*	Part I.C. Clinical expert report
4. Chemistry, MFG, controls	
A. *CMC*	
1. Drug substance	
1.1 Description, including physical and chemical characteristics and stability	Part II.C
Stability report	Part II.F
1.2 Manufacturer	Part II.C
1.3 Method of manufacture and packaging and in-process controls	Part II.C

		(Open Part of DMF)
	(DMF reference)	
1.4	Specifications and analytical methods	Part II.C
	Impurities	Part II.C
	Reference Standard	Part II.C
	Methods Validation	Part II.C
	Batch Analysis	Part II.A.4
	Development pharmaceutics	
2.	Drug product	
2.1	Components	Part II.B
2.2	Compositions	Part II.C
2.3	Specifications and analytical methods for inactive components	Part I.C
2.4	Manufacturer	Part II.B
2.5	Method of manufacture, packaging procedure and in-process controls	Part II.B
	– Validations of process, e.g. sterilizer, lyophilizer	Part II.B
	– Container specifications	
2.6	Specifications and analytical methods	Part II.D.E
	– Batch analysis	Part II.E.2.2
	(DMF reference)	Not required
2.7	Stability data	Part II.F
	a. Stability protocols for drug product	
	– Stability protocol for pre-NDA products	
	– Stability protocol for marketed drug products	
	– Statistical analyses for determination of drug product expiry periods	
	b. Summary of stability data and proposed expiry	
	– Stability reports including:	
	• Stability data for each marketed drug product	
	• Analytical procedures	
3.	Supporting information	Including in Part II
	Environmental assessment	Part II.H.
B.	*Samples*	
	Drug substance	
	Reference standard	Part I
	Impurities	
	Degradation products	
	Drug product	

Continued

Table 8. *Continued.*

NDA	MA
C. *Methods validation package*	Not required
Specifications	
Methods of analysis	
Flow chart of synthesis	
Methods validation reports	
Chromatograms	
Not required	Package Insert
	Translations Part IB
5. Non-clinical pharmacology and toxicology	Narrative summaries can be included in EC MA
A. *Overall pharmacology summary*	Not required
Overall ADME summary	
B. *Table of contents and cross references*	Part III.F. +
C. *Pharmacology studies*	Tabulated Study Reports
	Part III.A. +
D. *Acute toxicity studies*	Tabulated Study Reports
	Part III.A +
E. *Multidose toxicity studies*	Tabulated Study Reports
	Part III.H. +
F. *Special toxicity studies*	Tabulated Study Reports
	Part III.B. +
G. *Reproduction studies*	Tabulated Study Reports
	Part III.D. +
H. *Mutagenicity studies*	Tabulated Study Reports
	Part III.G. +
I. *ADME studies*	Tabulated Study Reports
6. Human pharmacokinetics and bioavailability section	
A. *Tabulated summary of studies*	Part IV.A.2. Optional
B. *Summary of data and overall conclusions*	Part of Clinical Export Report
C. *Drug formulations*	Part II.A.
D. *Analytical methods*	Part II.A.

E. *Dissolution profile*	Part II.C.
F. *Individual study reports*	Part IV.A.
1. Pilot studies	
2. Bioavailability/bioequivalence studies	
3. Pharmacokinetic studies	
4. Other *in-vivo* studies	
5. *In-vitro* studies (dissolution profile)	
7. Microbiology section	
8. Clinical section	
A. *Index to clinical section*	
1. Index	Optional
2. List of all investigators; location of documents	Not required
3. INF #s	Not required
B. *Background/overview of clinical investigations*	Not required
C. *Clinical pharmacology*	Not Required
1. Table of all studies/list of investigators/location of documents	Part IV.A.
2. Overall summary of ADME studies	Part IV.A1.
3. Early dose tolerance studies	Not required
Overall Summary of Subsection C.3.	Part IV.A.
4. Short-term studies of therapeutic response including dose-response studies	Not required
Overall Summary of Subsection C.4.	Part IV.A
5. Pharmacodynamic properties other than that related to effectiveness	Not required
Overall Summary of Subsection C.5.	Part IV.A.1.
6. Special studies	Not required
7. Overall summary of clinical pharmacology	
D. *Controlled clinical trials*	
1. Table of all studies/list of investigators/location of documents	Not required
2. Placebo-controlled studies	

Continued

Table 8. *Continued.*

NDA	MA
a. Completed	Part IV.B
i. Domestic with case reports (includes statistical reports)	
ii. Foreign with case reports (includes statistical reports)	
Roster of ERC/RC, qualifications	Not required
Description of Research Facilities	
iii. Published, no case reports	
Foreign, no case reports	
b. Ongoing with interim results	
c. Incomplete, no longer active	
3. Dose-comparison concurrent control	
4. No treatment control	
5. Active control	
6. Historical control	
E. *Uncontrolled clinical trials*	
F. *Other studies and information*	
1. Tables of all studies and information included in section	Not required
2. Controlled studies of uses other than those claimed in the application	Not required
3. Uncontrolled studies of uses other than those claimed in the application	Not required
4. Commercial marketing experience and foreign regulatory actions	Not required
a. List of countries in which drug approved/approval applied for	Part I
b. Copies of approved labelling abroad; explanation of differences in dosage	Not required
c. Reports from foreign Regulatory Authorities	Not required
d. Epidemiologic Studies	Not required

  e. Spontaneously reported AEs
  5. Published literature; any other information not included elsewhere — Not required / Part IV.B

G. *Integrated summary of efficacy* — Condensed for clinical expert report
H. *Integrated summary of safety*
I. *Overdose (and drug abuse)*
J. *Integrated summary of benefit/risks* — Part of clinical expert report

9. Safety updates — Not required

10. Statistical — Part of Part IV
A. *All controlled studies (Key to approval)*
B. *All safety all protocols*

11. Tabulated case reports — Part IV

12. Case reports — Not routinely required
All deaths — All Protocols
All dropouts due to AEs — All Protocols
Studies key to approval

13. Patent information — Not required

14. Patent certification — Not required

16. Debarment certification — Not required

17. Field copy certification — Not required / Part I.A. / Administrative data including clinical tests, the ingredients of the drug, the results of animal studies, how the drug behaves in the body, and how it is manufactured, processed and packaged.

Table 8 details the discrete sections of the NDA and allows comparison of these sections with those in the European marketing application dossier.

CONCLUSION

Under the guidance of ICH and driven by commercial requirements, the development of a pharmaceutical product is currently performed within a global context. This chapter confirms the status of regulatory affairs professionals as integral members of the project team involved in drug development. Their contribution reflects a profound understanding not only of their own country-specific regulatory requirements, but also of those in other countries or regions where the product is ultimately to be marketed. The process of bringing clinical trials to a successful conclusion will be facilitated and expedited if other clinical research professionals are also aware of the regulatory requirements that apply in specific countries/regions.

Simultaneously, the increasing globalisation of the pharmaceutical industry has been paralleled by the development of correspondingly global medicinal product regulations. These will lead to greater harmonisation of the processes of drug development, drug review and marketing authorisation.

REFERENCES

EudraLex (1998). *The Rules Governing Medicinal Products in the European Union. Volume 3C: Medicinal Products for Human Use. Efficacy – Clinical Guidelines*, European Commission, Brussels.

3

Ethical issues

David Talbot and Joan Perou

Ethics cannot be grafted on to a trial – it must be built in from the outset. Ultimately an ethical attitude must pervade the approach to clinical investigation, its establishment and follow-through.
Explanatory memorandum (June 1997) to proposed European Clinical Trials Directive

INTRODUCTION

Ethical issues deserve respect and consideration because they are an important part of clinical research and researchers have a duty to uphold them. Historically, the vast body of clinical research has been conducted by members of the medical profession who have been considered by the public to be trustworthy and reliable. However, there have been instances where the public's trust has been severely shaken and, during the last decade in particular, the topic of misconduct in clinical research has unfortunately become all too common (*see Chapter 24*). Ethics is defined as the discipline of describing behaviour, practices, thinking and moral values generally agreed to be acceptable to society. In the present context, ethical issues are those that determine whether a piece of clinical research conforms to accepted guidelines and rules on ethics. The aim of this chapter is to describe some of the common ethical issues to be faced when conducting clinical trials.

The existence of ethical issues in the conduct of clinical research was recognised in England as long ago as 1803 in *Percival's Medical Ethics* (Leake, 1927). Little changed for the next century until 1900 in Germany when The Directive on Human Experimentation was issued by the Prussian Minister for Religious, Educational and Medical Affairs (Vollmann and Winau, 1996). Following the well-publicised medical research horrors that emerged at the Nuremberg trials, during the course of which it was revealed that Nazi physicians had undertaken experiments on prisoners without consent and without regard for their human subjects' well-being, the Nuremberg Code was published in 1947 (US Government Printing Office, 1949). The Nuremberg Code emphasised for the first time the principles of informed consent. The World Medical Association (WMA) developed further the ethical principles laid down in the Nuremberg Code. Its deliberations eventually found expression in the Declaration of Helsinki, so called because it was during the annual assembly of the WMA in Helsinki in 1964 that the Declaration was agreed and published.

DECLARATION OF HELSINKI

The Declaration of Helsinki is the fundamental document in the field of human ethics and it underpins the principles of ethical decision-making in biomedical research throughout the world. The purpose of the Declaration is clearly stated in its introduction: 'The World Medical Association has developed the Declaration of Helsinki as a statement of ethical principles to provide guidance to physicians and other participants in medical research involving human subjects.'

The Declaration has undergone five subsequent revisions during WMA assemblies in Tokyo (1975), Venice (1983), Hong Kong (1989), Somerset/Republic of South Africa (1996) and – the current version – Edinburgh (2000). The full text of the current version of the Declaration of Helsinki is reproduced in Appendix I. The clear principles established in the 1964 version have been retained throughout the subsequent revisions. Although the WMA has adopted many other declarations, statements and guidelines concerning the ethical conduct of physicians, both before and since, the Declaration of Helsinki remains the cornerstone ethical reference for global medical research. It is not a legally binding document, although its principles have been incorporated into law in some countries, and it is often included as an appendix to research contract documents. The Declaration of Helsinki is a multicultural, multilingual declaration made by physicians for physicians. It confirms the role of the physician above that of the investigator. It is not a guideline or a set of rules, but is intended to be a set of principles defining the standards that should apply to biomedical research worldwide.

The Declaration of Helsinki comprises 32 paragraphs divided into three sections: Introduction; Basic principles for all medical research; and Additional principles for medical research combined with medical care. The basic principles are now listed in 18 paragraphs and can be summarised as follows:

- It is the duty of the physician to protect the life, health, privacy and dignity of the human subject.
- Medical research involving human subjects must conform to generally accepted scientific principles.

- Effects on the environment and the welfare of animals used for research must be considered.
- Each experimental procedure should be fully described in a protocol and be considered by an ethical review committee.
- The research protocol should contain a statement of the ethical aspects.
- Medical research should be conducted by scientifically qualified persons supervised by a clinically competent medical person.
- Predictable risks and burdens should be weighed against foreseeable benefits for the subject and others.
- Physicians should cease any investigation if the risks outweigh the potential benefits.
- The importance of the objective should outweigh the risks and burden to the subject, especially in healthy volunteer studies.
- Medical research is only justified if there is a reasonable likelihood that a population will benefit.
- The subjects must be volunteers and informed participants.
- The right of research subjects to safeguard their physical and mental integrity and privacy must be respected.
- Each potential subject must be adequately informed, and his/her freely given consent obtained, preferably in writing.
- Subjects in a dependent relationship with the researcher should be consented by an independent physician.
- For legally incompetent subjects, the investigator must obtain consent from a legally authorised representative.
- Where the legally incompetent subject is able to give assent to decisions about participation in research, that assent should be obtained in addition.
- If research is intended on subjects who cannot consent, it must be justified to and approved by the review committee.
- Results of all trials conducted according to these principles should be accurately published or otherwise made available.

Questions have been raised concerning the ownership of the Declaration of Helsinki. It is now used by many groups of people in addition to physicians, for example, clinical trial subjects, other researchers, governments, regulatory authorities, health care providers, and pharmaceutical manufacturers. At a workshop meeting in London in September 1999, there was general agreement that although the Declaration of Helsinki is clearly a WMA document, the values and principles that it represents are not 'owned' by the WMA but are 'shared' by the world community (Nicholson, 1999).

Strict interpretation of paragraph 29 of the Declaration that 'a new method should be tested against ... the best current prophylactic, diagnostic, and therapeutic methods' leads to problems when sub-optimal therapy is included in comparative study designs, e.g. placebo in hypertension studies, Phase I studies with cytotoxic agents, and choice of control group in human immunodeficiency virus (HIV) studies. Indeed, the development of all new treatments for conditions where a treatment is already licensed can be challenged on these grounds. Research designed to develop a less costly alternative to an expensive medicine for Third World use, e.g. short-duration zidovudine in perinatal HIV transmission, could also be considered to be in breach of the Declaration. Considerable discussion also surrounds the interpretation of 'best current' diagnosis and therapy. Does this mean worldwide or only in the country where the research is being conducted?

Unlike the Declaration of Independence, the Declaration of Helsinki is not a historical document, and therefore can be changed. It can be argued that the revisions to the original 1964 Declaration have not improved it, and may actually have made it worse. The broadly held view is that it should be regarded as a set of guiding principles upon which local rules are based. The principles should be formulated as clearly as possible, allowing for translation, because the field of research ethics is more complex than medical ethics in general. However, despite all these criticisms, the Declaration remains the fundamental guiding principle in research ethics.

GOOD CLINICAL PRACTICE

Good clinical practice (GCP) is: 'A standard for the design, conduct, performance, monitoring, auditing, recording, analyses, and reporting of clinical trials that provides assurance that the data and reported results are credible and accurate, and that the rights, integrity, and confidentiality of trial subjects are protected.'

The above statement is found in section 1.24 of the ICH GCP guideline which is now the most widely accepted GCP guideline in Europe and beyond (ICH Guideline, 1996). This document became effective in Europe in January 1997 and provides a unified standard for the European Union, Japan and the United States to facilitate the mutual acceptance of clinical data by the regulatory authorities of those jurisdictions. The first principle of ICH GCP (section 2.1) is that: 'Clinical trials should be conducted in accordance with the ethical principles that have their origin in the Declaration of Helsinki and that are consistent with GCP and the applicable regulatory requirement(s).' There have, in the past, been other versions of GCP guidelines, but the ICH guideline for the first time has the potential to become the global standard because it has attracted considerable interest from outside the ICH region. The benefits of a global standard would be enormous, in terms of cost savings alone, quite apart from all the moral and ethical benefits of not having to repeat clinical trials over again in each country simply to obtain a licence to sell the drug locally.

The ICH GCP document itself is very comprehensive. It includes specific sections listing the responsibilities of the institutional review board

(IRB)/independent ethics committee (IEC) (Section 3), the investigator (Section 4) and the sponsor (Section 5). In addition, there are sections detailing the format and content of a standard clinical trial protocol (Section 6) and investigator's brochure (Section 7). The guideline also specifies the essential documents for the conduct of a clinical trial, their purpose, and where (and by whom) they are to be retained.

The ICH GCP guideline is an excellent attempt to unify GCP standards but it requires a legal framework to give it the necessary 'muscle' to ensure that it is adhered to by investigators, sponsors and ethics committees. Although most sponsor companies have been working to ICH GCP since its implementation, investigators and ethics committees have not always agreed with the additional documentation they were required to provide. Until recently they were able to point to the guideline status of ICH GCP in mitigation. While this attitude may have been strictly correct in many respects, it would have been unwise for sponsor companies to recruit investigators with this mindset into regulatory studies. Ethics committees also needed some convincing on this count and often did not provide sponsor companies with the additional documentation required under ICH GCP since they felt that they were not legally obliged to do so. However, the European Clinical Trials Directive has signalled the end to such resistance (European Parliament and Council Directive, 2000); once implemented into local law, it will provide the legal status that is so urgently needed for ICH GCP.

INSTITUTIONAL REVIEW BOARDS AND INDEPENDENT ETHICS COMMITTEES

According to section 3.1.1 of the ICH GCP guideline: 'An IRB/IEC should safeguard the rights, safety, and well-being of all trial subjects. Special attention should be paid to trials that may include vulnerable subjects.'

IRBs are the North American equivalent of IECs in Europe. Section 3 of the ICH GCP guideline is devoted to the subject of ethical review and refers to both IRBs and IECs throughout. It defines the responsibilities, composition, functions, operations and record keeping of IRBs/IECs. It stipulates that the committee (or board) should have a 'reasonable number' of members, at least five, who collectively have the qualifications and experience to review and evaluate the science, medical aspects and ethics of the proposed trial. Such a committee should have at least one member whose primary area of interest is non-scientific, and one member who is independent of the institution/trial site. Regarding its function, the committee should have written operating procedures, and maintain written records of its activities and minutes of its meetings to comply with GCP. All protocols submitted should be considered at announced meetings, and only members who are present for the discussion may vote. An investigator who is a member of the ethics committee may give information to the committee on any aspect of the proposed trial, but should not participate in the deliberations or vote/opinion, and must declare an association with the ethics committee in writing in order to satisfy auditors that no bias was involved.

The ICH GCP guideline lists the documents that are to be provided to an IRB/IEC: these include the investigator's brochure, protocol, informed consent form, subject information leaflet, and safety information on the investigational product. The IRB/IEC must review the documents and decide whether or not the research proposal is ethical. The guideline states that ethical review should be completed 'within a reasonable time' (section 3.1.2) and that the committee should document its views in writing. The committee should consider the qualifications of the investigator and the suitability of the site, and should conduct 'continuing review of each ongoing trial at intervals appropriate to the degree of risk to the human subjects, but at least once per year' (section 3.1.4). Where the research proposal involves non-therapeutic research, or where the protocol indicates that prior consent of the subject/legally acceptable representative is not possible, the ethics committee should determine that the proposal adequately addresses relevant ethical concerns. The IRB/IEC should review both the amount and method of payment to subjects to ensure that this is neither coercive nor unduly influences the trial subjects. Moreover, payments should not be wholly contingent on completion of the trial by the subject.

As to its procedures (section 3.3), the IRB/IEC should determine its composition and the authority under which it is established, schedule its meetings, and provide expedited review and approval/favourable opinion of minor changes in ongoing trials that already have the approval/favourable opinion of the IRB/IEC. No subject should be admitted to a trial before the IRB/IEC issues its written approval/favourable opinion, and no deviations or changes to the protocol should be initiated without the written approval/favourable opinion of the IRB/IEC. There are two exceptions to this rule. First, where an immediate change to the protocol is necessary for reasons of subject safety, in which case the ethics committee can be informed after the change has been implemented (within 3 days). Secondly, where only logistical or administrative changes are required (e.g. a change of telephone number in the protocol), the ethics committee then only needs to be notified. All other changes to the protocol, however minor, need to be approved by the committee before being implemented.

For the system to work, it is important that both the investigator and the IRB/IEC communicate promptly with each other regarding deviations or changes from the protocol. In addition, all adverse drug reactions that are both serious and unexpected, and any new information that may adversely affect the safety of the subjects or the conduct of the trial must be promptly reported to the ethics committee. Once the review has taken place, the IRB/IEC should communicate its decision to the investigator in writing, listing fully all documents received and reviewed. To fulfil audit/inspection requirements, a statement of the ethics committee's compliance with GCP should also be provided to the investigator and sponsor company.

In the UK there are approximately 250 local research ethics committees (LRECs), most of which are based around hospitals and institutions. LRECs do not currently operate within a legal framework, although this will change when the European Clinical Trials Directive is fully adopted. Until the 1990s few guidelines existed on how LRECs should operate. As a result, LRECs were left to develop their own working practices and these vary widely across the UK. Some LRECs meet monthly, some bi-monthly and some rarely meet, but merely pass the protocol around the membership for comments which are considered by the Chair of the LREC.

Researchers frequently complain that it is extremely difficult to obtain any uniformity in the LREC approval process: not only do working practices vary enormously, so too do opinions on research proposals. In addition, considerable variation exists in the quality of the documentation received from LRECs and in the administration fees charged. Many LRECs still refuse to supply lists of members, standard operating procedures (SOPs) and a full list of documents reviewed, all of which are essential prerequisites for sponsor companies attempting to conduct studies to ICH GCP. Prior to the introduction of the multicentre research ethics committee (MREC) system (see below), each centre in a multicentre trial had to receive approval from the LREC before the investigator could proceed with the research. For large multicentre trials this was a very time-consuming process that could take many months to accomplish.

Sponsor companies were therefore very optimistic when the MREC system was introduced in the UK in October 1997. This step was taken in advance of the European Clinical Trials Directive which states in Chapter II, Article 5: 'For multicentre clinical trials limited to the territory of a single Member State, Member States shall establish a procedure providing for the adoption of a single opinion for that Member State.'

There are 10 MRECs across the UK and they currently review research proposals for clinical trials that would normally require submission to five or more LRECs. Additionally, once proposals have been approved by the MREC, LRECs have to consider them for local acceptability. It was hoped that this system would improve the significant delays that researchers experience in receiving approvals for multicentre studies. However, while there are some advantages, there is criticism that it has become a time-consuming, two-tiered system because subjects cannot be recruited into clinical trials at local centres until the research proposal has also been 'considered' for local acceptability by the LREC.

The advantage of the MREC system is that MRECs do have standard application forms and SOPs, they publish meeting dates and work in accordance with ICH GCP. They also provide the necessary GCP documentation to researchers and use experienced administrators who assist researchers with enquiries and information. In addition, the Research Ethics Committee Central Office (COREC) has been in operation in London since June 2000: this provides support regarding ethics review to LREC and MREC members as well as to sponsor companies and researchers.

In many UK hospital trusts, ethics committee approval is also conditional upon approval to carry out the study being granted by the trust's research and development (R&D) department. R&D departments in trusts review research proposals in a very different way from ethics committees. They will want to satisfy themselves that the proposed research will not impinge upon the trust's resources, or cost the trust money, and that it is not likely to incur any litigation due to its nature. However, this additional R&D approval, although relevant, is a further time-consuming step for researchers already burdened with administrative procedures before their clinical trial is able to start. Unfortunately, this is another 'nail in the coffin' for clinical research in the UK, as more and more sponsor companies are taking their research elsewhere in Europe to countries where it is possible not only to obtain good quality data, but also to complete the studies earlier because of more efficient approval processes.

Some Member States have very good administrative systems in place for ethical review. In France, for example, a single committee known as the Comité Consultatif de Protection des Personnes dans la Recherche Biomédicale (CCPPRB) has the authority to approve a study and all proposed French centres and investigators in a single meeting.

However, to minimise start-up times for multinational studies, sponsor companies must select countries with care. Times from ethics committee submission to approval vary considerably between countries. Countries with good reputations for prompt review (typically 1 month) are Belgium, the Czech Republic, Denmark, Estonia, Finland, Greece, Lithuania, and Sweden. At the opposite end of the review time scale (typically 3 months) are Austria, France, Germany, Hungary, Ireland, Italy, Spain and the UK.

Language is an important issue in many European countries. To conduct a multinational trial in just six European countries can require translations of some documentation into more than six languages. For example, Austria will accept applications in German, but Belgium requires French and/or Dutch – depending on centre location. Some ethics committees in Germany will require subject documents in Turkish; some Italian areas require documents in German; in Spain, translation of documents into regional languages such as Catalan is required; and trials involving Swiss sites can require documentation in three languages – German, French and Italian. Formal translations, with back-translation required in some countries, all add to the cost of performing multinational studies in Europe. It will be interesting to see how the implementation of the European Clinical Trials Directive, which includes proposals for a maximum review time of 60 days, will impact on approval timelines.

Another factor affecting ethical review in Europe is the need to submit an insurance or indemnity document. Some committees also require draft case record forms (CRFs), quality of life (QoL) questionnaires, or details of pre-clinical work and pharmaceutical formulation and manufacturing, rather like the UK Clinical Trial Exemption (CTX) scheme.

INFORMED CONSENT

Regardless of country, the primary purpose of ethics committees is to protect subjects, especially vulnerable subjects, and one of the most important documents reviewed is the informed consent form. This is often in two parts: written information describing the clinical trial, and a form which the subject signs to document that he/she has given consent to take part in the study.

Before a subject receives medical treatment or undergoes a medical procedure, he/she must give consent. For a doctor even to touch a subject without consent constitutes an assault. In a clinical trial context, it is even more important to obtain informed consent for a research procedure, and to document that this has been freely given. Consent is valid when freely given, provided that the subject understands the nature and consequences of what is proposed. The degree of understanding of what is proposed will depend on the subject's education and intelligence, as well as on the skill with which the proposals are explained. Informed consent is defined in section 1.28 of the ICH GCP guideline as: 'A process by which a subject voluntarily confirms his or her willingness to participate in a particular trial, after having been informed of all aspects of the trial that are relevant to the subject's decision to participate. Informed consent is documented by means of a written, signed and dated informed consent form.'

Section 4.8 of the ICH GCP guideline explains in detail the investigator's responsibilities to obtain informed consent from each trial subject. It states that:

- The ethics committee must approve the written information sheet and informed consent form.
- The information must be up to date, and subjects who have already consented must be similarly informed of any new information.
- The investigator, or trial staff, must not unduly coerce a subject to participate.
- The subject's legal rights must be maintained.
- The subject, or subject's legally acceptable representative, should be fully informed of all pertinent aspects of the trial, including the written information given approval/favourable opinion by the IRB/IEC.
- The written information should be as non-technical as practical and as understandable as possible.
- Ample time and opportunity must be allowed for the subject to ask questions and digest the information.

The ICH GCP guideline makes it clear in section 4.8.8 that the written informed consent form should be signed and personally dated by the subject (or the subject's legally acceptable representative), and by the person who conducted the informed consent discussion.

The term 'legally acceptable representative' appears throughout the ICH GCP guideline section on informed consent. It is offered as an alternative when the subject is unable to give consent. Under UK law, however, the term is unacceptable because no adult can consent on behalf of another. This greatly complicates the issue of obtaining consent from an individual who is incapable of consenting and yet may benefit from the research on offer. Subjects who are unable to give written consent are often referred to as 'vulnerable groups', and such groups may include people who are mentally impaired, unconscious, illiterate, or geriatric. Researchers must decide exactly how it is proposed to obtain consent in trials to which subjects from vulnerable groups are to be recruited, and each individual study must be designed to take account of the ethical and emotional needs of those prospective subjects. Usually, researchers should define in the protocol exactly how they intend the consent procedure to be conducted, and special care needs to be taken when designing consent forms. It is extremely important that ethics committees should review/approve whatever procedures the researcher proposes. For example, for trials in dementia, it is important that an independent witness ensures that the consent procedure is carried out satisfactorily to the level of the subject's understanding. If the subject is unconscious and yet thought likely to benefit from the treatment on offer, it might be appropriate for two doctors to sign the consent form to confirm that the subject, although unable to give consent, may benefit from the research treatment (and therefore has a right to be included). Trials should include unconscious subjects only if the research cannot be performed on subjects who are able to give consent.

For consent purposes, children are also classed as a 'vulnerable group'. For clinical trials including children, the age at which a child may give consent/assent to enter a trial varies between countries (and between states in the USA), and in some cases has never been clearly defined. Local law may also define if one or both parents must sign consent. Under English law, consent may be given on behalf of a child by the parent, but parents can only consent to minimal increased risk for their child. Effort must be made to fully inform the child up to his/her maximum level of understanding. The child's views must always be respected and the child's assent should be obtained if he/she is of an age where this is possible (this is often considered to be from school age upwards). This process may involve the use of written information sheets and consent forms appropriate for different ages of children to be enrolled, in addition to the information sheet and consent form prepared for parents. Parents may also not understand that the child needs to be part of the decision process. Relatively few trials have been performed in children because of the difficulties with informed consent, the practicalities involved, and the ethics of conducting experimental research on children. However, the regulatory agencies are now encouraging the investigation of drugs in children because problems have resulted from extrapolating results from adults to children, and some diseases and adverse effects are specific to children.

In legal terms, as soon as a child reaches the age of majority (18 years in England and Wales, and 16 years in Scotland), whatever their mental capacity, no other person has authority to grant consent on their behalf. The difficult age is when children are approaching the age of majority. Under the Children (Scotland) Act 1995 (section 15(5)(b)), a parent's right to act as a child's legal representative in relation to the giving of consent applies only where a child is incapable of consenting on his or her own behalf. Children under 16 are able to give their full consent to treatment, provided that they meet the Gillick criteria of competence, namely that they have been counselled, have shown maturity and understanding, and are thought by the physician to be capable of expressing their own wishes. However, there is a difference as far as 'consent to treatment' and 'consent to research' is concerned, and therefore children under the legal age of consent should not be allowed to participate in clinical research without the additional consent of a parent/guardian (Kennedy and Grubb, 1994).

Some confusion persists over who can actually take responsibility for the consent process. ICH GCP allows the investigator to delegate the taking of consent. However, the Declaration of Helsinki refers only to a 'physician' taking consent. This point has been the subject of much heated debate. Some have argued that the Declaration of Helsinki is 37 years old and that study nurses/teams did not exist when it was written. The investigator conducted all aspects of the study alone, so the requirement to have help with the consent process was not relevant. On the other hand, quality assurance (QA) personnel point out that the Declaration is a 'living document' that has been amended several times and this point has not been changed or clarified. QA personnel therefore usually expect to see consent forms signed off by a medically qualified person. It is widely agreed that study nurses play an important role in the study team and subjects often find nurses more approachable during the consent process than investigators. It would therefore be unfortunate if study nurses in particular were to be excluded from the consent process. The general opinion is that while study nurses, and other members of the study team, may take part in the consent process (such as explaining study procedures, giving study information and answering any related questions), responsibility for enrolling a subject at the centre lies ultimately with the investigator. The investigator should ensure that the subject has fully understood what he/she is consenting to and should then sign and date the consent form. If study nurses are going to take part in even a small part of the consent process, space should be provided on the consent form for them to sign, in addition to the investigator (cf. section 4.8.8 of the ICH GCP guideline).

The written information that a sponsor is obliged to provide to the subject is extensive. Section 4.8.10 the ICH GCP guideline lists 20 different items of information (the elements of informed consent) that must be included in the information sheet. A further element for inclusion is mentioned in section 4.3.3: the agreement of the subject for his/her family doctor to be notified of the subject's participation in the trial. In addition, the European Data Protection Directive (Directive 95/46/EC, 1995), implemented into UK law on 1 March 2000, requires the sponsor company to include details of which data relating to the subject are being processed by the sponsor company and the locations to which these data are likely to be transferred.

It is important that the subject receives a copy of the informed consent form and written information. Any new information that becomes available during the course of the trial should also be promptly passed on to the subject, after approval by the ethics committee. Ethical issues sometimes arise, for example, when results of another trial with the same test compound become available, or information is published on another treatment being used in the same indication. New information could render it unethical for a placebo-controlled trial to continue.

The volume of written information to be provided for subjects, in the attempt to inform them fully, is therefore considerable. The comprehension of that information will differ widely between subjects. Many potential subjects approached to take part in a clinical trial are ill, and the last thing they want is to have to take decisions about the type of care they are about to receive. Can patients make such decisions when they are ill? Simply to tell a patient that there is no obvious best treatment for his/her condition may in itself be harmful. The ICH GCP guideline states that the subject must be allowed ample time to decide whether or not he/she wishes to participate in a trial. However, some countries have imposed minimum time limits between providing subjects with information and asking for their consent to participate. In Ireland this is referred to as the six-day rule because a full 6 days must elapse between the subject being informed about the trial and his/her agreement to take part. In Germany, a minimum 24-hour period is usually required between information being given and the obtaining of consent. Where acute studies are to be performed, exemptions must be sought from such restrictions. The level of detail a subject wishes to receive will also vary, and the investigator and site staff should tailor information to suit each subject, giving verbal information as required, to meet individual needs. However, this should not be used as an excuse to minimise information on potential risks, especially with anxious individuals.

Wherever possible, trials with no direct anticipated benefit for the subject, e.g. Phase I or human pharmacology studies, should include only subjects who can personally consent, sign and date the informed consent form. The only exceptions are likely to be in cases where the trial objective cannot be met by including subjects who can consent personally, the foreseeable risks are low, the negative impact on the subject's well-being is minimal, the trial is not prohibited by law, and the ethics committee approves the inclusion of such subjects. For example, some non-therapeutic research may need to be carried out in children, or in seriously traumatised patients in Accident and Emergency departments. Whatever the practical challenge to obtaining informed consent, it remains essential that the procedures to be followed and the written information to be given are carefully reviewed by an ethics committee.

Ethical issues are also discussed in ICH Topic E4: *Dose-Response Information to Support Drug Registration* with reference to the problem of dose-finding studies in life-threatening diseases (ICH Guideline, 1994). Is it ethical to give less than the maximum tolerated dose, especially where effective salvage treatment may not be available and permanent damage may result? Studies in vulnerable populations are referred to in ICH Topic E8: *General Considerations for Clinical Trials* (ICH Guideline, 1997) and will be discussed in greater detail below. Blinding a trial to minimise bias may also raise ethical issues, as discussed in ICH Topic E9: *Statistical Principles for Clinical Trials* (ICH Guideline, 1998). Is it ethical to blind a comparison between surgery and a drug treatment? This could be a very relevant comparison to make, but the inclusion of a control group receiving dummy surgery in addition to the drug is somewhat extreme, and may be unrealistic. Placebo-controlled trials may be unethical in serious illnesses if a therapeutic treatment has been shown to be efficacious. Once a trial is under way, one of the main reasons for stopping it early is that it may be unethical to continue. For example, the incidence of adverse events, or more likely the risk–benefit ratio may prove to be unacceptable. Alternatively, an interim analysis may reveal that the statistical power of the study will be inadequate to detect the probable difference. Decisions of this nature may be taken by an independent data monitoring committee. This is not an ethics committee, but rather a committee of scientific experts acting independently of the conduct of the study: they may be unblinded to a degree and can advise the study sponsor or take such decisions autonomously.

ETHICAL ISSUES IN CLINICAL TRIAL DESIGN

Almost all aspects of clinical trial design are potentially associated with ethical issues. The difference between therapeutic and non-therapeutic research has already been mentioned with respect to informed consent in vulnerable subject groups. Methods of subject recruitment, diagnosis, randomisation, blinding, analysis of drop-outs, and use of concomitant medication may all raise ethical questions. Issues are also present in clinical trials that determine which designs are ethically acceptable to perform.

The simplest design is a non-comparative study, usually open, in which the test treatment is given and its effects are measured. Both the investigator and the subject know which treatment is being given. Such trials are criticised on the grounds of bias: the investigator may have pre-conceived ideas about how well (or how badly) the treatment may work, and non-comparative trials lack a control group which is required for scientific validity (is the observed effect attributable to chance alone?). A better design is the controlled clinical trial in which the test treatment is compared in some way with another treatment. The comparison may be with the response of other patients with the same disease (i.e. historical controls) or it may be a parallel-group study (but this may lead to a bias in treatment allocation or measurement of response).

The gold standard for comparing two treatments is the randomised, double-blind, parallel-group study. However, the concept of withholding information from the subject and investigator in order to achieve double-blinding stands in conflict with the principle to fully inform the subject, as required by the Declaration of Helsinki and GCP. The information withheld may extend far beyond the identity of the treatment given in order to maintain investigator blinding. For example, certain types of adverse event or clinical effect may be associated with a particular treatment, e.g. a reduction in pulse rate with beta-blockers, or changes in blood test results characteristic of certain treatments. Knowledge of such effects could unblind the study for individual subjects. Is it therefore ethical to perform the clinical trial at all? Is it better to give an unproven treatment to hundreds of patients to find out which treatment is best, or to give the treatment to patients without knowing how effective it is? In any blinded trial, investigators should be provided with the means to unblind each individual subject in an emergency.

It is rare for subjects to be recruited to clinical trials as rapidly as planned, and monitors frequently put investigators under pressure to improve recruitment rates. It has been argued that such pressure might encourage inclusion criteria to become compromised. With monitors performing source data verification (SDV), it may now be impossible to include a subject just outside the eligible age range, but it is still possible to stretch the meaning of soft inclusion criteria such as 'moderate' disease severity where no precise definition for the term 'moderate' exists. Encouraged by the attractiveness of payments for work done, investigators may also be less than fully honest with information concerning the potential risks associated with participation, or they may be over-enthusiastic regarding potential benefits for the subject. Such issues underline the importance of thorough pre-study evaluations of prospective trial sites to ensure that the investigator has adequate time, resources and subjects available (*see Chapter 11*). It is therefore imperative to seek to select investigators without preconceived ideas about the relative merits of the treatments being tested.

Randomisation

Randomisation is used wherever possible to allocate treatment in order to eliminate investigator bias as a result of preconceived ideas about the

effectiveness or safety of a particular treatment. Influenced by such precon-
ceptions, the investigator might otherwise give the 'preferred' or best treatment to the more severe cases, or assume that the new treatment is more
effective and allocate it preferentially to the more severe cases, thereby creating an imbalance between the treatment groups. However, considering the
ethics of randomisation for the individual patient, it can be argued that
randomised treatment allocation may not select the best treatment for a given
individual. If the trial works, it will have proved that some patients received
an inferior treatment. However, not to have performed the trial may have
denied future patients a more effective treatment. As stated above,
randomised treatment allocation removes the investigator's ability to select
the best treatment for a particular patient. This is probably ethically acceptable if no standard treatment of choice is available for such patients. In many
situations, however, a treatment is already licensed, and in those circumstances the researcher must believe that the new treatment is as good as the
licensed treatment before the trial begins. If it becomes obvious during a
clinical trial which treatment is best, consideration may be given to stopping
the trial early. Such subjective assessments are notoriously difficult: statistical significance may be achieved, but is the difference clinically significant?
If there is a likelihood that a trial could be stopped early, an interim analysis should be planned in the protocol from the outset. If a clinically significant difference is not shown, such an analysis can also indicate whether it is
worthwhile completing the study. Alternatively, it may show that the treatments are so similar that completing the study is unlikely to demonstrate a
difference. It is unethical to expose too many or too few patients to a new
treatment, but it is also unethical to stop a study early before a result has
been obtained. The randomised trial may not be ideal, but it remains the
cornerstone of clinical trial design today.

Withdrawals

An important ethical principle of clinical research is that subjects are free to
withdraw from a study at any time. Such subjects, together with those
withdrawn by the investigator, can pose a problem at the analysis stage.
Subjects who do not complete a study can, for example, be withdrawn from
subsequent analyses, or their last data can be carried forward, or a subject
who drops out can be replaced. Each approach has its merits but in general
it is advisable to minimise the number of drop-outs as they can bias treatment
effects positively by inclusion or negatively by exclusion. Subjects who 'guess'
their assigned treatment in a blinded trial and who then decide to continue or
withdraw on this basis can undermine the success of the trial. This is even
more of a risk in open studies. It is important to ensure that subjects are
willing to participate in the first place, and that they understand what is
expected of them, thus making early withdrawal less likely.

Whether a trial is designed to demonstrate a difference between two treatments, or merely to show that two treatments are equivalent or that one treatment is not inferior to another can have ethical consequences. If a trial designed to show a difference is successful, there can be a measure of confidence that a true difference probably exists. However, if a trial designed to show no difference indeed detects no difference, it is not possible to be certain that the trial was capable of finding a difference, even if one truly exists. Insensitive rating scales, insufficient subject numbers, general carelessness and missing data tend to support the 'no difference' conclusion. Such trials should therefore be avoided if possible, and given careful ethical consideration if proposed. It is clearly unethical to perform any study that is unscientific.

Concomitant medication

Another aspect that can affect the scientific validity of a trial is concomitant medication, i.e. that given before the study treatment starts or during the study treatment phase itself. Is it ethical to halt a subject's medication for a wash-out period to make him/her eligible for a trial? If the subject is unlikely to suffer any long-term ill effects, for example, in mild hypertension or acne, such action is ethical. If, however, there is a significant risk that a satisfactorily controlled subject could suffer harm by the withdrawal of existing medication, an alternative trial design should be sought. The subject's consent must always be obtained before any therapy adjustments are made to make a prospective subject eligible for inclusion in a clinical trial.

In most trials the use of concomitant medication may confound any treatment effect, with the result that the use of such medication should be restricted, thus detracting from optimal subject care. Rigorous clinical study protocols can restrict the freedom of investigators to give the best possible care to trial subjects. The ethical impact of this scientific requirement can be minimised by utilising tight eligibility criteria during Phase II and early Phase III studies, when the aim is to measure the size of a treatment effect, and by allowing more concomitant medications in later phase trials, when the aim is to evaluate the treatment in a situation approximating more closely to real life. This strategy may also permit the detection of common drug interactions that might otherwise remain undetected until the treatment is administered more extensively. The use of concomitant medication is an example of potential ethical conflict with scientific perfection in clinical trial design, but careful planning and risk assessment can minimise the ethical disadvantage to each trial subject while maximising the scientific gain for society as a whole.

Volunteer studies

When an investigational product is administered to a trial subject and that subject is not expected to derive any therapeutic benefit, the subject is commonly referred to as a healthy volunteer. Such trials are often described as Phase I or human pharmacology studies, and usually represent the first experience with a new drug in human subjects. They usually involve relatively young, healthy adults, but may include special populations such as healthy elderly subjects, for example, if the objectives of the trial are to determine how the elderly body handles the investigational product and to identify the product's effects in an elderly population. Such trials raise special ethical issues in addition to those already described concerning therapeutic trials. The Declaration of Helsinki still applies in such cases, and the rights, safety and well-being of the trial subject must take precedence over the interests of science and society as a whole.

If the subject is to derive no therapeutic benefit, it is clear that only a very low level of risk is acceptable. It can be argued that no risk is acceptable and, as recently as 25 years ago, volunteer studies were prohibited by law or at least very unpopular and difficult to perform in certain countries (e.g. France and Germany). Interestingly, there is currently no requirement in the UK for regulatory approval to conduct a volunteer study: this is on the grounds that the investigational product does not have a proven effect at this stage, and therefore has not been classified as falling under the UK Medicines Act. The European Clinical Trials Directive has harmonised these requirements between Member States, and it is likely that regulatory permission will be required to conduct such studies in the UK in the near future. Laws already exist in the USA covering volunteer studies.

The method of volunteer selection and recruitment is very important in such studies. There have been cases where the 'volunteers' were all students of the professor organising the research. This does not mean that all students are barred from being healthy volunteers, but the method of recruitment must be seen to avoid any form of coercion or pressure from the organisers of the research. Because they can hardly be said to volunteer freely, the recruitment of prisoners is also discouraged.

In most Phase I studies volunteers are paid for their participation. This is another area of potential ethical conflict. Financial rewards must be determined before the study commences, must be set at a level that does not 'bribe' participants, and must be approved by the appropriate ethics committee. The payments need to be realistic to offset the time taken, restrictions placed on freedom of choice (e.g. diet) and any discomfort experienced by the volunteers taking part in the study. For many studies, volunteers are housed in purpose-built accommodation so that conditions are standardised, checks and examinations may be performed easily and frequently, and samples taken as required. Such centres maintain registers of volunteers to ensure that an individual does not volunteer too frequently. In the UK the prospective volunteer's general practitioner (GP) should be informed and checks should be run to exclude anything in the medical history that would put the subject at increased risk by participating in the proposed trial, and to identify any prescribed medication that might influence the outcome. Volunteers can expect a thorough pre-trial medical screening, to ensure that they are as healthy as possible before they participate in the trial and that any underlying medical problems are identified. They do not have to be in perfect health, but the effect of any pre-existing condition must be taken into consideration. When evaluating the ethics of such trials, it is imperative that the risks to the individual are kept to an absolute minimum. No-one should be allowed knowingly to volunteer to put their health at risk for the benefit of a sponsor. In certain situations where the substance to be tested is toxic, an ethically acceptable risk–benefit ratio may only be achieved by conducting the study in the target patient population.

Use of placebo

In placebo-controlled studies, subjects are randomly assigned either to the active treatment being evaluated or to an apparently identical treatment with no intended activity, a placebo. Such studies are usually double-blind, and placebo is included as the control treatment in the trial design. Most placebo-controlled studies seek to demonstrate a difference in effectiveness in favour of the active treatment being evaluated, but they may also be used to demonstrate a lack of difference in terms of safety. The scientific justification for the use of placebo as a control allows for changes in the disease course, subject or investigator expectations, concomitant therapy, subjective assessments or other factors confounding treatment, so that any difference observed between the two groups can be attributed to the test treatment. The inclusion of a placebo control group also allows a distinction to be made between adverse events due to active treatment and those due to the disease. The fact that the patient is in a clinical trial and receiving 'treatment' is known to produce a measurable beneficial effect – the placebo effect – the size of which varies between diseases and types of trial but can range from 10 to 50%. The use of placebo allows a robust trial to be conducted and if a difference in favour of the test treatment is demonstrated, the data can be submitted to the regulatory authorities as part of a marketing authorisation application (MAA).

When a potentially beneficial new treatment is tested in a condition for which no licensed treatment yet exists, there is usually no ethical issue associated with the selection of placebo as the control group treatment. However, if an effective treatment already exists, the use of placebo has to be considered carefully. If the withholding of treatment places the patient at significant risk of serious harm or irreversible morbidity, the use of placebo is probably unjustified. As mentioned earlier, strict interpretation of paragraph 29 of the Declaration of Helsinki, which states that subjects should receive the best current prophylactic, diagnostic and therapeutic methods, calls into question the use of any sub-optimal comparative therapy at any time. If there is no significant health risk associated with withholding or delaying effective therapy, the use of placebo can probably be justified. In such situations it is important that subjects are fully informed about available therapies, and about any expected consequences of delaying treatment, and that their participation is entirely voluntary. The availability of a known effective therapy may vary internationally, making it ethically justifiable to conduct a placebo-controlled study in one country but not in another.

Ethical acceptability can also be positively influenced by good study design and appropriate selection of the subject population. For example, studies can be designed with several control groups, only one of which is allocated to placebo, thus reducing the proportion of subjects receiving placebo. In a simple five-arm study comparing three different dose levels of a new active treatment with a known active treatment and placebo, the proportion of subjects receiving placebo would be one in five. If the sensitivity for the comparisons between active treatments is increased by doubling the proportion of subjects in these groups, the chances of an individual subject receiving placebo can be reduced to one in nine. Whether a trial is ethical depends on the precise circumstances in that particular case. It is probably ethical to use placebo control in a short study in mild hypertensive patients, but not in patients with moderate or severe hypertension. Where a placebo control is used in more severe illness, ethical requirements can be satisfied if all patients receive the best available standard care, and the new treatment or placebo is given as additional therapy. Such designs require that existing treatment is not fully effective, and they may be appropriate in oncology, epilepsy or heart failure trials, for example.

Placebo-controlled studies can be made ethically acceptable either by reducing the number of subjects exposed to placebo alone, or by reducing the duration of exposure to placebo, for example, by making effective rescue medication available if a subject's condition reaches a predetermined level of pain or blood pressure, or if some baseline variable changes by a predefined amount during the study. The use of placebo control and the modifications to trial designs to make them more ethically acceptable are discussed in greater detail in ICH Topic E10: *Choice of Control Group in Clinical Trials* (ICH Guideline, 1999).

Not every study involving the use of placebo generates significant ethical issues. Placebo may be used to achieve blinding, for example, when comparing tablets of different appearance (the 'double-dummy' technique). The only ethical issue here is that subjects are required to take more tablets than otherwise necessary, although this is probably a minor consideration because the trial is still an active control design. Of greater concern are trial designs incorporating placebo run-in or wash-out phases, or in which placebo is used to blind the comparison of treatment courses of differing durations. In such circumstances the researcher must be convinced that to leave the subject without treatment for these periods of time will not cause any long-term irreversible damage. The ethical issues are in fact the same as having placebo as the control treatment for the whole study.

Publication

It may not be obvious that there are ethical issues surrounding the final stage of a clinical trial. It is generally accepted that the results of a clinical trial must be reported clearly and fairly. The report may be submitted to a regulatory authority as part of an MAA. The ethics committees and regulatory bodies that approved the clinical trial initially will require summaries of the report. If the trial is successful, the sponsor and investigators are bound to want to publish the results to achieve maximum impact. However, the situation may be different if the results are neutral, or potentially damaging for the sponsor. According to the Declaration of Helsinki, the trial was only ethical in the first place if it was designed to improve diagnostic, therapeutic and prophylactic procedures and to enhance understanding of the aetiology and pathogenesis of the disease in question. Thus, an ethical duty exists to the subjects who took part in the trial that the results should be published. Negative results can be useful, although it is admittedly difficult to publish negative or neutral results.

CONCLUSION

In the light of the foregoing discussion, the abiding impression could be that it is impossible to conduct clinical research in an ethical manner. However, many trials continue to be successfully planned, set up, conducted and reported. Highly trained and experienced people throughout the world are now able to successfully plan entire clinical development programmes and individual clinical trials in the face of many ethical challenges. The development of innovative treatments based on gene therapy and other new technologies will bring its own special challenges to the ever-changing field of ethics in clinical research. However, with the support of organisations like The Institute of Clinical Research, the future for ethical health care research remains promising.

REFERENCES

Directive 95/46/EC (1995). On the protection of individuals with regard to the processing of personal data and on the free movement of such data.

European Parliament and Council Directive (2000). Common Position adopted by the Council with a view to the adoption of a Directive of the European Parliament and of the Council on the approximation of the laws, regulations and administrative provisions of the Member States relating to the implementation of good clinical practice in the conduct of clinical trials on medicinal products for human use. (Procedure number: COD 1997/0197. Common Position document date: 20 July 2000.)

ICH Guideline (1994). *Topic E4: Dose–Response Information to Support Drug*

Registration, International Federation of Pharmaceutical Manufacturers Associations, Geneva (Issued as CPMP/ICH/378/95).

ICH Guideline (1996). *Topic E6: Good Clinical Practice – Consolidated Guideline*, International Federation of Pharmaceutical Manufacturers Associations, Geneva (Issued as CPMP/ICH/135/95).

ICH Guideline (1997). *Topic E8: General Considerations for Clinical Trials*, International Federation of Pharmaceutical Manufacturers Associations, Geneva (Issued as CPMP/ICH/291/96).

ICH Guideline (1998). *Topic E9: Statistical Principles for Clinical Trials*, International Federation of Pharmaceutical Manufacturers Associations, Geneva (Issued as CPMP/ICH/363/96).

ICH Guideline (1999). *Topic E10: Choice of Control Group in Clinical Trials*, International Federation of Pharmaceutical Manufacturers Associations, Geneva (Reached Step 4 in July 2000).

Kennedy, I and Grubb, A (1994). *Medical Law*, Butterworth, London.

Leake, CD (1927). *Percival's Medical Ethics: or, a Code of Institutes and Precepts Adapted to the Professional Conduct of Physicians and Surgeons (1803)*, Williams & Wilkins, Baltimore.

Nicholson, R (1999). Revising the Declaration of Helsinki: a fresh start. *Bull Med Ethics* **151**, 13–17.

US Government Printing Office (1949). *Nuremberg Code: Trials of War Criminals before the Nuremberg Military Tribunals under Control Council Law No. 10, Vol. 2, Nuremberg, October 1946 – April 1949*, US Government Printing Office, Washington DC, pp. 181–182.

Vollmann, J and Winau, R (1996). The Prussian regulation of 1900: early ethical standards for human experimentation in Germany. *IRB: A Review of Human Subjects Research* **18**, 9–11.

4

Liability and indemnity in clinical research

Angus Donald

EUROPEAN COMMUNITY GOOD CLINICAL PRACTICE GUIDELINES

The European Community has laws governing the data that are required to be submitted in support of an application for a marketing authorisation for a medicinal product. In an amendment to Directive 75/318/EEC, Directive 91/507/EEC (Part 4, Clinical Documentation, B, 1.1) states that such data which come from clinical trials must conform to 'good clinical practice'. The EC has issued guidelines (CPMP, 1991), which are not legally binding but need to be observed in practice, on what it considers to be good clinical practice (GCP). These guidelines specify in section 2.3j that it is the responsibility of the sponsor to provide:

... adequate compensation/treatment for subjects in the event of trial-related injury or death, and provide indemnity (legal and financial cover) for the investigator, except for claims resulting from malpractice and/or negligence.

Section 9 of the Annex to these guidelines further states: 'Patients/healthy volunteers taking part in a clinical trial should be satisfactorily insured against any injury caused by the trial. The liability of the involved parties (investigators, sponsor/manufacturer, hospital/clinics, etc.) must be clearly understood before the start of a trial of the medicinal product containing an active ingredient'.

In Chapter II, Article 4 the European Clinical Trials Directive states that:

... the ethics committee shall consider, in particular: ... f) provision for compensation in the case of injury or death attributable to a clinical trial; g) any insurance or indemnity to cover the liability of the investigator and sponsor.... (European Parliament and Council Directive, 2000).

It is unclear whether self-insurance by a sponsor, something often encountered in larger companies, is prohibited. The most common form of compensation is through *ex gratia* payments (given as a favour, where no legal obligation exists).

The legal background

Much of what follows is dependent upon the matrix of contractual or other legal relationships between the different parties involved in clinical research, and so it is important to understand the legalities of these arrangements. There should always be a contract in existence between the sponsor, contract research organisation (CRO), if any, and investigator. There will typically be a contract between a healthy volunteer research subject and CRO or sponsor, usually based on an extended consent form. There will usually only be a contract between a patient research subject and an investigator if the former is a private patient.

Civil liability to compensate a research subject who is injured as a result of being involved in clinical research by means of a payment of money (damages) might arise under one of three legal bases: breach of contract, negligence or strict liability as producer (or in some cases, supplier) of a defective product.

A research subject who is unfortunate enough to suffer injury as a result of participation in clinical research might encounter difficulties or complexities when seeking to bring a claim under any of these three heads. First, a patient volunteer may not have a contract with anyone, but even a healthy volunteer may have difficulties, such as establishing the details of which contractual term might have been broken since the terms of the contract might be vague or minimal. Secondly, the chances of succeeding in a claim of negligence or strict liability for a defective product in the context of clinical research are extremely slim. In addition to the usual problems of delay and cost associated with involvement in the legal system, the research subject should have been warned that he or she was taking part in research, should have been informed about the procedures which would be involved and the general risks which might be encountered, and should have consented to take part on this basis.

In view of these difficulties, the pharmaceutical industry has devised specific mechanisms with the purpose of allowing injured research subjects to be compensated where this is justified. Specific legislation has recently been enacted in France, Ireland and Portugal, and other countries may follow (Hodges, 1991, 1992). The Netherlands (Het medisch wetenschappelijk onderzoek met mensen: Decree of July 1999, regulating obligatory insurance for medical research involving human subjects) and Poland (Ministry of Finance Decree, 28 July 1990, Group 13, Section 2) have enacted decrees which dictate the amount of insurance required and necessitate that clinical trial insurance be taken out in their own country.

In the UK there was considerable public concern following the deaths in 1985 of two students (one in Cardiff and the other in Dublin) who were healthy volunteers in drug trials. One developed a neurological lesion shortly after the administration of an influenza vaccine, and the other suffered a heart attack after administration of beta-blockers. More recently, the first death of a volunteer receiving experimental recombinant gene therapy has been reported in the USA. Death was caused by multiple organ systems failure secondary to a severe immune system reaction and this case has led to serious questions being raised by the US Food and Drug Administration (FDA).

The Association of the British Pharmaceutical Industry (ABPI) has developed a self-regulated approach based on in-house guidelines. These have worked well and there are different sets of guidelines relating to healthy (non-patient) and to patient volunteers.

ABPI Guidelines for Medical Experiments in Non-Patient Human Volunteers (1988 and amended 1990)

The undertaking by the sponsor to compensate an injured non-patient research subject is contractual, based on an extended consent form signed by the subject. The ABPI Guidelines (section 11.7) state that:

The agreement should clearly record the obligation the pharmaceutical company or research establishment has accepted in terms of financial rewards for participation and compensation in the event of injury. In particular, the volunteer should be given a clear commitment that in the event of bodily injury he will receive appropriate compensation without having to prove either that such injury arose through negligence or that the product was defective in the sense that it did not fulfil a reasonable expectation of safety. The agreement should not seek to remove that right of the volunteer, as an alternative, to pursue a claim on the basis of either negligence or strict liability if he is so minded.

Essentially:

a volunteer can reasonably expect that compensation will be paid quickly and that any dispute regarding who will finally bear the cost of the compensation paid to him will be resolved separately by the other parties to the research (section 11.8).

A model agreement is attached to the Guidelines which provides that, in the event of the subject suffering any significant deterioration in health or well-being caused directly by participation in the study, compensation will be paid by the company. The amount of compensation is to be calculated with reference to the amount of damages commonly awarded for similar injuries by an English court if liability is admitted, provided that such compensation may be reduced to the extent that the subject is partly at fault and responsible for the injury.

ABPI Clinical Trial Compensation Guidelines (1991)

There is usually no contract between a sponsor and a patient in research. Ethics committees generally require that a sponsor should undertake to abide by the ABPI Guidelines, but this is voluntary and without legal commitment.

Under the Guidelines (section 1.2), the sponsor should pay compensation:

... when, on the balance of probabilities, the injury was attributable to the administration of a medicinal product under trial or any clinical intervention or procedure provided for by the protocol that would not have occurred but for the inclusion of the patient in the trial ...

1.4   Compensation should only be paid for the more serious injury of an endur- ing and disabling character (including exacerbation of an existing condition) and not for temporary pain or discomfort or less serious or curable complaints.

1.5   Where there is an adverse reaction to a medicinal product under trial and injury is caused by a procedure adopted to deal with that adverse reaction, compensation should be paid for such injury as if it were caused directly by the medicinal product under trial ...

4.1   The amount of compensation paid should be appropriate to the nature, severity and persistence of the injury and should in general terms be consis- tent with the quantum of damages commonly awarded for similar injuries by an English Court in cases where legal liability is admitted.

4.2   Compensation may be abated, or in certain circumstances excluded, in the light of the following factors (on which will depend the level of risk the patient can reasonably be expected to accept):

    4.2.1   the seriousness of the disease being treated, the degree of probabil- ity that adverse reactions will occur and any warnings given;

    4.2.2   the risks and benefits of established treatments relative to those known or suspected of the trial medicine.

The Guidelines include provision for arbitration by an independent expert in the event of any difference of opinion.

Compensation is excluded in certain circumstances, including those where the injury was caused by another licensed medicinal product which was admin- istered as a comparison with the product under trial, or where a placebo has failed to provide a therapeutic benefit. It appears disingenuous that a patient who would not have received this treatment but for his/her participation in the study (or has treatment withheld and receives placebo) is not covered by these Guidelines. Equally, injury due to withholding active treatment is not covered. While companies will often provide compensation in these situations to avoid adverse publicity, it appears wrong that this is not accounted for and places the public at the mercy of company finances. Compensation should not be paid, or should be abated, to the extent that the injury has arisen through a significant departure from the agreed protocol, or through the wrongful act or default of a third party, including a doctor's failure to deal adequately with an adverse reaction, or through contributory negligence by the patient.

Research ethics committees

It should not be forgotten that each party involved in clinical research owes a duty of care to patient volunteers. The UK National Health Service (NHS) local research ethics committee (LREC) is formally a sub-committee of the health authority. There can be no doubt that, as such, the health authority is legally responsible for the decisions of the committee. The authority *and* each individual member of the committee owe a duty of care to all those who participate in research approved by the ethics committee. Although there has as yet been no case in England where an ethics committee has been sued by a research subject, it is important to recognise that ethics committees have direct legal responsibilities to research subjects (Brazier, 1990).

Marketed products

There are separate guidelines relating to injury arising from clinical trials on marketed products covered by a product licence. *Guidelines on Post-Marketing Surveillance 1988* are issued by the Joint Committee of the ABPI, BMA, CSM and RCGP, and a *Code of practice for the Clinical Assessment of Licensed Medicinal Products in General Practice 1983* has been jointly agreed between the BMA, RCGP and ABPI. These documents make no mention of compensation issues and these remain to be resolved under the general law.

Insurance for research injuries

Product liability policies for marketed products may cover claims arising in respect of research products, for which separate policies are available. According to the European GCP guidelines (CPMP, 1991), it seems to be a requirement that insurance should be available for compensation or treatment in respect of injury or death attributable to a clinical trial but it is unclear whether self-insurance by a company is prohibited (Hodges, 1993; Donald, 1996).

Indemnities

According to section 2.3j of the European GCP guidelines, a sponsor should indemnify an investigator in relation to any claim for compensation or treatment which may be made against the investigator by a research subject in the event of trial-related injury or death, except for claims resulting from malpractice or negligence of the investigator or his staff (CPMP, 1991). In the UK a standard form indemnity for clinical studies in relation to research carried out by or involving NHS or NHS Trust employees or facilities has been agreed between the ABPI and the Department of Health.

This standard form provides that, if a claim should be made, the sponsor indemnifies and holds the health authority and its employees and agents harmless against all claims brought by or on behalf of research subjects taking part in a study arising out of or relating to the administration of the product(s) under investigation or any clinical intervention or procedure provided for or required by the protocol to which the subject would not have been exposed but for his/her participation in the study. The sponsor also agrees to operate in good faith the appropriate ABPI compensation guidelines. As is normal in relation to indemnity provisions, the sponsor may control the defence of any litigation brought against the health authority or investigator.

The Consumer Protection Act 1987

The Royal Commission on Civil Liability and Compensation for Personal Injury 1978 (The Pearson Report), whilst not feeling that strict liability was appropriate, bemoaned the state of affairs in the UK where reliance is placed on *ex gratia* payments for volunteers in medical research (Pearson Report, 1978). It appears that little has changed since that time and that volunteers are still at risk. The most significant advance in terms of product liability was the introduction of Directive 85/374/EC in 1985, which was incorporated into legislation in the UK in the Consumer Protection Act, 1987. This imposes strict liability on a producer for products marketed after 1 March 1988, and includes among the definition of producers those who import products into the EC.

Of greatest importance to the pharmaceutical industry is the incorporation of a 'Development Risks Defence' (section 4(1)(e)). This means that the manufacturer will not be liable if it can be shown 'that the state of scientific and technical knowledge at the relevant time was not such that a producer of products of the same description as the product in question might be expected to have discovered the defect if it had existed in his products while they were under his control'.

This defence was permitted to be incorporated into national legislation in the EC Directive and has been incorporated to differing extents in different countries. For example, Germany has not incorporated the development risks argument, preferring not to become a testing ground for new drugs. The arguments are that, without this defence, pharmaceutical companies will be unable to insure against unforeseeable risks and this will stifle drug development. Unfortunately, the reverse situation, as offered in the UK, allows for little protection of subjects involved in research and marks a return to the system of *ex gratia* payments.

Claims under the Consumer Protection Act 1987 have a 10-year limitation period (Limitation Act 1980) which, in terms of long-term side-effects, may be a disadvantage to a claimant, especially if the latter is affected as a foetus. This limitation would have done nothing to remedy the effects of the thalidomide disaster, which was one of the primary reasons for the introduction of legislation. This 10-year period should be noted in relation to archiving and should be the minimum period in the UK, as opposed to the definition adopted in sections 4.9.5, 5.5.8 and 5.5.11 of the ICH GCP guideline (ICH Guideline, 1996).

The Consumer Protection Act 1987 includes references to the avoidance of liability through adequate warnings and instructions. This is not merely to a reasonable standard, but to the standard of an expert in the field. The burden of proving that the knowledge was not available is placed on the defendant (pharmaceutical company) and is an ongoing duty, so that companies need to maintain a competent drug surveillance department.

Postscript

Although the UK has been slow to follow, other countries, notably Germany (German Pharmaceutical Pool), Sweden (Swedish Pharmaceutical Insurance Scheme) and New Zealand (New Zealand Accident Compensation Scheme, Acts 1972–1975) have introduced extensive compensation schemes to avoid disputes. However, the New Zealand scheme does have the same drawbacks as the ABPI compensation guidelines detailed above (Peart and Moore, 1997).

ACKNOWLEDGEMENT

The author wishes to acknowledge C.J.S. Hodges who wrote the corresponding chapter in the second edition of *Handbook of Clinical Research* (Lloyd and Raven, 1997).

REFERENCES

Brazier, M (1990). Liability of ethics committees. *Professional Negligence* **6**, 186.

Committee for Proprietary Medicinal Products (CPMP) Working Party on Efficacy of Medicinal Products (1991). *Good Clinical Practice for Trials on Medicinal Products in the European Community*, (111/3976/88–EN Final), European Commission, Brussels.

Donald, AE (1996). Liability and indemnity. *Clin Res Focus* **7**, 9–12.

European Parliament and Council Directive (2000). Common Position adopted by the Council with a view to the adoption of a Directive of the European Parliament and of the Council on the approximation of the laws, regulations and administrative provisions of the Member States relating to the implementation of good clinical practice in the conduct of clinical trials on medicinal products for human use. (Procedure number: COD 1997/0197. Common Position document date: 20 July 2000.)

Hodges, CJS (1991). Developments in compensation, insurance and indemnity for research injury in the European Community. *Pharm Med* **5**, 135–147.

Hodges, CJS (1992). Harmonisation of European controls over research: ethics committees, consent, compensation and indemnity. In: Goldberg, A and Dodds-Smith, IC (Eds), *Pharmaceutical Medicine and the Law*, The Royal College of Physicians of London and the Faculty of Pharmaceutical Medicine of the Royal Colleges of Physicians of the UK, London, pp. 63–89.

Hodges, CJS (1993). Is insurance necessary to protect the subjects of clinical research? *Regulat Affairs J* **4**, 7–12.

ICH Guideline (1996). *Topic E6: Good Clinical Practice – Consolidated Guideline*, International Federation of Pharmaceutical Manufacturers Associations, Geneva (Issued as CPMP/ICH/135/95).

Lloyd, J and Raven A (1997). *Handbook of Clinical Research*, Churchill Communications Europe, London.

Pearson Report (1978). *Royal Commission on Civil Liability and Compensation for Personal Injury*, Her Majesty's Stationery Office, London.

Peart, N and Moore, A (1997). Compensation for injuries suffered by participants in commercially sponsored clinical trials in New Zealand. *Med Law Rev* **5**, 1–21.

5

Clinical trial design

Julia Lloyd-Parks

'Have nothing in your homes that you do not consider useful or beautiful.'
William Morris

INTRODUCTION

Clinical trials are the foundation upon which the whole of clinical research is built and without a good design a clinical trial may fail to achieve its aim. The effects of poor design can have major implications. For example, 'the past 30 years of poorly designed clinical research on prostate cancer have left us without reliable answers in key clinical issues' (Denis *et al.*, 1997). While this criticism is aimed particularly at one disease area, the message is important throughout clinical research.

Before a clinical trial may proceed, it will undergo numerous reviews that will include a review of the trial design and a consideration of its applicability to the situation. A good trial design will ensure that the trial is given approval to proceed, from regulatory agencies, from ethics committees, from the sponsor company and, of course, from the investigator. A good design will ensure that the trial set-up is achievable, that the investigator will recruit subjects and that the trial will be completed – all within the target timescale. The resulting report may then be presented (within a submission dossier) to regulatory agencies for approval of a drug, a new indication, or a new formulation.

Failure of a trial's design to achieve any of these steps may have consequences that are more far-reaching than the failure of one trial alone. One trial is part of a whole programme that defines the life of a drug. A failure in one part of that programme may lead at best to a delay in reaching targets or to redesign of the programme, or at worst to its cancellation. A major consequence of this is the cost, in money, time and resources, and in the loss of a potentially useful drug, which may have been chosen for development in preference to another.

Decisions made as a consequence of the result of a trial, *whether positive or negative,* must be taken with the confidence that the result is true. This is where the trial design is most important – any doubt as to the validity of the result indicates a problem in design. These considerations are encapsulated in the following sentence taken from section 6.4 of the ICH good clinical practice (GCP) guideline: 'The scientific integrity of the trial and the credibility of the data from the trial depend substantially on the trial design' (ICH Guideline, 1996).

The purpose of this chapter is to discuss the elements that must be considered in the design of a clinical trial, particularly with reference to Phase II and Phase III studies.

THE PHASES OF A CLINICAL DEVELOPMENT PROGRAMME

The trials carried out in the development of a drug can be split into four phases. These phases are helpful to gain a generalised view of drug development, and each phase requires a different approach to trial design. However, the definition of the phases is essentially arbitrary. It is also important to remember that the phases overlap. Phase I studies may still be ongoing when Phase II has started, for example. This may depend on how strictly Phase I is defined.

One important point to note for those carrying out trials is that the ICH GCP guideline applies to studies of all phases.

Phase I

Clinical studies in Phase I are the first experiments carried out in humans. Healthy volunteers are usually studied in these trials, but this may not be appropriate to all therapies, for example, cytotoxic agents. The primary objective of these studies is to gather safety data, but they are also concerned with defining a dose that might be effective, and with investigating the absorption, pharmacokinetics, metabolism and excretion of the drug (i.e. the pharmacokinetic/pharmacodynamic profile). This type of study is described in *Chapter 6*.

Phase II

In Phase II the drug is administered to trial subjects with the target disease, and it is these trials that may be defined as 'therapeutic pilot studies'. The aim of Phase II is essentially to demonstrate pharmacological activity and to assess short-term safety in subjects suffering from the target indication.

Studies in this phase will involve small numbers of subjects, and the information collected about each subject during the course of the trial and its follow-up will be very detailed. Phase II studies allow a determination of appropriate dose regimens and dose/response relationships.

Throughout Phase II the clinical development programme will identify milestones or targets; at these points key decisions will be made, for example, whether or not to continue the programme into Phase III, or whether there is a need for a modification or tighter definition of the Phase III programme.

Phase III

It is likely that Phase III will start before all Phase II studies have been completed. The decision to proceed to Phase III will have been made once efficacy has been established, no gross safety problems are found to exist, and the appropriate dose is defined.

Studies carried out in Phase III are much larger than those in Phase II. The reasons for the increasing size are manifold and are related to the objectives of the drug development programme. The efficacy of the drug must be compared with currently used treatments, and a more accurate estimation of the occurrence of adverse events must be made. During Phase III the use of the drug should be as close as possible to its ultimate clinical use, which is likely to be very different from the intense monitoring of the Phase II trial.

There is sometimes a further subdivision of Phase III into IIIa and IIIb. Essentially, this separates studies completed before submission of a licence application (IIIa) from those ongoing at that time, or that are started after submission but before approval (IIIb). Phase IIIb studies are therefore subject to the clinical trial applications for non-licensed products, but may be comparative studies against a therapy used in only a small market. Phase IIIb also includes studies of new indications for licensed drugs or new populations for licensed drugs.

Phase IV

Phase IV studies are those performed after approval of a drug for a product licence (*see Chapter* 7). They are sometimes carried out to answer questions specific to one particular market, or to enable physicians to gain experience of a new drug under controlled conditions. They tend to be carried out in very large numbers of subjects and many fewer data are collected for each subject than in Phase II and Phase III. Nevertheless, Phase IV studies can be vital to establish a large comparative safety database for a drug. The most widely used type of Phase IV study is post-marketing surveillance (PMS).

TRIAL DESIGN

The design of any given clinical trial will be dependent on many contributing factors. The fundamental factor in the design is clearly the target indication, the influence that this will have on the objectives of the trial, the options for clinical measurement, and the circumstances in which the trial is to be carried out. Bearing in mind that the individual trial is part of a larger clinical development plan, some of the influencing factors may already be defined, and there may be standards set by the programme plan that must be included in the design. These must be considered, where appropriate.

For a trial to make a credible contribution to its governing development plan, the result must not be biased by any outside influence. One fundamental objective of design is to ensure the absence of any bias. The result achieved must be clearly representative of the drug's effect.

SOURCES OF BIAS

A major cause of bias in the interpretation of a drug's activity appears when any or all of the people involved in the clinical trial hold preconceived expectations of that activity. A precept required at the outset of any trial is that the investigator assumes impartiality, and this is embodied in the adoption of a null hypothesis that the trial will reveal no difference (*see Chapter 16: Statistics*). This 'therapeutic equipoise' should be held by the investigator, the subject and the sponsor's representatives. However, the absolute requirement for sharing all known information about the drug at the time of establishing a trial is likely to unbalance this impartiality.

The way that this will introduce bias may be reflected in the investigator's choice of subjects to be treated with the trial product. For example, concerns about a potential adverse effect may lead the investigator to select a study population that may have a lower risk of experiencing the adverse effect in question. In the case where an investigator is unconvinced of efficacy, the population selected may be those subjects who exhibit a less severe form of the target disease.

In the case of a comparative study, an investigator may select which subject will receive which drug, perhaps on grounds similar to those cited in the previous paragraph. Such a selection strategy may yield results that cannot be transferred to a real patient population. This could be particularly dangerous if the basis for selection is not documented.

Another source of bias relates to the nature of the target indication. Many diseases are cyclical in nature, having periods of flare-up and remission. One such example is rheumatoid arthritis. Other diseases that are self-limiting will improve even without treatment, for example, certain infections or injuries. The result of a trial for a treatment of such diseases will be biased by the stage of the disease at which the treatment is introduced. This makes it difficult to separate the effect of the test treatment from the natural history of the disease.

The choice and method of use of clinical measurements is also a potential source of bias. This is illustrated particularly where the measurement method is subjective, for example, in the assessment of pain. The individual subject's response to a question about a sensation will be influenced by the way in which the question is asked and by the choice of words available. Both these influences may be affected by the observer's and the subject's preconceived idea of the trial or treatment, and may be further compounded by existing relationships between the interviewer and the subject. A willingness to please can bias the result towards efficacy, or some other concern may lead to a more negative response.

The conclusion to be drawn from this short discussion of bias is that control must be introduced into any test of a drug. This is the ultimate aim of the trial's design, to control the sources of bias. We will now discuss the elements of clinical trial design that will enable bias to be avoided and controlled.

THE ELEMENTS OF TRIAL DESIGN

In this part of the chapter the objective is to describe the elements that make up a clinical trial, and to suggest how these should be considered when designing a trial, or reviewing a design. It will become obvious that the person designing a trial is reliant upon information from many sources: the statistician, the regulatory experts, the clinical trial supplies/packaging group, the data processing group, the preclinical pharmacologists, the medical experts and the investigators.

Although this chapter is too short to provide an account of all possible clinical trial designs, Table 1 summarises those elements of trial design that will be considered in some detail. It is important to obtain input from all available sources, and in particular, to be aware that not all designs are applicable

Table 1. Summary of elements to be considered in clinical trial design.

Types of control
- Active control
- Placebo control

Patient population
- Indication being treated
- Concurrent diseases
- Concomitant medication

Indication for treatment

Randomisation

Levels of blinding

Types of trial design
- Parallel
- Cross-over
- Other trial designs

Duration of dosing

Methods of clinical measurement

to all situations. A particular therapeutic area may have specific trial designs that have become standards.

Types of control

A first rule is that, to enable a conclusion to be made from the results of a scientific study, there must be a *control group*. The purpose of the control group is to provide a yardstick against which to measure the efficacy and safety of the drug under investigation, and the control may be an untreated group or a group receiving an active treatment or a placebo.

Historical controls are employed in *retrospective* studies, which utilise data from medical history, either from the literature or from records of the same institution. These studies are mostly used in Phase IV, the prime example being the case-control study.

Studies are also carried out *prospectively*, and it is these that are considered throughout this chapter. In a prospective study the control group is studied as part of the trial in question; all subjects, in the study groups and the control groups, are entered into the study over the same time interval and experience the same conditions of treatment. The comparator group therefore 'controls' sources of variability due to the situation, so that any differences between the groups can be attributed with confidence to the difference between the treatments received by the groups. The situation in which the study is carried out may introduce variability due to geographical location or the season of the year. Alternatively, outcome may be affected by elements of the social or political environment.

Choice of active control

The choice of comparator for the control group is greatly influenced by, and greatly influences, trial design. This, combined with the constraints imposed by the characteristics of the test compound, makes selection of the comparator a question of vital importance when considering the design of a study. The following are some of the points, both theoretical and practical, to consider when choosing the comparator.

1. Objective of the study. In simple terms, the objective of most studies is to investigate the efficacy and safety of a compound under test. In order to maintain clarity of design it is paramount that every study has one primary objective that is stated in the protocol. In cases where efficacy has not yet been established, it may be that a placebo is the most appropriate comparator. A comparison against a non-pharmacologically active compound will undoubtedly provide the answer to questions of efficacy. However, the use of placebo is fraught with ethical issues and practical trial management issues, the comparative importance of which will depend on the disease being treated and the treatments currently available. The use of placebo will be addressed separately later.

Assuming that the compound has been shown to possess efficacy, the objectives of later studies (Phase III onwards) will be to compare the extent of efficacy and safety with that of currently used therapies. These studies will be used as a major component of the regulatory submission, and therefore input from the regulatory department is most important. These colleagues will be able to provide information as to what is accepted as the best current treatment against which all new treatments must be compared. As a further source of valuable input, the marketing department will provide information as to the most widely prescribed current treatment. It will be valuable for future marketing to have a comparison against such treatment(s). This means that although the stated scientific objective of any study will be an assessment of efficacy and safety, in order to maximise the benefit of a study to the development programme, these secondary objectives must be considered when selecting a comparator.

The objective of the study then is linked to the phase of the development programme.

2. Countries where the study is to be carried out. This is an area where thorough research is needed, particularly in multicentre, multinational studies. The vagaries of the regulatory process may mean that a drug that has been suggested as a potential comparator may not be approved for sale or, if approved, may not be marketed in countries scheduled for participation in the clinical trial. In these cases there may be regulatory obstacles to running the study in that country. A further source of variation between countries can be found in the different formulations and dosing instructions that are registered in different countries. This may be particularly true for older drugs that have many generic forms.

3. Registration status of the potential comparator. For the reasons stated above, when discussing the objective of the study, regulatory and marketing considerations suggest that it is most productive to choose an active comparator that is established and marketed. This will also have practical benefits.

To use two unlicensed drugs in a study increases the complexity of set-up for two reasons. From the regulatory point of view, full information about both drugs would have to be submitted to the licensing authority, and it would be highly unlikely that a competitor company would make their preclinical information available to another company. From the practical point of view, it would be very difficult to obtain supplies for use in a comparative study from the manufacturer of a future potential competitor.

Included under this heading is the status of the drug in terms of exclusivity. While a patent is still current for any drug, it is likely that the drug will be available only from the original manufacturer or its licensees. Since the ideal study design may be considered to be double-blind, and marketed formulations are often identifiable, perhaps by unique markings on a tablet, it is difficult to ensure a double-blind supply of medication. Sometimes simple encapsulation of a tablet may be possible, but any manipulation (e.g., grinding a tablet to fill a capsule) will mean not only extra work for the clinical trial supplies department but also, as a minimum, dissolution studies to ensure that this manipulation has not affected the characteristics of the formulation. This might necessitate the use of a double-dummy design. Placebos matching the active treatment must be obtained, and this will undoubtedly be from the patent holder and will take time.

When a patent is no longer current, generic forms will be available and their manufacturers will frequently supply their active formulation with matching placebos, perhaps more quickly than in the on-patent situation.

Consideration of these practical factors must necessarily be accommodated when designing the study, as delays may mean that the trial fails to achieve its schedule and this will have implications for the whole development programme.

4. Dosing regimens of the potential comparator. It has already been stated that for a study to have full value for registration and marketing, the study drug should be compared with a known and established active treatment. To increase this value, the active comparator should be used in the way in which it is known to be active. Therefore, it is not advisable to use a dosing regimen different from that registered or in common use. To do so would create specific problems that would need to be taken into account in the trial design. Examples of such problems might be that the comparator has a once-daily dosing regimen while the test drug has a twice-daily regimen; alternatively, one of the two may be formulated to be long-acting or slow-release. Differences in dosing frequency may reflect a difference in the pharmacokinetic properties of the two drugs. A further, more complex, situation related to pharmacokinetics might arise if one of the drugs has a very long or a very short half-life; this may affect how a subject is withdrawn from the drug, a factor that is of particular significance in a cross-over trial.

Dosing instructions for established drugs will reflect their pharmacodynamic activity; for example, withdrawal of the drug may have to be gradual to avoid precipitating a worsening of symptoms. In designing the trial so that its level of blindness is maintained, clear instructions must be included to take account of issues such as these.

5. Marketing input. The marketing department will offer input as to the most appropriate comparator for its purposes. In some cases there may be reasons for carrying out trials late in Phase III to allow comparison with drugs that are specific to only one country: treatment of some diseases shows a marked specificity to individual countries.

The placebo-controlled trial

The ethical issues raised by the use of a pharmacologically inactive control were discussed in *Chapter 3*. We will address here some of the practical issues that are prerequisites for designing a placebo-controlled trial.

Essentially, all these points must be considered for any trial, but they are particularly pertinent to designs involving a placebo control, and include:

- withdrawals due to inadequate efficacy;
- selection of an appropriate population of trial subjects; and
- sample size.

The ideal placebo is a formulation of the excipients from the test medication, and will be identical in appearance to the test medication.

Treatment with placebo is sometimes efficacious, and can also produce significant adverse reactions. The extent of these effects varies between different indications. For example, in patients with angina, exercise tolerance has been shown to increase by about 10% in the placebo group compared with 22% in the active treatment group (Weihrauch and Gauler, 1999). In contrast, in patients with diabetes, placebo produced no effect on blood glucose levels. Placebo-induced adverse effects also vary between indication groups. Weihrauch and Gauler (1999) conclude that placebo treatment cannot be considered as 'non-treatment' and that the effects of placebo must be known before the effects of active treatment can be assessed.

The placebo effect is particularly apparent when the clinical measurement is subjective. This is illustrated clearly by trials of analgesics in which it can be expected that about 25% of the placebo group will record some measure of pain relief following a single dose (McQuay *et al.*, 1982). This finding highlights two points. First, it is why the placebo group was included. It must be assumed that this finding is due to the placebo effect plus the background rate of 'recovery' against which the test treatment is to be judged. Secondly, it also means that 75% of placebo patients do not achieve any pain relief, and so the study design must specify how those subjects will be handled.

In preparing the design, clear instructions must be given to the investigator (who has to treat the subject) on how that subject should be treated in the clinic, including specification of any rescue medication. This will depend on how the subject's results will be analysed statistically. In the example of the single-dose analgesic trial, in the event of withdrawal due to inadequate pain relief, the result of the last pain assessment (i.e. at the time of withdrawal when pain severity was great) might be carried over for all subsequent assessment times, and this assumes a worst-case scenario for the analysis.

The investigator could therefore be instructed to withdraw the subject from the study, and the subject will be given the most appropriate standard treatment. The net result of including such substitution will be that the subject's data will contribute a value of 'no response' to the analysis of the placebo group.

In gathering information to assist in designing the study, one of the most valuable pieces of information for the statistician will concern the level of difference between treatments that will be considered as significant. Since the placebo response may be considered to be the least expected, the sample size required to demonstrate efficacy of the test treatment will be smaller than for a comparison with another active treatment. Accurate characterisation of the placebo response will include an assessment of the spontaneous improvement of the disease, for which reference may be made to previous clinical trials.

Patient population

It is important carefully to define the patient population from which the study participants will be drawn. This is to avoid the bias that derives from a non-defined, perhaps investigator-specific, selection strategy. In early Phase II the entry criteria for a study may be very restrictive, and throughout the development programme these criteria will evolve as the drug's characteristics are discovered. For example, Phase I trials may have studied healthy volunteers, probably with a restricted age range, usually between 18 and 45 years. As further studies are completed in older (and possibly in younger) subjects, the newer study protocols may be extended to include these age groups. By the end of Phase III the studies should include a population that is representative of the wider patient population who will potentially receive the licensed drug; the trial results should have generality. Within one study the protocol should define clearly which subjects are eligible for entry, so that the differences between groups may be reliably ascribed to treatment differences, and not to variability between subjects.

The following are some of the points to consider when preparing the inclusion and exclusion criteria:

- nature and history of the disease being treated,
- concurrent diseases, and
- concurrent medication.

In the effort to achieve uniformity in the population of study participants, there must always be consultation with the investigators who are to carry out the trial. Otherwise there is a risk of limiting the selection criteria to such an extent that the trial may not be feasible.

Nature of the disease being treated

Variability is inherent within any population or sub-population. In a study of an antihypertensive therapy, simply enrolling any subject with elevated blood pressure will introduce a wide range of variability into the trial. This may have consequences for the response that is being measured, as this will also be variable. Expressed in terms of the actual blood pressure, subjects with severe hypertension could display improvement of a greater magnitude than those with mild hypertension. Therefore, the disease severity should be specified. In particular, terms such as mild, moderate or severe must be clearly and objectively defined in the protocol. Using the example of hypertension, this may be expressed in terms of a diastolic blood pressure between x mmHg and y mmHg. Continuing with this example, caution must be exercised to ensure that information is gathered for all three grades of severity to avoid unnecessarily limiting the final registration of the drug to one of these categories only. (However, there may be cases where the conclusion is that the new agent is an effective antihypertensive drug only in patients, for example, with severe hypertension.)

A large variability in disease severity will necessitate a greater sample size. Other sources of variability due to disease may derive from the time since disease onset or diagnosis, and response to previous treatment.

Concurrent diseases and concomitant medication

It is unlikely that the patient population suffering from the target disease will present with no concurrent diseases. This fact will undoubtedly affect the interpretation of trial results and therefore must be considered in the criteria for selecting study participants. In the early phases the decision to include or exclude subjects with specific diseases will be based on preclinical pharmacology; the knowledge base can then be extended in the light of the results of Phase I and Phase II trials.

Concurrent diseases may influence the efficacy and safety of the drug through, for example, metabolic interaction, but the necessity for medication to treat a concurrent disease may confound the interpretation of the result. Hence concurrent diseases and concomitant medication need to be considered together.

Influence of the indication on trial design

Certain of the elements that are considered when designing a trial will be influenced by the natural history of the disease being treated. For example, the onset and progression of the disease will affect the duration of the trial, the timing of each subject's treatment, and the number and timing of assessments.

A neat classification of disease might be between acute and chronic, each having implications for trial design. Acute indications, for example, infections or musculoskeletal injuries, will require a short treatment period, and during that period it is expected that a cure (or at least an improvement) would be effected. These types of disease also display spontaneous remission within a certain time after onset. Additionally, the signs and symptoms are not constant, and indeed may initially increase in severity. Therefore, the known profile of the disease may dictate that the study treatment period is one week, that subjects should enter the study within one day of onset, and that assessments be carried out daily for the first four days, to detect any signs of efficacy in the early stages. In comparison, the signs and symptoms of some chronic diseases will be stable over long periods of time. This may dictate, for example, a study of six months' duration, with monthly assessments carried out for efficacy. (More frequent assessments at the start of the treatment period will be necessary in early phase studies to monitor safety.)

This rather simplistic approach to chronic disease may be confounded when study participants are already receiving treatment that may necessitate a wash-out period. Any withdrawal of previous therapy must be carefully considered, so as not to destabilise the subject without clinical justification. If a wash-out period is used, the trial design should incorporate repeat assessments of the variable under study (e.g. blood pressure) to provide a stable baseline against which to assess efficacy.

The nature of the disease may, however, dictate that withdrawal of any current therapy is not clinically justifiable. There are several ways to continue clinical development despite this hurdle. The first is to use only subjects who are newly diagnosed with the condition. This will mean that the number of subjects available for the study will be reduced compared with the total population suffering from that disease. One implication is a longer trial and another is the need to access a large population from which to recruit such subjects. Alternatively, the need to withdraw treatment can be avoided by designing a trial where the test treatment is added to the current treatment. This implies that current therapy is inadequate and that there is still measurable improvement to be gained, either in terms of efficacy or safety. This type of add-on trial may be used, for example, in epilepsy. There is a need for adequate knowledge about the potential for interaction between treatments. In this situation a placebo may be the most appropriate comparator. Following a trial that proves efficacy and safety of the combination treatment, it may be appropriate to design trials that investigate the potential for decreasing the dose of the standard medication, while still maintaining efficacy. This is a particularly appealing approach when the standard therapy has an adverse event profile that is clinically undesirable. This type of trial is frequently referred to as a 'sparing' trial, and examples appear in the use of systemic corticosteroids, anti-rejection treatments, and narcotic analgesics.

Some diseases may be cyclical in nature, exhibiting periods of exacerbation and remission; one example in this category is rheumatoid arthritis, and many clinical trials featuring this condition are described in the literature. The anticipated length of the cycle between the two extremes of disease will influence the time at which subjects can be entered into the study in order to ensure a standardised population. It will also influence the treatment period within the study because the remission of the disease itself may inflate the apparent treatment effect.

Some diseases are seasonal, the most obvious example being hay fever. To complete a study within one season will require careful planning, with particular consideration given to sample size and the necessity for many centres.

Randomisation

We have now established two foundation stones for the development of a trial's design. A control group will be included, and the study population has been defined. Within that definition of subject characteristics, however, there will still be variability. For example, ages may range from 18 to 65 years, both men and women may be included, and more than one grade of severity may be allowed. This will provide an opportunity for the introduction of bias because an investigator may consider that all 18- to 30-year-olds should receive treatment A. This would mean that the two treatment groups will not be comparable, i.e. any difference in efficacy or safety may be due to more than just the drug. To overcome this, subjects are allocated to treatment using a method called randomisation. In a randomised trial successive subjects are assigned to a treatment in a predetermined but random manner.

The most common practice when randomising subjects is to assign equal numbers to each treatment group – simple randomisation. However, there are situations where unequal randomisation may be appropriate (Peto, 1978). By allocating more of the subjects to a new treatment, more experience of its effects can be gained, particularly if the comparator is a well-known standard. A further advantage is that fewer subjects are needed for a placebo/active comparison than for an active/active comparison.

In cases where there are differences in the nature of the disease, for example, relating to severity or site, there may be different responses to treatment. Randomisation should ensure that each treatment group contains a sample of subjects with the same extent of variability as the defined population. However, if a marked degree of difference in the response is predicted, *stratification* can be employed.

This means that separate randomisation lists are prepared for each of the different disease categories or strata, so that there will be an equal number of subjects receiving each of the treatments within each of the disease categories. Examples of the use of stratification might be to separate subjects with mild or severe pain in an analgesic trial, where the response might be different, or to separate subjects with a first or second renal transplant in a study of an immunosuppressant drug because the risk factors for rejection might be different. Each stratum may then be analysed separately, if deemed appropriate. Advice is required from the medical expert and the statistician to ensure that use of stratification is appropriate.

In a useful review, Kernan *et al.* (1999) conclude that stratification is important in small trials in which known clinical factors may have a major influence on prognosis, hence affecting treatment outcome, and also in large trials when interim analyses are planned with small numbers of subjects. Another method that can be used to produce treatment groups that are well matched for several variables is adaptive randomisation or *minimisation*. With the increasing availability of interactive randomisation systems via telephone or the Internet, sophisticated randomisation methods may be easily incorporated into clinical trial designs.

Levels of blinding

An *open* study is one in which both the subject and the investigator are aware of the identity of the treatment given. Open studies are appropriate where knowledge of the treatment received does not enable the subject or investigator to influence the results of the study, for example, in pharmacokinetic studies. In a comparative study, however, when treatment is given in an open manner, the sources of bias are many. The subject or the investigator may feel eager to please and their assessment of efficacy and reports of adverse events may favour the new treatment. Conversely, despite informed consent, they may have a negative attitude to the new drug and provide an entirely negative opinion. Even if assignment to either treatment is randomised, the investigator may select which subject receives which treatment on the basis of preconceived ideas about its performance, considered in conjunction with the subject's individual case. The drop-out rate might also be biased because subjects and investigators may be more cautious with a new treatment than with the familiar standard.

To avoid these biases, the majority of clinical trials are carried out in a 'blind' manner. There are two primary levels of blinding: a *single-blind* study is one in which the subject does not know which treatment has been administered; and a *double-blind* study is one in which neither the subject nor the investigator knows which treatment has been given. The latter is generally considered the preferable type of study. In designing such a study it must be remembered that there may be decision points for which the investigator in clinical practice would need to know the identity of all drugs administered. Contingency must be built in to accommodate this, either by disclosing the treatment or by providing some type of decision tree. An example of such a contingency in the event of failure might be the use of a specified rescue medication that is known not to interact with either of the blinded treatments, to avoid breaking the blind.

Maintenance of the blind nature of the study is vital to preserving the impartiality of the investigator. It is at the study design stage that full consideration must be given as to how this blind will be maintained, especially if there are differences in the presentation of the various treatments.

A further level of blinding may be appropriate, in addition to the subjects and the investigators and their staff. It is conceivable that representatives of the sponsor may unwittingly influence the investigator because they are aware of the treatment allocations. This may become apparent to the investigator because of a particular focus at monitoring visits. It is therefore appropriate that monitoring staff should not become aware of treatment allocation, and it may be necessary to consider the use of an independent committee to monitor safety reports, where necessary.

Types of trial design

The most frequently used designs for prospective clinical trials are the *parallel* study and the *cross-over* study, although many other alternative designs are possible (Palmer and Rosenberger, 1999). It is helpful to review the available literature of published trials carried out in the area of clinical interest to establish what alternatives are applicable. Several textbooks also contain descriptions of clinical trial designs (Altman, 1991; Pocock, 1983).

Parallel and cross-over trials

In a parallel study each subject is assigned to receive one or other of the treatments, and the subjects are studied 'in parallel'. In a cross-over study each subject will receive a course of each of the treatments under study.

The choice of one of these two designs over the other demands careful consideration. Selection of the cross-over design may be appealing because each subject acts as his/her own control, and in the context of clinical treatment this may be helpful in identifying which treatment is best for that particular subject. However, the application of that result to the general population cannot be extrapolated from the results of that particular subject's individual cross-over trial. Nevertheless, cross-over designs may be excellent models for demonstrating efficacy in Phase II studies, or for investigating phenomena such as drug interactions.

One practical issue to consider is subject (and perhaps investigator) compliance with the protocol. A typical cross-over study may have two treatment periods of 4 weeks each, with one wash-out week at the beginning and one in the middle. For a comparable parallel study, each subject will be in the trial for 5 weeks (one wash-out week plus four treatment weeks). The cross-over study will clearly necessitate more subject visits – invariably more than they would make in the normal course of treatment. This increases the probability of subjects dropping out, or even not entering. The visit schedule is clearly more of a burden and such considerations must be discussed with the prospective investigator when planning the design.

The choice of a comparator for a cross-over study must be made carefully. For example, the side-effect profile is an important factor. A cross-over comparison between drugs with such different side-effect profiles as a beta-blocker (bradycardia) and a calcium entry blocker (tachycardia) may cause a double-blind study to become unblinded, therefore leading to the potential for bias.

Careful consideration of such issues will ensure that the cross-over design is used in an appropriate way. Statistical advice is of paramount importance at the design phase, and the final analysis must investigate the possibility that differences observed between treatments may be due to 'period effects' rather than to genuine treatment differences.

In the clinical trial situation, use of the cross-over design may mean that the number of subjects in the study will be smaller than in a parallel design (*see Chapter 16* for a discussion of the issues of statistical power). This reduction in subject numbers is useful in some of the less prevalent diseases, or where time to trial completion is important.

The first issue that must be considered when designing a successful cross-over study is the nature of the disease being treated. The cross-over design is only appropriate if the disease is relatively stable (e.g. hypertension). In a self-limiting disease, such as an infection or an injury, there will be improvement over the period of the study and this will bias the results obtained for the later treatment periods; therefore a cross-over design is not appropriate.

In a disease characterised by cyclical periods of activity and remission (e.g. rheumatoid arthritis), the underlying natural history of the disease may again affect the treatment results – either adversely or positively. This type of bias can be taken into account by planning the randomisation method in advance. The number of subjects receiving treatments in the sequence A then B should be the same as that receiving B then A.

In the case of a cyclical disease, knowledge of the cycle length will influence the duration of treatment. Environmental factors must also be considered. Is it sensible to have a cross-over study of an antihistamine in hay fever if the subject will not receive the second treatment until late in the pollen season?

Whether the disease is of variable character or not, there is always a need to establish the baseline measurement of the primary efficacy variable (e.g. blood pressure or pain) at entry into each treatment period. For the second and subsequent periods this will require a wash-out between treatments, in order to avoid the carry-over of activity from the first drug received. The duration of the wash-out period should be at least five times the half-life of the drug. When including such a period, the ethical and/or practical consequences for the subject of a treatment-free phase must be considered. If a wash-out period cannot be implemented, it might be possible to transfer the subject straight from one treatment to the other and to ignore the first day's or week's results in the analysis. However, if one of the treatments is a novel drug, there will be an unknown potential for interaction.

Other trial designs

Ethics are a prime consideration in the design of clinical trials. It is a basic principle that no subject should be harmed by receiving a drug that is known to be inferior. Hence it may be considered appropriate in some instances to review the incoming data to avoid prolonging a trial where efficacy has been established beyond doubt. Analyses carried out to assess between-treatment differences while a trial is ongoing are called *interim analyses*. Interim analyses may not be as extensive as the final analysis, and may be based solely on safety reports.

There are major statistical complications to be overcome if interim analyses with significance testing are required in a trial. The use of repeated significance tests increases the chance of detecting a treatment difference at the conventionally accepted level of 5%, and the possibility of reporting a false-positive error is increased. As a consequence, a significance level that is more stringent than $p < 0.05$ must be chosen. This will influence the sample size in the study, and statistical input is vital in this context. Most importantly, interim analyses should always be planned from the outset, and stopping rules should be developed at that time. Interim analyses are discussed by Pocock (1983).

A type of trial design that uses repeated analyses is the *sequential design*. With this design groups of subjects are studied in parallel, with analyses carried out repeatedly, for example, after receipt of each subject's data, until a clear difference is shown between the treatments. Alternatively, it may become clear that no difference will be revealed. The advantage of this design is that the total trial length may be reduced, as fewer subjects would be needed. This type of trial is useful for rare diseases, particularly where a rapid response to treatment is likely to be shown by each subject. Certain practical problems are posed when planning a sequential trial with analysis after each subject. A *group sequential design*, where analysis is carried out after treatment of blocks of subjects, may be easier to plan, particularly in a multicentre trial.

The cross-over design is a type of *within-patient comparison*; a further design of this type is the *within-patient paired comparison* in which treatments are compared in the same subjects at the same time. This type of design will eliminate much of the variability, such as that due to timing of treatment, but its use is limited to treatments that may be administered to different parts of the anatomy independently. An example would be topical treatment of psoriasis in circumstances where there is no systemic absorption of the active compound.

A further variation on this type of design is the *matched pair design* where pairs of subjects are treated with the alternative treatments. The pairs will be matched for age, sex and those prognostic factors appropriate to the indication (Altman, 1991).

Duration of dosing

The factors that will determine the most appropriate duration of dosing are the pharmacokinetics and mode of action of the drug and the natural history of the disease being treated. However, beyond these clinical and scientific considerations there are many practical issues.

Particularly in early Phase II, available toxicology data may support only a limited duration of dosing. A drug development programme will include substantial chronic animal toxicology studies running in parallel with the clinical phases, and results from these studies may extend the permissible duration of dosing as they become available. Consultation with the regulatory department will ensure that a study plan is within the regulations for clinical trials in the candidate countries. Some countries require a shorter period of animal dosing to support human dosing than others, and trials may be completed sooner by conducting them there, but the ethical requirement for adequate safety data must be considered to be paramount.

Before designing a study of any length it is essential to ensure that sufficient supplies of the drug will be available. Any alteration of the dosing period may have far-reaching consequences; for example, an increase of the study period from 2 to 4 weeks doubles the amount of drug required. Consultation with the clinical trial supplies department is essential to ensure that the trial can be supported. This is particularly important in Phase II, at a time when the drug is not yet being manufactured in large quantities. Another issue concerning clinical trial supplies is the expiry date/retest date. At very early stages of development, the stability data for the test drug may provide only a short shelf-life and subjects may require new supplies. The visit schedule might have to accommodate visits for further supply, and the packaging should be planned to be synchronous with the supplies. This is a particular problem for trials with long treatment periods.

Methods of clinical measurement

The assessment method must be standardised so that the results from all subjects may be pooled, and therefore the trial design will specify which method will be used and at what time intervals throughout the study. It may appear obvious to state that the measurement method chosen must be relevant, but in ensuring relevance, the following factors should be considered.

The method chosen must have been validated as being accurate and reproducible in the given situation. For a quantitative measurement such as blood pressure, the use of standardised equipment, e.g. the sphygmomanometer, is clearly most appropriate. For an assessment of a more subjective parameter, e.g. depression, there may be many rating scales available, or there may be proposals to use a new scale. In such a situation it is advisable to use a scale for which there is documented information about its specificity to provide an assessment of the depression. Without appropriate assurance of the validity of a new scale in the same population, it could be unwise to use any novel instrument to support claims of efficacy for a new treatment. It is advisable to use new scales in parallel with established ones.

Assessment methods used for the management of patients in routine clinical practice may not be appropriate for repeated use in clinical trials. This type of situation sometimes leads to the development of scales specifically for use in trials. For example, in the assessment of depression, standard rating scales such as the Hamilton Rating Scale for Depression (Hamilton, 1967) were felt to lack sensitivity in consistently detecting differences between drugs. A new scale was therefore developed and validated for this purpose (Montgomery and Asberg, 1979).

Having confirmed that the method is suitable for assessment of the given parameter, the practical feasibility of the measurement method must be addressed. The time required to carry out the measurement should be determined because outpatient visits may be brief. Frequent, repeated inpatient measurements may be very time-consuming; for example, studies of analgesic efficacy following administration of a single dose will require the time of a devoted observer, or a subject in the immediate postoperative period may have difficulty responding. The statistical implications of such repeated measures should also be considered.

The timing and circumstances of the assessment should be standardised when considering the design of a trial. Even the result of an apparently objective and quantitative measurement such as blood pressure will be influenced by circumstance unless a standard procedure is specified. For example, the subject should have been sitting for 10 minutes before two blood pressure readings are taken, and the mean of the two readings is then used for analysis. This type of instruction will control many of the biases caused by local circumstances. Additionally, the time of day for the measurement may be standardised to avoid the introduction of additional variability due to diurnal variation. There is a further cause of bias that can be controlled, namely observer bias. In the case of blood pressure, this may be due to number preferences, or 'rounding' when reading the pressure. The use of a device such as a random zero sphygmomanometer is one way to avoid this pitfall. The device introduces a random baseline, which is subtracted from the numbers initially recorded to obtain the true blood pressure.

The choice of measurement method will affect other aspects of the trial design because of the statistical implications. The accuracy of the measurement, reflected by the variability about the mean, will be needed for the calculation of the sample size. Additionally, the statistician will require information about what is considered to be a clinically significant difference according to the key measurement method. The sample size chosen should be such that, given the variability, a significant difference will be detected.

Regulatory authorities such as the Food and Drug Administration (FDA) and the World Health Organization (WHO) have published guidelines on preferred and acceptable clinical measurement techniques in many areas of drug development.

Colleagues in different, but related, specialist disciplines now frequently demand that extra measurements be added into a trial. Examples include quality of life (QoL) assessments, pharmacoeconomics (PE) and pharmaco-kinetics, all of which are covered in more detail elsewhere in this book. There are advantages in including extra measurements into a study, as this might reduce the number of subjects who need to be treated, but it is unwise to attempt to achieve too much with a single trial. Extra measurements are often time-consuming, and the clinical setting of the original trial may not be appro-priate for gathering this additional information. It will need careful discussion to ensure that combining many objectives into one trial does not compromise the primary objective.

Quality of life and pharmacoeconomics

In response to the increasing demands of governmental health care policies worldwide, the pharmaceutical industry is investigating the impact of new treatments on aspects other than disease severity.

The assessment of QoL is becoming common and may be used to identify benefits of one treatment over another when their effect on the disease is equal. An example of this may be the comparison of a beta-blocker and an ACE inhibitor in the treatment of high blood pressure. The two do not differ to any clinically significant extent in terms of lowering blood pressure, but subjects receiving the ACE inhibitor feel better. QoL assess-ment scales have been developed to assess what 'feeling better' means, in an attempt to quantify apparently subjective endpoints. In some cases the scale may identify which drug displays the most acceptable adverse effect profile.

As with all measurement methods, the scale chosen must be appropriate for the situation; it should be meaningful for the disease being studied, and should be practical to administer in the given trial situation.

PE is a field that has grown in response to pricing policies of health care purchasers, usually governments. The cost of pharmaceuticals is an obvious target for price control, as the other elements of health care are not so clearly defined. Hence the need to demonstrate the benefits achieved by a new treat-ment in relation to cost, as well as the savings made elsewhere in the health care process or in society at large.

Pharmacokinetic sampling

The topic of pharmacokinetics is dealt with in *Chapter 6*. In designing Phase II and Phase III trials, the pharmacokinetics of the test treatment will be known. However, the early pharmacokinetic studies will have been conducted intensively in small numbers of subjects. In parallel with broadening the target population for the safety and efficacy assessments so that Phase III closely approximates to the target population, there has been a recent development in pharmacokinetics known as population pharmacokinetics.

The aim of population pharmacokinetics is to collect a small number of samples for drug concentration assay from a large number of subjects, in order to identify the extent of variability in the population. This may have implications, for example, in dosing. Basic demographic details of the subjects need to be recorded: age, weight, race and, depending on the type of drug, metabolic status. The samples, perhaps only two or three, would be collected at target times associated with one dose. The modelling of the pharmacokinetic parameters will take account of variability around the target times, but the accurate times in relation to a dose must be recorded.

The incorporation of such testing into a trial design should ensure that it does not interfere with the primary objective, which is probably an efficacy assessment. Additionally, it must be practically feasible. This type of sampling may be carried out in long-term studies, and if the subjects are outpatients or the trial is carried out in a general practice setting, the availability of adequate time and facilities should be established.

DESIGNING A MULTICENTRE TRIAL

The need to increase the number of subjects who have received a new treatment prior to marketing approval, combined with the need to study these increased numbers in a limited time, means that many trials, in particular in Phase III, will be carried out at more than one centre. Such trials are called multicentre trials. The aim of this chapter so far has been to discuss ways of avoiding or controlling bias in the results of a trial by carefully choosing the elements in its design. The introduction of more than one investigational site multiplies the ways in which bias can be introduced. Some of the elements discussed above will be re-addressed here to highlight points that will require additional consideration when several people are involved, not only at the investigational site but also in the sponsor organisation.

Multicentre trials may be carried out in one country only, or in more than one. The multinational, multicentre trial has been chosen for this discussion.

Choice of comparator

In cases where an active comparator is necessary for the study, it must be one that is registered in all the target countries, both for the indication required and at the same dosage. This is not always the case. Advice from regulatory experts will be necessary to investigate ways of overcoming any restrictions such a lack of standardisation may impose. Packaging and formulation may also need to be reviewed carefully to ensure that the study will comply with regulations in all countries. The comments so far have addressed the regulatory impact. Differences in clinical practice are more difficult to tackle. For example, the standard treatment in one country may not be considered efficacious or safe in another, and is therefore disqualified from use as a standard comparator.

The placebo-controlled trial

There will undoubtedly be as many different views about the suitability of a placebo-controlled trial as there are centres in the study. Therefore, the ethical issues must be clearly addressed in the earliest stages of study preparation.

Patient population

Differences in clinical practice may emerge when discussing the population of study participants. There may be differing opinions as to what defines a particular disease, and also what severity of disease demands which type of treatment. Clarity in defining the study population is most important. This may require prolonged discussion in order to identify sufficient numbers of subjects according to a common definition.

Concurrent diseases and concomitant medication

While concurrent diseases may be easy to control by excluding certain subjects, the use of concomitant medication is difficult to standardise. Different formulations and different dosage regimens will be used, and often entirely different treatments. To address this issue, it must be clear what influence any concomitant medication will have on the primary objective of the study. In certain situations it may be impossible to change a hospital protocol that is well established and used by all staff members. A most valuable way to resolve clinical differences is to arrange a meeting of the investigators to discuss ways to compromise, where necessary.

Clinical measurement

The use of clinical measurement methods must be standardised at all centres. An example will serve to illustrate how detailed the instructions must be. While a tape measure may be used to record the circumference of a swollen ankle, each individual may take the measurement at a slightly different place. Therefore, the distance from the tibial tubercle to the measurement point, and the position of the subject, should be specified. To avoid diurnal variation, the time of day of measurement should be stipulated. To control for environmental factors – the weather, or the fact that the subject was driven to the clinic rather than driving him/herself – the uninjured ankle is also measured, and the difference between the two is used in the analysis. This may seem a long 'protocol' for something relatively simple, but it is necessary to achieve standardisation.

For subjective assessment methods there are even more sources of potential inconsistency. The way that a question is asked will influence the answer, even within one culture. When this is extended to a multinational study, many problems arise. This is also related to language. The example of a four-point verbal rating scale of 'none', 'mild', 'moderate' and 'severe' may produce a different distribution of results across Europe, with Scandinavians perhaps recording a preponderance of 'mild' and 'moderate' and southern Europeans a higher proportion of 'severe'.

Rating scales may be validated in the language for which they were developed, but for use in another language they must first be translated, and then validated again, as the subtleties of the assessment may be lost in a different language or culture.

CONCLUSION

The importance of clinical trial design cannot be overestimated because every element in a clinical trial is influenced by its design. Every study team member should have a role in design development. Poor planning at the design stage can result in costly R&D losses, in terms both of budget and resource. Marketing pressures should not be allowed to compromise careful and timely consideration of trial design; every effort must be made to ensure that the clinical trial is consistent with its scientific objective and is not open to criticism because of poor design. This short review should be used alongside other chapters in this book to ensure that all options for clinical trial design and management are utilised practically to bring about a successful conclusion.

At the time of writing, the impact of genetic research on clinical research, and therefore on clinical trial design, is unclear but inevitable. Knowledge acquired through genomics may enable us to predict more clearly which subjects are likely to benefit from certain classes of drug, and which subjects are likely to experience side-effects. The implication may be that subjects selected to participate in clinical trials will display less variability: while this may lead to a reduction in subject numbers required, it may also have an impact on the generisability of the data obtained. However, genetic research still has to clear a number of hurdles (e.g. informed consent and the Human Rights Act) before any radical changes can take place.

REFERENCES

Altman, DG (1991). *Practical Statistics for Medical Research*, Chapman & Hall, London.

Denis, L, Norlen, BJ, Holmberg, L *et al.* (1997). Planning controlled clinical trials. Prostatic cancer. *Urology* **49** (Suppl 4A), 15–26.

Hamilton, M (1967). Development of a rating scale for primary depressive illness. *Br J Soc Clin Psychol* **6**, 278–296.

ICH Guideline (1996). *Topic E6: Good Clinical Practice – Consolidated Guideline*, International Federation of Pharmaceutical Manufacturers Associations, Geneva (Issued as CPMP/ICH/135/95).

Kernan, WN, Viscoli, CM, Makuch, RW, Brass, LM and Horwitz, RI (1999). Stratified randomization for clinical trials. *J Clin Epidemiol* **52**, 19–26.

McQuay, HJ, Bullingham, RES, Moore, RA, Evans, PJD and Lloyd, JW (1982). Some patients don't need analgesics after surgery. *J Roy Soc Med* **75**, 705–708.

Montgomery, SA and Asberg, M (1979). A new depression scale designed to be sensitive to change. *Br J Psychiatry* **134**, 382–389.

Palmer, CR and Rosenberger, WF (1999). Ethics and practice: alternative designs for Phase III randomized clinical trials. *Controlled Clinical Trials* **20**, 172–186.

Peto, R (1978). Clinical trial methodology. *Biomedicine* **28** (special issue), 24–36.

Pocock, SJ (1983). *Clinical Trials: A Practical Approach*, John Wiley, Chichester.

Weihrauch, TR and Gauler, TC (1999). Placebo – efficacy and adverse effects in controlled clinical trials. *Arzneimittelforschung* **49**, 385–393.

6

Early phase studies, pharmacokinetics and adverse drug interactions

Tim Mant and Elizabeth Allen

Phase I studies

INTRODUCTION

Phase I studies may be defined as the initial investigations of drugs in man. The subjects are usually healthy, male, adult volunteers. The development of new drugs in animals and patients is under strict legal control, but no legislation currently governs the conduct of healthy volunteer drug studies in the UK, although guidelines and recommendations have been published by the Royal College of Physicians (RCP) in 1986, the Association of the British Pharmaceutical Industry (ABPI) in 1988, and the Association of Independent Clinical Research Contractors (AICRC) in 1989. The ICH Harmonised Tripartite Guideline for Good Clinical Practice (ICH Guideline, 1996) also covers many aspects of early phase studies. With the advent of the European Clinical Trials Directive, it is envisaged that Phase I study regulation and the need for prior approval will be brought into line with the requirements for later phase studies.

With the world's continuing demand for more efficacious, safer drugs, increasing dissatisfaction with animal experiments and the escalation in cost and bureaucracy associated with Phase II and Phase III studies, more precise, predictive data are required from Phase I studies. Technological advances in non-invasive techniques to measure drug response, greater understanding of mechanisms and more sensitive investigations to detect 'subclinical' toxicity have enabled major decisions to be made earlier in the development process.

Relationship of studies in animals to Phase I studies in man

Before a drug can become available for general administration, evidence of safety and efficacy must be presented to expert committees established by government. There is a natural and proper reluctance to expose human subjects to any risk by the administration of new drugs. However, the only alternative would be to find laboratory tests that predict the actions and tolerability of a new drug in man. Some *in-vitro* models are used to study drug passage across human tissue barriers. Cell cultures offer opportunities to study drug metabolism and cellular responses *ex vivo*. However, most laboratory studies involve the use of experimental animals. Animal studies are conducted to investigate the pharmacology, toxicology and pharmacokinetics of new chemical entities (NCEs). The types of preclinical studies are listed in Table 1. Not all these studies will be completed by the time human studies commence (Ritter *et al.*, 1999). The timing of toxicology studies to support human studies is described in ICH Topic E4: *Dose–Response Information to Support Drug Registration* (ICH Guideline, 1994).

Table 1. Preclinical studies.

- Pharmacology[a]
- Acute toxicity[a]
- Repeated-dose toxicity (2 weeks)[a]
- Mutagenicity[a]/genotoxicity[a]
- Carcinogenicity
- Reproductive testing

[a]Minimum requirements before human exposure to a new chemical entity (NCE), according to EU guidelines.

While other mammals have the same general circulatory pattern, organs, tissues and sub-cellular fractions as man, the responses to drugs in laboratory animals may differ from the responses in man in a completely unpredictable way. Inter-species pharmacokinetic differences may be quantitative (for example, the half-life of phenylbutazone in man is 72 hours while in the rat and dog it is 6 hours) and qualitative (for example, parahydroxylation of amphetamines is a very minor metabolic pathway in humans but a major metabolic pathway in rats).

The most problematic difficulties in using laboratory experiments, instead of observing drug actions in man, are associated with the direct pharmacodynamic effects on the organism, since there are gross and well-established inter-species differences. Penicillin is highly toxic to the gastrointestinal tract of the guinea pig and readily produces haemorrhage, but is relatively well tolerated in man. Also, certain types of drug activity can only be investigated in man because they require detailed subjective reporting; for example, changes in mood, arousal and perception. Even gross effects such as alterations in sleep, appetite and physical energy are very difficult to observe in experimental animals. The investigator in a Phase I study must be cognisant of the preclinical results and their interpretation before exposing humans to the NCE (see Table 2).

Table 2. Preclinical data review.

- Pharmacology/Toxicology/Toxicokinetics
- Identify target organs
- Mechanisms of toxicity
- Mode of death
- Seek expert help to assess significance
- Design protocol/assessments accordingly
- Be prepared for anything

The tenuous relationship between the effects of drugs in animals and man therefore requires that man be the final experimental animal. Because only an indication of the possible efficacy or toxicity of a drug can be obtained from animal studies, the early studies in man must be conducted cautiously and initially must use very low doses.

Aims of Phase I studies

Phase I investigations represent the first time in the development programme when drugs given to man and they are carried out to establish data on human tolerance, pharmacokinetics and pharmacodynamics. In the majority of cases it is an advantage that the volunteers are healthy adults. With some types of drug, which may be predicted to have unacceptable harmful effects in healthy volunteers, e.g. anti-leukaemia drugs, patients for whom there may be a therapeutic benefit are invited to participate. Drug effects are determined by history, clinical examination, clinical measurements (such as blood pressure, electrocardiography (ECG), electroencephalography (EEG), psychometric tests) and laboratory studies (including blood and urine examinations). With all drugs, a broad spectrum of safety tests is always carried out, but with individual agents, additional tests may be appropriate (such as coagulation studies, endocrine function tests or continuous 24-hour cardiac monitoring) (*see Chapter 13*).

To assess tolerability, a dose-ranging schedule is applied in which successive volunteers are exposed to increasing drug doses. In this way an indication of the maximum tolerated dose may be obtained. Clearly, it is important to determine whether the estimated therapeutic dose can be exceeded without mishap. Occasionally, dose escalation is terminated because the projected cost of manufacturing the drug becomes prohibitive.

Increasingly during Phase I studies, useful information other than safety data will be obtained; for example, determination of the appropriate route of administration. The sampling of body fluids (e.g. blood, urine and saliva) during the course of single- and multiple-dose studies will provide useful information on the pharmacokinetic profile of the parent drug and metabolites. However, this will be dependent on the development of reliable and sensitive assay methodology.

Some classes of drug can only be assessed therapeutically when given to sufferers from diseases peculiar to man (for example, schizophrenia, rheumatoid arthritis and asthma). However, the efficacy of certain types of agent can be predicted from studies in normal subjects – as with hypnosedatives, general anaesthetics, drugs acting on the autonomic nervous system, and anticoagulants. Although such early observations on pharmacodynamics are valuable indications of proof of concept and of therapeutic dose ranges, they do not replace later work in the target patient population. However, if correctly designed, studies using pharmacodynamic assessments as 'surrogate' markers of potential toxicity or efficacy will help to plan the initial therapeutic Phase II studies with greater safety and economy of time.

SELECTION OF VOLUNTEERS

The usual practice for Phase I studies is to recruit volunteers from males between the ages of 18 and 35 years, who are not on current medication, do not abuse alcohol or other drugs and show no clinically significant haematological or chemical pathological abnormality. However, it is difficult to find completely 'normal' individuals (Joubert et al., 1975). This is partly a consequence of the adoption of a 95% normal range in many laboratory tests, a practice which ensures that 5% of the population will be considered abnormal. Thus, if 20 separate, independent tests are made on 100 individuals, 64% will show one or more abnormal results. Tables have been published of the expected distribution of abnormal results for tests utilising various percentile limits to define normality (Schoen and Brooks, 1970). The possibilities of laboratory error and inappropriate normal ranges of values must also be considered. It is important, therefore, for the investigators to use clinical judgement in their interpretation of laboratory tests.

Subjects must be screened for serological evidence of past or present hepatitis. It is recommended that human immunodeficiency virus (HIV) screening be performed and investigators must ensure that volunteers fully understand the meaning of both positive and negative results (Jagathesan et al., 1995).

With ever-increasing numbers of studies in apparently healthy volunteers, it is also becoming clear that clinical observations which have hitherto been regarded as indicators of disease may occur in normal subjects. Thus, although complete right bundle branch block occurred with an incidence of 1.2–1.3 per 1000 in studies of the ECGs of healthy flying personnel between the ages of 19 and 29 years, this finding seems only very occasionally to indicate clinically relevant disease (Rotman and Triebwasser, 1975; Adamson et al., 1998). With more sophisticated monitoring, even more 'abnormalities' may emerge. Thus, 24-hour ambulatory ECG monitoring showed that 23% of 120 normal subjects had episodes of ST-segment changes, a finding that is often interpreted as indicating myocardial ischaemia in patients with ischaemic heart disease

(Quyyumi *et al.*, 1983). Many of the healthy young men who volunteer for drug studies are athletes. Mid-systolic murmurs, cardiomegaly, sinus brady-cardia, sinus arrhythmia, wandering atrial pacemakers, first-degree heart block and second-degree heart block of the Möbitz type 1 variety (but not type 2) are all more commonly reported in athletes. The phenomenon of the athletic heart syndrome has been well reviewed by Huston *et al.* (1985).

In a similar way, repeated examinations of the urine of young (18–33 year-old) men for microhaematuria revealed a cumulative incidence of 38.7% after an average of 12.2 yearly examinations per person. Careful investigation and follow-up of these individuals suggested that this is a 'normal' finding (Froom *et al.*, 1984).

The US Food and Drug Administration (FDA) has recognised this problem and has defined 'normal subjects' as those 'who are free from abnormalities which would complicate the interpretation of the data from the experiment or which might increase the sensitivity of the subject to the toxic potential of the drug' (Food and Drug Administration, 1977). Thus, although not normal practice, individuals with mild but stable illnesses, such as hypertension or arthritis, could be considered for Phase I studies. Indeed the wisdom of exces-sively rigid exclusion criteria can be questioned, for it may be desirable to include otherwise healthy subjects with diseases for which the candidate drug may be indicated.

Although it is well recognised that there are pharmacokinetic and pharmacodynamic differences between elderly and young subjects (Ritter *et al.*, 1999), it is unusual to perform the first studies of an NCE in the elderly because they tend to provide a less homogeneous population due to concur-rent illnesses and concomitant medications; they are also considered to be at greater risk from deleterious drug effects. Since the elderly are more likely to be the 'target population' than the young, it is essential that any differences are determined; however, this is usually done when sufficient human safety and pharmacokinetic data are available to support less stringent inclusion/exclusion criteria and less 'in-patient' supervision. Women of child-bearing potential are also underrepresented in early clinical studies. This is due largely to concerns over potential harm to the foetus, and if women of childbearing potential are used for such studies, it is essential that the risk of pregnancy is minimised.

The setting of exclusion criteria is clearly not an easy matter and will vary for different drug types. Potential epileptogenic drugs, such as tricyclic anti-depressants, should not be given to subjects with a history of epilepsy, faint-ing attacks or head injury or with a family history of epilepsy. Screening for such a study might include an EEG, but as 5–10% of the non-epileptic popula-tion exhibit an EEG abnormality, this alone would lead to the exclusion of up to 10% of otherwise satisfactory volunteers. However, there is no doubt concerning the wisdom of excluding anyone with a history of asthma and wheezing in investigations of beta-adrenoreceptor blocking drugs.

Individuals taking other medication or who may be abusing alcohol or drugs of dependency must be excluded from Phase I studies. Not only is the chance of adverse reactions greatly increased during drug administration, but analytical, safety and kinetic measurements may also be distorted. Hence, it is common practice to carry out a toxicological screen on urine taken at study entry and on random samples taken while the study is in progress. Cigarette smokers are commonly admitted as volunteers; in many units they are allowed to smoke during the study on the grounds that the physiological and psychological disturbances produced by withdrawal of nicotine are more disruptive than its pharmacological actions. However, it is important to note that the smoking of a single cigarette within an hour of a pulse rate measurement, a blood pressure reading or an ECG recording can produce changes that can mask the cardiovascular actions of the drug under study. The effect of smoking on hepatic drug metabolism must also be remembered when recruiting subjects and interpreting results. If the preclinical studies indicate effects on heart rate and blood pressure or suggest that the drug may be metabolised by cytochrome P-450$_{1A2}$ (CYP$_{1A2}$), smokers should be excluded from the early studies (non-smoking can be confirmed by urinary cotinine estimation).

It is not necessarily sensible, although usually requested, to restrict the use of caffeine, since its withdrawal is associated with headache, yawning, tiredness and dysphoria which may confound the interpretation of drug effects (Silverman et al., 1992). Hence, if caffeine is to be restricted, it would be best to exclude subjects who frequently consume caffeinated drinks.

Individual dietary habits can also alter drug disposition and may need to be taken into consideration when interpreting results (Kappas et al., 1978).

Enzyme polymorphism, such as acetylator status and CYP$_{2D6}$ activity, can greatly alter drug kinetics, effects and toxicity. Only in special circumstances is it usual to select subjects on this basis. Where preclinical studies indicate oxidation to be a significant component of the total elimination process, the influence of the 'poor oxidation (metaboliser)' phenotype should be investigated in early studies of the drug. If the drug is predicted to have a narrow therapeutic index and its metabolism is related to CYP$_{2D6}$ activity, slow metabolisers (approximately 8% of Britons) may be expected to experience greater exposure to drug than subjects with normal CYP$_{2D6}$ activity. Hence, poor metabolisers may be excluded (by genotyping or phenotyping at screening) and only studied first at a dose lower than that shown to be well tolerated in people with normal enzyme activity.

While the importance of somatic characteristics as criteria for volunteer selection is widely accepted, the possible effects of psychological factors are less well recognised. Thus, not only does the level of neuroticism affect responses to centrally-acting drugs but there is also evidence that the rate and extent of absorption of diazepam, for example, is greater in subjects with a high level of neuroticism, probably due to enhanced gastric motility (Nakano *et al.*, 1979). Stress may also affect the absorption of drugs such as indomethacin (Leopold *et al.*, 1980).

Informed consent

One aspect of volunteer selection that has both scientific and profound ethical importance is the desirability for the volunteer to understand the precise nature of the study and what is expected of him/her. It is the investigator's responsibility to explain in terms that are fully comprehensible to volunteers: the purpose and description of the research study; the tests to be performed before, during and after drug administration; any possible risks and side-effects associated with administration of the drug; and the investigative procedures. It is important to discuss even the possibility of rare idiosyncratic reactions and volunteers must always be allowed the opportunity to ask questions of the investigator, either in a group or in private. The explanation of the study must include reminding volunteers of their responsibility to disclose their full medical history, to comply conscientiously with the protocol and to report any symptoms that may occur during or after the study. It must be explained to volunteers that they have the right to withdraw voluntarily from the study at any stage. Details must also be explained concerning the compensation available in the event of injury as a result of the research project. Volunteers should also be informed that it is possible that taking part in the study may affect their personal insurance. Only a small minority of the population understands drug toxicity and the statistical nature of biological phenomena; hence a lengthy explanation in layman's terms is essential.

Most anti-cancer drugs are too dangerous to be given to healthy volunteers and it is more appropriate that patients with cancer are invited to participate in Phase I studies with these agents. The type of patient enrolled will have disease that is considered unsuitable for currently available therapy. It is still desirable that these patients should have relatively normal organ function and should not have received extensive prior therapy that may confound study assessments or make evaluation of the study medication difficult. In addition, patients should be expected to survive for at least two months so that toxicity can be evaluated. From the patient's point of view, participation may offer therapeutic hope and indeed benefit. However, many anti-cancer drugs produce toxicity, which is at best unpleasant (e.g. vomiting) or at worst life-threatening (e.g. bone marrow depression). There is always an ethical dilemma in the presentation of risks and benefits of participation to the patient. This is illustrated by the fact that when 200 cancer patients were tested, one day after signing consent forms for chemotherapy, surgery or radiotherapy, only 60% understood the purpose and nature of the procedure and only 55% could list even one major risk or complication (Cassileth *et al.*, 1980). One identified problem which overlaps with the difficulties of using unsophisticated normal subjects in Phase I studies is that of presenting complex data concerning drugs and risks in a form that is easily assimilated by the average person. This applies particularly for individuals, such as cancer patients, who are going through a very difficult time in their personal lives. A study of 60 informed consent forms from five national cancer clinical study groups in the USA (Morrow, 1980) showed these to score 35–46 ('difficult') on a readability scale on which the *New England Journal of Medicine* scored 23 ('very difficult'), *Newsweek* scored 63 ('fairly easy') and *The Amazing Spider Man* scored 99. Many of these consent documents required university-level education in order to be understood, a background possessed by only 28% of the US population. Information for subjects must therefore be simplified and preferably read and corrected by patients and lay individuals rather than by medical staff. This issue has been recently covered by Eisenhauer *et al.* (2000) in their review of Phase I oncology study design.

Place of investigation

There are no statutory regulations concerning the facilities required for Phase I studies in the UK, although a 'registration' scheme exists through the AICRC, involving an on-site inspection every 2 years. The AICRC is a voluntary organisation. The Medicines Control Agency (MCA) offers a voluntary inspection service and it is predicted that MCA inspection and licensing of clinical drug research units will become mandatory in the UK. In France the law dictates that all laboratories conducting Phase I studies must undergo inspection in order to be licensed; no studies can be performed if the appropriate licence is not granted.

The first administration of drugs to man should take place in a specialised unit devoted to such studies. The staff should include clinical pharmacologists (who are also physicians) and nurses experienced in carrying out Phase I studies. The unit must have facilities for resuscitation – in particular, emergency drugs and equipment for defibrillation – and all staff should be trained in cardiopulmonary resuscitation. In our opinion, volunteers should not normally be allowed home on the same day after receiving a new drug; they should spend at least one night under observation, or longer if it is likely that pharmacodynamic effects are present beyond this time. This means that nursing care must be continuous during the entire period the volunteers are in the unit and medical staff must be on call during this time.

Since a particular dose of a drug cannot be administered until the results of all important investigations relating to the previous dose of the drug are known, facilities such as chemical pathology and haematology departments must be near enough to enable rapid evaluation.

The work involved in a Phase I study is facilitated by access to a computer with validated database and word processor programs. Even in a simple study, many thousands of labels are needed for the various samples, and the results of clinical and laboratory investigations for each subject must be recorded daily. Such data handling facilities permit daily data review and early warning of possible hazard.

Proximity to a general hospital is a great asset and will be required for some studies, giving access to specialised departments and personnel, for example, echocardiography, cardiac catheterisation, nuclear and computer-assisted tomographic scanning, or endoscopic examination.

Ethics committee

In the UK there is no statutory requirement for the protocols of Phase I studies in normal subjects to be examined by the Committee on Safety of Medicines (CSM). Phase I studies require permission from an independent ethics committee, or research ethics committee (REC), which is usually local to the Phase I unit or may even be an internal committee of the unit itself. Ethics committees should be properly constituted, should follow the *Guidelines on the Practice of Ethics Committees in Medical Research Involving Human Subjects* (Royal College of Physicians, 1996), and comply with ICH guidelines.

The REC should protect research subjects (both volunteers and patients) from exposure to unethical risk, while facilitating ethically acceptable attempts to identify new and better treatments. Phase I studies have no intention to directly benefit healthy participants; hence it is essential the REC is satisfied that any risks are minimal (Royal College of Physicians, 1996). In addition to the protocol, the REC must consider the investigator's current curriculum vitae, any payment to subjects, written background information/consent documents, any advertising material and the investigator's brochure. The REC must be informed promptly about any additional emerging information that may affect the ethics or safety of the study, and about any serious adverse events (SAEs) that occur during the course of the study, or other studies being performed concurrently. This subject is discussed in greater detail in *Chapter 3*.

Insurance and compensation

The manufacturer of the drug is responsible for ensuring that adequate arrangements exist for compensation of subjects in the event of mishap. As well as ensuring that there is insurance to cover for negligence, there should also be a separate 'volunteer accident policy' which pays compensation without consideration of legal liability, once it has been established that the volunteer's injury resulted from participation in the study. In addition to these arrangements, it is recommended that the investigators themselves should be insured by a medical defence society.

Payment of volunteers

Although it may be considered a privilege to be allowed to participate in research that has scientific interest and could also help in the treatment of illness, it would be unreasonable for the volunteers to suffer financially because of their altruism. On the other hand, any payment should not be so large that it could be considered an inducement in itself to act as a volunteer. By contrast, 'it could be argued that a participant without the wit to demand a (reasonable) fee ... is unlikely to be fit to give informed consent' (Editorial, 1984). One basis for payment can be to consider the loss of earnings potentially incurred by a shift worker (e.g. an ambulance driver) during the period of the study and to add a quantum for discomfort and inconvenience. The amount of payment for a study is considered by ethics committees and should be stated on the volunteer consent form.

Volunteer motivation

Experimental subjects are usually recruited by word of mouth or by advertisement in academic institutions and in places of work, newspapers and periodicals. A potential concern over the recruitment of students, hospital staff and employees of drug firms is that of coercion.

It is often extremely difficult to determine the motives and rewards that encourage a person to behave in a particular fashion. The decision to volunteer involves much more than the transfer of accurate information concerning the drug and its risks followed by the exercise of individual free will. Ayd (1972) offers the reminder 'that many people, including physicians and scientists, indulge in more dangerous avocations than offering to take part in a medical research project'. He classified volunteers' motives into financial, psychological and spiritual and found that in those for whom financial rewards are *not* the most compelling, a mild psychopathy is common, with obsessive and schizoid personality types predominant. In certain circumstances, recruitment of a high proportion of a certain category of volunteers could result in a psychologically unrepresentative sample. Findings obtained from such a group would not be readily generalised to a population with a more normal personality mix. Interestingly, a study of prisoner volunteers in the USA found that such subjects had significantly higher IQ scores than prisoners who did not volunteer (Cudrin, 1969). At present it would be imprudent to generalise any of these findings to all volunteer groups. In the case of patient volunteers, an additional (and perhaps more compelling) reason for participation is the hope that they might obtain therapeutic benefit from the new drug.

In our view there is little doubt that financial reward is the commonest reason for young healthy volunteer participation in studies, a conclusion corroborated by a study by Hassar *et al.* (1977). They interviewed two groups of volunteers from a university and the pharmaceutical industry and found financial reward to be the paramount motive, although this incentive was not liable to cause volunteers to take part in a study in which the perceived risk, or inconvenience, was excessive.

It is important to prevent, if possible, the emergence of 'professional volunteers'. Apart from registration both of volunteers and institutions, as practised in France where a French National Insurance number is a prerequisite for participation, it is difficult to see how this can otherwise be easily accomplished. Certainly we would wish to place an (admittedly arbitrary) limitation on volunteer participation in studies to no more than three per year. In our experience it is most unusual for long-term unemployed persons to volunteer for a study because, in the UK, they lose a proportion of their unemployment benefit.

Protocols

It is unthinkable (i.e. people sometimes think of doing it!) that a study be undertaken without having first produced a detailed protocol. This is the only way the work can be planned, agreed and performed in a uniform and reproducible manner by all those concerned with the development and testing of the drug. It is the document to which the ethics committee can refer about any detail regarding the study. Development of the protocol should be an interactive process between the sponsor (usually a pharmaceutical company) and the investigators. General information should include the study title, name, address and contact numbers of sponsor, sponsor's medical representative, monitor, investigator, research unit and any laboratories involved in the study. The following should be included in a protocol for any clinical drug investigation:

1. *Introduction.* This should include general and scientific background information about the study and the medicinal products/devices being used. At this stage the information will be based almost entirely on animal experiments.
2. *Objectives and purpose.* Much of this is self-evident in a Phase I study, but any particular action in man that is to be specifically investigated/ assessed should be stated, including pharmacokinetic investigations.
3. *Study design.* This should include a detailed description of the design of the study. The primary end-points should be defined. A description of whether the study is to be placebo-controlled, blinded and, if appropriate, of parallel/cross-over design, and a description of the method of randomisation and blinding should be included (as well as procedures for breaking the study blind). The proposed doses and dose escalation procedure to be employed should be stated. The expected duration of subject participation should be included. Any stopping rules or discontinuation criteria should also be defined.

4. *Investigational product.* A description of the investigational product(s) detailing formulation type, labelling requirements, storage conditions, method of dispensing and administration, and full accountability procedures.

5. *Selection and withdrawal of subjects.* This specifies inclusions, exclusions, e.g. body mass index range, number of subjects to be enrolled, when and how subjects should be withdrawn.

6. *Study procedures.* Procedures to be followed should be described in detail and divided into pharmacokinetic assessments, pharmacodynamic assessments and safety assessments. It is important that the order and timing of the study procedures are feasible and enable the protocol objectives to be met; it is unrealistic to expect a subject to have blood samples taken, and to have respiratory rate, lying and standing blood pressure, pulse and temperature measured every 15 minutes for 24 hours. Such protocol requirements are indicative of inexperience in clinical investigations.

   Pharmacokinetic assessments should state the type and volume of samples to be obtained (e.g. blood, urine, saliva), sampling times relative to dosing, details of how the samples are to be processed and then stored until required for analysis, and where and how samples are to be analysed.

   Pharmacodynamic and safety assessments should include details of the methods to be employed and assessment times relative to dosing. The information provided should be as unambiguous as possible. For example, 'resting blood pressure' is not a sufficient description: clear instructions should be provided concerning the type of blood pressure measurement device to be used (normal mercury-in-glass sphygmomanometer, random zero sphygmomanometer, automated sonic blood pressure device), which Korotkoff sounds are to be recorded, how many readings are to be taken and at what time delay, and finally the subject's posture during measurement.

   The reporting of adverse events should be clearly defined in terms of recording and classification, with particular attention to procedures for reporting any SAEs. Although much can be planned in the protocol, the investigators will have to use their judgement in many instances of unexpected pharmacological activity or toxicity. It is important that such events be investigated thoroughly, even if it is decided to withdraw the volunteer from the study.

7. *Treatment programmes.* A flow chart will help to clarify the scheme of administration of the drug, dose frequency, the days when the drug is to be administered, and when dose changes are permitted. Permissible concomitant medication (if any) should be defined. If concomitant medication is required to treat adverse effects or incidental illness, it should be specified how and to whom this should be reported.

8. *Statistical considerations.* Phase I studies are exploratory, often involving the first administration of an NCE or biological entity to man. Because there may be no previous human data, sample sizes are therefore

sometimes determined from previous experience with Phase I studies rather than from any statistical calculations.

9. *Ethics considerations.* Informed consent – details of the informed consent procedure and a copy of the informed consent document that the volunteers are required to sign – must be included in the protocol. The protocol must also include details of the ethical review and approval procedure, i.e. the documents to be reviewed and who will be responsible for obtaining approval.

10. *Data handling and record keeping.* This section should describe how and where data should be recorded, processed, stored and archived.

11. *Finance and insurance.* The sponsor's policy in terms of indemnity and insurance cover for the investigator(s) and study participants should be clearly specified.

12. *Publication policy and confidentiality.* Because the data collected during Phase I studies may be of a sensitive nature, this section should clearly define who will be the 'owners' of the data/information produced, who will be responsible for any resulting publications, and the level of use that an investigator may make of the data collected.

13. *References.* A comprehensive list of all relevant references should be appended.

DESIGN OF STUDY

Types of study

Phase I studies are usually carried out in two stages: single rising dose and repeated administration.

Stage 1: single rising dose

Each volunteer is given a single dose of the drug or placebo. The initial dose to be used in man is usually determined from results obtained in animal studies. Even though several species of animals may be used to investigate the doses of a new drug which produce pharmacological actions, toxicity and death, extrapolation of animal data to man is hazardous. In view of this, the usual practice in man is to start with about 1–2% of the dose (per unit weight) that produced any effects on animals. The route of administration in the volunteers should be the same as that used in the animal work. According to James (1976), it is usual to start with 2% of the scaled dose that is effective in animals. Dollery and Davies (1970) suggest a starting dose of 1–2% of the maximum tolerated dose in animals. Vaidya and Vaidya (1981) suggest using the following three different methods for evolving a starting dose in Phase I studies:

- 10–20% of the maximum tolerated dose in the most sensitive species of animal tested;
- examination of animal data to assess the doses which produce the pharmacodynamic action relevant for its proposed therapeutic role in man; and
- scrutiny of the effective and safe doses in man of closely related compounds.

We would add:

- finding the minimum blood concentration in animals which produces a pharmacological effect (C_E) and significant acute toxicity (C_T); we would not start with a dose higher than that predicted to produce a blood concentration of $C_E/10$ in man.

In the past, 10–12 volunteers were often used for this type of investigation, with pairs given the same dose simultaneously. In recent years, studies have tended to become more extensive. Commonly, at each dose level, eight to 12 volunteers are admitted to the research ward: two or four of these receive placebo and six to eight the drug under investigation.

Screening is usually carried out within 2–4 weeks before drug administration. Meticulous screening is important, not only to minimise risk but also to facilitate interpretation of the results.

Typically, the volunteers are admitted on the morning of the day before drug administration, and physical examination, blood tests, urinalysis and clinical tests (such as ECG) are repeated to confirm continued eligibility. Enquiry is made about current symptoms, administration of medication and alcohol intake. Blood and/or urine tests are carried out for drugs of abuse. The next morning an indwelling cannula is inserted into a vein and blood is taken as a baseline (blank) for pharmacokinetic measurements. The drug is then given and blood and urine samples are taken at various intervals, according to the kinetic properties of the drug predicted from the preclinical data. At the same time urine is collected for drug analysis over appropriate intervals, e.g. 0–4, 4–12 and 12–24 hours. It is our practice to monitor continuously the ECG of subjects during the first 4–6 hours after drug administration. Dosing should be performed at approximately the same time of day for each dose increment because circadian changes in drug disposition can occur (Reinberg and Smolensky, 1982); the volunteer's posture should also be standardised.

Usually 24–48 hours after drug administration, the final samples of blood and urine are collected for pharmacokinetic studies. A physical examination is carried out after asking about subjective changes and safety check samples have been taken to repeat the baseline blood and urine tests performed before drug administration. Similarly, special clinical tests, such as an ECG, are repeated and reviewed before discharge. Volunteers should return to the unit 4–7 days after the dose for further follow-up, including a blood count and biochemical screen to help exclude delayed effects. It is important that, if necessary, volunteers and the facilities should have the flexibility for extending admission.

The next group of volunteers in the study should not receive the drug until the results of the previous group's safety tests are known. The doses in each group may be increased either by doubling the dose used in the previous stage or by smaller or larger steps. The dose increments should be influenced by the dose–response curve in preclinical studies. In the protocol design it is often valuable to allow some flexibility, such as the option to repeat a dose level to confirm or refute a possible drug effect or to allow more conservative dose increments. Such decisions require full communication between the investigator and the sponsor to discuss ongoing results. Any changes in design not allowed in the original protocol must be approved by the ethics committee.

How far the increments should proceed is determined mainly by the appearance of toxicity, or the attainment of a predetermined effect. If data from previous animal work showed that a particular blood concentration was associated with a serious toxic effect (e.g. convulsions), this should also be used as a guide as to how far to proceed with this stage of the Phase I study. If such toxic levels are known, the peak blood level of the human subjects should be measured before the next experiment. Apart from the appearance of toxicity, the attainment of blood concentrations regarded as adequate can be used as an indicator to stop further dose increases. In the absence of knowledge about drug levels, the appearance of toxicity that interferes with normal daily activities is the signal to stop increasing the drug dose. For example, once complete anorexia and severe nausea are experienced, nothing can be gained (apart from non-cooperation) by inducing vomiting at higher doses.

With an oral drug it is prudent to repeat a dose level in a new group of subjects to investigate the effect of food on bioavailability. This is usually a randomised, two-way, cross-over design, with all subjects taking active medication; the drug is given following an overnight fast on one occasion and following a standard meal on another.

Repeated administration

Only when single-dose administration has been investigated can multiple-dose studies begin. In this type of study, drug or placebo is given repeatedly, as inpatient treatment, for one or more weeks. Many such chronic Phase I studies last for 14 days – but drugs which are normally given for a shorter time in therapy are tested for a shorter interval (e.g. antibiotics for 5–7 days). On the other hand, anticonvulsants (which may be used for several years) may be tested in Phase I for 4 weeks or more, until steady-state blood concentrations are reached.

The interval between doses is usually approximately one half-life, but it is desirable to aim at what can be easily accomplished: thus, once-daily or eight-hourly administration can always be attained, but administration every 27 hours or 5.5 hours is not practical and would not mirror clinical use.

As with the single rising-dose study, screening is carried out within 2–4 weeks of the start, and these tests and examinations are all repeated when the subjects are admitted to the ward on the day prior to the start of drug administration, at intervals during the study, before discharge and 4–10 days after the final dose.

Kinetic data are obtained by taking blood and urine samples after the first and last doses in the study at the times determined from the single-dose study. In addition, information about accumulation and attainment of steady-state blood concentrations is provided by taking blood samples each day immediately *before* drug administration (trough samples). Attempts to record peak concentrations after each oral dose are generally less valuable because of variations in drug absorption, even in the same individual, and the unlikelihood of obtaining a blood sample at the precise time of the peak blood level.

The doses to be investigated in the chronic limb stage of the Phase I studies are determined by the results of the single rising-dose study. If pharmacokinetic data have been generated from the latter, then the highest repeated doses administered are of such a size as to give steady-state blood levels below those producing toxicity in the single-dose study, unless tolerance is predicted.

The size of chronic Phase I studies is variable but, as a general rule, groups of eight to 12 volunteers (some of whom take placebo throughout) are used. The results of tests from each group are analysed before the next group is given the drug. Typically, three to five such groups are investigated, i.e. 24–30 subjects are used in all. As well as 'standard' single and multiple rising-dose studies, additional studies may be required; for example, to investigate changes in formulation/dosage regimen, possible relevant interactions or unanswered pharmacodynamic questions arising from the earlier studies. While exposing healthy subjects to minimal risk, each Phase I programme must provide sufficient information to allow the decision to be made either to proceed with drug studies in patients or to stop further drug development.

Route of administration

The intended final (or routine) route of administration should normally be used. Oral administration in patient therapy is generally safer, cheaper and more convenient than injections, and this is therefore the route of first choice in Phase I; however, it might also be useful to give the drug intravenously to allow the effects of maximum absorption to be predicted. All intended routes of administration, and all preparations likely to be used in clinical practice, should be investigated. However, no route of administration should be used that has not been previously tested in animal species. Absolute bioavailability can be calculated in a two-way cross-over design. In some cases the route of administration will be governed by the properties of the drug itself; for example, peptides and other substances likely to be destroyed in the gastro-intestinal tract will generally be given by injection.

Blood sampling

Before any pharmacokinetic samples are taken, the collection (e.g. volume of plasma or serum required) and timing of blood samples must be discussed with the pharmacokineticist. It is important to avoid over-zealous sampling, in order to prevent the appearance of anaemia.

Repeated samples over the course of several hours are most conveniently taken using an indwelling venous cannula. In all cases the time the sample is taken (not the time it should have been taken!) should be recorded. Such devices do not impair a subject's mobility and in our experience only rarely produce complications, such as phlebitis. The cannula is kept patent between samples by flushing with heparin saline unless (as in studies on anticoagulants) heparin could interfere with the action of the drug under investigation or interfere with the laboratory test on the blood samples. To avoid contamination, the saline/heparin saline must be removed before any kinetic or other sample is taken. Staff must be obsessional concerning safety with needles and avoidance of contamination. Subjects with blood-borne disorders should generally not be used, unless required for specific Phase I studies, for example, in the case of HIV-positive or hepatitis B-positive patients.

Placebos

In Phase I studies, as in later phase studies, placebo administration acts as a control (Rosenzweig *et al.*, 1995). The need for placebo control is summarised in Table 3. Phase I studies usually involve parallel groups – active and placebo. The allocation of subjects to either group is determined by a formal randomisation procedure. The advantages of such a randomised design include:

● removal of potential conscious or unconscious bias in the allocation of subjects to a control or drug group;
● comparable groups so that variations between individuals will become balanced in both groups: thus, for independent covariates (detected and

Table 3. Need for placebo control.

● 'Background' adverse events and laboratory value variations can be determined by placebo administration.
● Common influences (e.g. lighting, temperature, air conditioning, diet, caffeine and tobacco withdrawal, group 'psychology', staff–subject interaction) may be excluded.
● Common 'placebo' symptoms (e.g. headache, dry throat, bruising at cannula site, drowsiness, lethargy, upper respiratory tract infection) may be evaluated.
● For parenteral studies the placebo should be the 'diluent'.

undetected), the overall difference will tend to be distributed equally in magnitude and direction between the two groups;

- statistical tests can be applied with greater confidence; in fact, if the randomisation is perfect, the validity of the statistical tests is guaranteed although the power is often limited due to the small numbers.

Cross-over designs are less commonly used in Phase I studies, although they are appealing because they are a form of controlled study in which the subjects can act as their own controls. They are randomised studies and the randomisation schedule determines the order in which the test substance and placebo or even different doses of the same treatment are to be taken.

Not only is a cross-over design economical in its use of volunteers from the pool of possible subjects, but individual variation is also reduced since the observed effects of the drug on one person can be considered to be largely due to the intervention alone. Such a reduction in individual variation generally enables smaller sample sizes to be used to detect differences between the drug-treated state and control state. Even the most objective tests (such as automated biochemical and haematological tests) require control groups to obviate the effects of batch-to-batch variations in laboratory conditions. A 'period' effect is a potential disadvantage of the cross-over design. If the 'wash-out' period is inadequate, effects may persist from an earlier dose. Also, if a subject has experienced a profound effect, this may alter his/her response through anticipation to subsequent doses.

Ideally, from a statistical point of view, volunteers should be allocated to placebo and active treatment groups with equal probability, so that eventually the test and control groups are of equal size. In practice, due to financial constraints, it is usual for allocation ratios to be between 1:4 and 2:3 so that more subjects receive the active drug than control. Thus it is possible to give a larger number of different drug doses and to increase the chance of detecting toxicity.

Investigation of efficacy

The main aims of Phase I studies are to determine something of the pharmacological properties and to find the maximum tolerated single or multiple dose of a new drug in man. Phase II studies are concerned with efficacy – in particular, they are used to determine whether the doses found to be well tolerated in Phase I are sufficiently effective to warrant further study. Stated in these terms, it is apparent that the two types of study cannot be combined without producing a protocol of formidable complexity. It is preferable in any type of biological research to carry out several simple experiments rather than one difficult experiment which may not yield clear-cut results. However, in the course of a Phase I study, particularly at steady state, a 'challenge test' or pharmacodynamic assessments may be included which may indicate a pharmacologically active dose, hence providing a proof of concept. Thus, at a certain dose, a hypnosedative will produce feelings of sedation in normal volunteers and may also prolong sleeping time, affect the sleep EEG and perhaps cause a hangover. Impedance cardiography provides a simple non-invasive and inexpensive way of measuring changes in cardiac output (Thomas, 1992). There are also standard methods for evaluating $\beta_1 + \beta_2$ adrenoceptor activity in man (Wheeldon et al., 1992). Analysis of coagulation parameters, e.g. activated partial thromboplastin time, prothrombin time and thrombin time, may indicate the likely effective dose range for anticoagulants. The efficacious dose of a general anaesthetic or neuromuscular blocker can be determined accurately while at the same time subjects are closely monitored for adverse effects in the absence of confounding factors such as surgery. Occasionally, a condition can be mimicked, e.g. ipecacuanha-induced vomiting is a model for $5HT_3$ antagonist anti-emetic efficacy (Minton et al., 1993).

Studies on the behavioural effects of drugs are very sensitive to environmental factors. It is therefore essential that such factors are controlled (Spealman, 1985).

In Phase I studies in patients, a more substantial component of efficacy investigation is built into the protocol. This may involve surrogate markers. For example, patients with mild asthma who are not on concomitant inhaled steroids may be included. If such patients show an early and late response to particular allergens, the effect of the potential anti-asthmatic agent on the response can be investigated (Frew and Holgate, 1995). Hence, if the drug is effective in reducing the response to allergens, it may be implied that it will also be effective in asthma.

ADVERSE EFFECTS

The appearance of a severe adverse event, such as a toxic reaction, is one of the major challenges in the testing of new drugs. If the adverse effect is the result of the drug under investigation, it is important to recognise this to prevent harm from subsequent administration of the agent. On the other hand, it would be a serious error to falsely attribute a harmful effect to a potentially useful drug. For example, a vasovagal episode may produce dramatic symptoms in the subject and long pauses on an ECG trace; drugs may precipitate or exaggerate such episodes. One of the commonest 'toxic' effects causing drugs to be withdrawn from a Phase I programme is an increase in liver transaminases (Rosenzweig et al., 1999). However, before such an increase is attributed to the test drug, other possible causes must be excluded, for example, viral infection, exercise and changes in diet, all of which can act to increase transaminase levels. Initially, interpretation of adverse effects is extremely difficult but in retrospect, with all the data available, it may be obvious. An investigator who is experienced in conducting healthy volunteer studies is invaluable not only in initiating an appropriate immediate response to the adverse effect but also in planning appropriate investigations and, following consultation with the sponsor, any subsequent changes to the protocol that may be required.

In normal circumstances, if any significant reaction occurs during a multiple-dose or continuous infusion study, the subject will usually be withdrawn from further dosing. However, subjective, clinical and laboratory tests should be continued in order to ensure that the subject's condition normalises prior to release from the research unit. Assessment of data and, if necessary, consultations with independent experts should be made in order to decide the possible role of the drug and whether the study should proceed. The identification of causality of adverse reactions is difficult and is often subjective and imprecise, the concordance rate between clinicians being around 50%.

Park *et al.* (1992) classified adverse drug reactions into four types: type A, in which the effects are predictable from the pharmacological actions of the drug; type B, in which reactions are idiosyncratic, in that personal factors are involved and the drug alone is not sufficient to cause the reaction in every individual; type C, in which reactions present as long-term effects, such as analgesic nephropathy; and type D, in which reactions are delayed consequences of drug administration – this category includes carcinogenesis and teratogenesis.

There can sometimes be surprisingly wide differences in the incidence of adverse effects between groups of subjects. We found that in two groups of normal individuals taking identical doses of a new antidepressant, the incidence of sedation was 0/8 and 6/8. Lasagna and von Felsinger (1954) quoted a five-fold increase in the gastrointestinal toxicity of quinacrine in Ohio State medical students as compared with Sing Sing prisoners. It is a sobering thought that in the very first study of iproniazid in tuberculous patients, four patients experienced severe headaches and hypertension. Unfortunately, the significance of this finding was overlooked until this side-effect was rediscovered after millions of patients had been treated with monoamine oxidase inhibitors for depression (Blackwell, 1973).

The type and severity of harmful effects cannot be anticipated with certainty before a Phase I study. Once a serious adverse event has occurred, even if the relationship with the drug is uncertain, it may be considered unethical to proceed with the study: a dilemma such as this is even more difficult. Because of this, it is essential for an immediate, full and rigorous investigation of serious toxicity to be made in this type of study.

In practice, serious toxicity is rare. A far more common problem is the interpretation of clinical measurements or laboratory data that show a deviation from the normal range. To decide whether such a change is due to the drug, statistical analysis of the results in the test and control groups is required but may be impractical due to small numbers. It is important not to be lulled into a false sense of security by the wide 'normal' ranges quoted by many laboratories. Within-subject comparison of data is mandatory: for example, if an individual's plasma creatinine increases from 60 to 120 µmol/l following drug administration, this may reflect a 50% deterioration in renal function, even though both values are within the laboratory's 'normal' range. Difficult decisions will have to be made in the early stages of a study, when only small numbers of subjects have taken the drug. Such problems underline the necessity for continuous examination of all data, and the importance of not proceeding with dose increments until the evidence generated from the previous step has been analysed. As with more obvious toxicity, considerable judgement is required to decide whether it is ethical to proceed; it is essential to err on the side of safety.

Risks

As with the administration of any drug at any phase of its development, there are risks in Phase I studies. Some are associated with procedures (e.g. venepuncture and injection of supposedly sterile materials) and are small; others are associated with the drug under investigation and are unquantifiable. Overall, the safety record of Phase I studies is impressive. Zarafonetis *et al.* (1978) reported on Phase I studies carried out on prisoners in the State of Michigan: 805 studies were conducted over the course of 12 years, involving 19 162 volunteers and occupying 614 534 subject-investigation days. During these studies, 64 significant medical events were encountered, of which 58 were thought to be adverse drug reactions and six were complications of the procedures carried out. Complete recovery occurred in all but two subjects. One (on placebo) suffered a myocardial infarction and one was left with a stiff hip following a septic complication of an injection. One way of expressing the risks from these data is to anticipate one significant adverse reaction every 26.3 years of individual subject participation in Phase I studies.

In the British Isles, two deaths were reported in 1985 in association with healthy volunteer drug studies but there have been none since. The first death involved a volunteer who had failed to disclose at screening that he had been diagnosed with schizophrenia and was taking a concomitant antipsychotic drug. He died almost immediately after intravenous administration of an antiarrhythmic agent. The second case involved a volunteer who developed aplastic anaemia after receiving three doses of midazolam (oral, rectal and intravenous). Based on worldwide experience with midazolam, it is most unlikely that this event was drug-related, although it can never be proved for certain. Unfortunately, the overall incidence of SAEs in healthy volunteer pharmacology studies is unknown since there is no mandatory database.

Sibille *et al.* (1998) reported their experience of adverse events in Phase I studies involving 1015 volunteers over 10 years. They concluded that adverse events in Phase I studies are very common, usually of minor intensity and rarely severe, even though exceptional life-threatening adverse events are possible. A survey conducted among members of the clinical section of the British Pharmacological Society to find out about the administration of drugs to healthy volunteers over the period October 1986–October 1987 obtained data in over 8 000 subject exposures to drugs. The authors concluded that the survey suggested the risk involved in these studies is very small, with only four moderately severe and three severe adverse reactions. The severe adverse reactions included a severe skin irritation and rash, anaphylactic shock after an oral vaccine, and perforation of a peptic ulcer after the administration of multiple doses in a non-steroidal anti-inflammatory drug (NSAID) study. All subjects made a full recovery, although the last-mentioned required surgery (Orme *et al.*, 1989).

In our own unit, which at present exposes over 1000 volunteers to experimental drugs each year, the most life-threatening adverse events in healthy volunteer studies have been:

1. Collapse, asystolic episodes and severe bradycardia following administration of an intravenous antipsychotic drug. The subject made a full recovery following external cardiac massage and intravenous atropine.
2. Anaphylactoid reaction following ingestion of an oral antibacterial drug. The subject made a full recovery following administration of adrenaline, hydrocortisone, chlorpheniramine and plasma expanders. There was no history of previous exposure to this class of drug.

Both cases illustrate the necessity of having trained medical staff and immediate availability of emergency drugs and equipment.

Although not concerned solely with Phase I studies, a telephone survey of 331 investigators conducted by the US Department of Health, Education and Welfare concluded that the risks of participation to volunteers in non-therapeutic research 'may be no greater than those of everyday life' (Cardon *et al.*, 1976). The dangers of testing new drugs must not be underestimated. Previous studies have usually gone well. Carelessness in any single facet of the study is an invitation to disaster; Dengler (1973) pointed out that using staff without specialised training leads to underestimation of the responsibility associated with Phase I work and is a potential danger to the volunteers.

Phase I units that belong to the AICRC have compulsory SAE reporting to an AICRC central database. Anaphylactoid reactions, skin reactions (in particular to photosensitising agents) and reactions to CNS compounds have caused particular concern. While indicating that the risk to an individual subject is low, the data available highlight how essential it is to have a careful study design together with well-trained, experienced and skilled staff working in good facilities. A compulsory national database with due regard to confidentiality is highly desirable, particularly with the wealth of novel, potent pharmacological agents currently being developed. If published or made available via the Internet, such a database may help to avert catastrophe.

If the investigator, pharmaceutical company or ethics committee considers that the risk of any healthy volunteer study is greater than minimal (i.e. greater than that of flying on a civil airline), the study must not proceed. Although it is anticipated that EU legislation will further protect the volunteer, the ultimate responsibility for safety will always lie with the clinical investigator.

Pharmacokinetics

INTRODUCTION

Pharmacokinetics is the study of the time course of drug absorption, distribution, metabolism and excretion. For most drugs the magnitude of pharmacological effect depends on the concentration of unbound drug or active metabolite at the site of action. An understanding of basic pharmacokinetic principles, coupled with knowledge of a drug's pharmacokinetic profile, is not only valuable in the rational planning of dose, dose frequency and route of administration, but also in explaining interindividual variability of drug response. For example, where there is little correlation between plasma drug (or metabolite) concentration and effect (as with corticosteroids, for example), detailed pharmacokinetic data are rarely beneficial. In contrast, if there is a close correlation between the two and the drug has a narrow therapeutic range (as with phenytoin, for example), an understanding of the drug's pharmacokinetics is critical in planning appropriate dosing regimens to maximise efficacy while minimising toxicity.

The objective of this section is to describe the derivation of the most important equations and to define the terms frequently used in pharmacokinetic reports. The starting point of pharmacokinetics is the plasma concentration–time curve, and no apology is made for using this to illustrate the principles involved. There is no substitute for practical experience, but it is hoped that this section will allow all those involved in clinical research to apply pharmacokinetic parameters and interpretations to their research programme. This exposition is necessarily concise, but some recommended textbooks are listed after the references at the end of this chapter.

The human body is a complicated combination of interacting systems. Drug absorption, distribution, metabolism and excretion occur simultaneously, and hence formulae to describe these processes are based on simplified assumptions in order to allow the mathematics to be intelligible to ordinary mortals. Fortunately, most physicians and scientists involved in pharmaceutical research and development (R&D) need to understand only the basic principles of practical pharmacokinetics in order to interpret the clinical implications of the pharmacokinetic data provided.

COMPARTMENTAL CONCEPT

Although the body is composed of a large number of 'compartments', it is possible to lump together organs and tissues into larger compartments that have no anatomical or physiological counterpart. The simplest pharmaco-kinetic model considers the body as a single well-stirred compartment, within which an administered drug distributes instantaneously and uniformly and from which it is subsequently eliminated (see Figure 1).

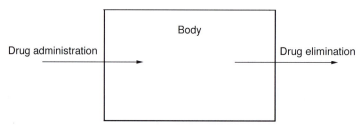

Figure 1. One-compartment model.

Many drugs are eliminated at a rate proportional to their concentration; such processes are described as 'first order'.

The volume of the compartment and the amount of drug administered determine the concentration of drug in the compartment. If the single compartment is the plasma, this provides the convenient proportionality constant known as the *apparent volume of distribution* (V_d) and defined by the equation:

$$V_d = \frac{A}{C} \tag{1}$$

where

    A = amount of drug in the body
    C = plasma drug concentration

The volume of distribution is most conveniently measured following an intra-venous bolus dose and extrapolating from the log–linear plot of a concentra-tion–time curve to estimate C_0 (see Figure 2). C_0 is the plasma drug concentration immediately after dose administration is complete and before drug elimination starts. At this time the amount of drug in the body is the total dose administered.

If a drug is confined to the plasma in a 70 kg man, its volume of distribu-tion would be 3 litres/70 kg body weight. However, drug distribution generally involves a variety of fluids and tissues. Tissue binding in particular may result in a volume of distribution many times the volume of the body; for example,

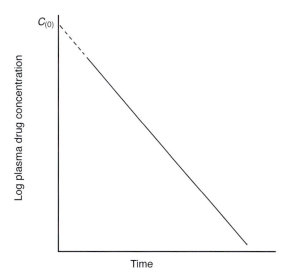

Figure 2. Hypothetical plot of a plasma concentration decline for a one-compartment model.

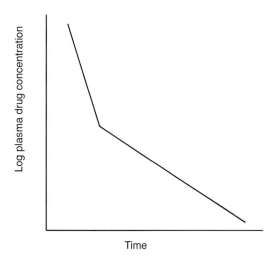

Figure 3. Hypothetical plot of a biphasic plasma concentration decline for a two-compartment model.

the volume of distribution of amitriptyline, which is highly lipid-soluble, exceeds 250 litres.

Examples of the value of this concept are the calculation of drug clearance (see below) and estimation of the dose required (the 'loading dose') to provide a desired plasma concentration:

$$\text{Loading dose} = \text{desired plasma concentration} \times V_d \tag{2}$$

A one-compartment model, although useful in explaining the concept of volume of distribution, rarely reflects reality. More commonly there is a biphasic fall in log plasma drug concentration following an intravenous bolus dose (Figure 3), which is more adequately explained by a two-compartment model (see Figure 4). This model involves a central compartment (V_1) and a more slowly equilibrating deep or peripheral compartment (V_2). The movement of drug between compartments is governed by first-order processes characterised by microconstants $k_{1.2}$ and $k_{2.1}$.

The initial rapid decline in plasma drug concentration is primarily due to drug distribution (α phase). During drug elimination (β phase) the drug concentrations in the central and peripheral compartments decline in parallel, as shown in Figure 5 (i.e. kinetic homogeneity is attained). The *half-life* ($t^{1/2}$)

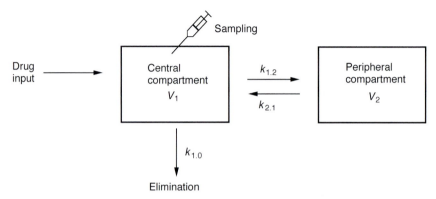

Figure 4. Movement between compartments is by first-order processes characterised by microconstants $k_{1.2}$, $k_{2.1}$.

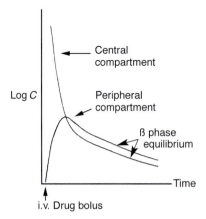

Figure 5. Changes in drug concentrations in central and peripheral compartments after an intravenous bolus injection.

for both the distribution (α) phase and the elimination (β) phase can be calculated from the log concentration–time plot but it is the elimination half-life ($t^1/_{2\beta}$) which is most useful and most commonly quoted.

The availability of computers and sophisticated pharmacokinetic programs has dramatically increased the scope of pharmacokinetics and reduced the mathematical labour. Once the pharmacokinetic data have been entered, parameters such as T_{max}, C_{max}, $t^1/_2$ and the area under the curve (AUC) can be rapidly computed, with individuals and dose levels compared. Some programs are even able to determine what model (e.g. two- or three-compartment) best fits the plasma concentration–time data.

CONSTANT RATE INFUSION

When a continuous intravenous infusion is administered at a fixed rate via a pump, and serial blood samples are taken from the contralateral arm during and after the infusion, a plasma concentration–time curve can be constructed (Figure 6). The plasma concentration rises to a plateau when the rate of drug input equals the rate of drug elimination. This is the *steady state plasma concentration* (C_{ss}). C_{ss} is dependent on the infusion rate and the clearance of drug from the body. *The clearance is the volume of plasma that is completely cleared of drug per unit time.*

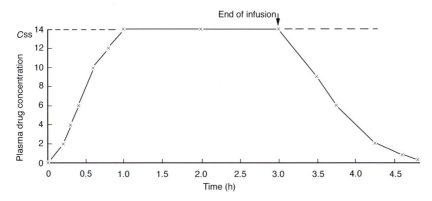

Figure 6. Constant rate infusion.

When the infusion is stopped, the plasma concentration declines, as shown in Figure 7, which represents a one-compartment model with first-order elimination showing an exponential decline. The time taken for the plasma concentration to halve is the *elimination half-life* ($t^1/_2$). After a second half-life has elapsed, the plasma concentration will be one quarter of C_{ss} and so on. The

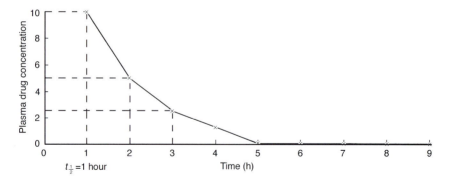

Figure 7. First-order decline in plasma concentration on stopping an intravenous infusion.

increase in plasma concentration after the start of the infusion is also exponential until C_{ss} is reached and is the inverse of the decay curve. Consequently, the half-life is used in practice to predict not only a drug's rate of elimination but also its rate of accumulation.

It is important to note that a drug exhibiting first-order kinetics has a single value for elimination half-life independent of the rate and route of administration, dose given and C_{ss}.

The elimination half-life helps to determine an optimal dose interval, whether the drug is given by intermittent injection or by multiple oral doses, since it indicates the time over which drug accumulates until C_{ss} occurs, after the start of a regular treatment regimen. This is approximately five times the elimination half-life. If a drug has a long $t^{1/2}$ (e.g. amiodarone has a $t^{1/2}$ of 20–100 days) and plasma concentration correlates with effect, a loading dose is necessary to reach C_{ss} more rapidly in order to produce the required clinical effect. Clearance and not $t^{1/2}$ must be used as a measure of the efficiency of drug elimination since $t^{1/2}$ is also dependent on volume of distribution.

ADMINISTRATION

Intravenous bolus dose

Following a single bolus injection of drug over 5–30 seconds into a vein, the decline in plasma concentration of drug plotted against time appears as shown in Figure 8 if the drug obeys first-order kinetics. The plasma drug concentration decreases most rapidly immediately after the injection as the drug undergoes distribution followed by elimination/metabolism. During the initial phase, distribution is normally the dominant cause of the decrease in plasma concentration. If the plasma concentrations are plotted on a logarithmic scale (Figure 9), the separation between a distribution (α)

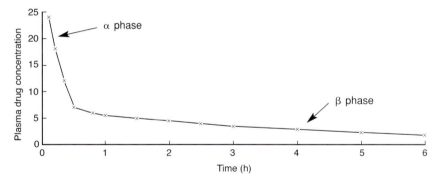

Figure 8. Plasma concentration of drug plotted against time following an intravenous injection.

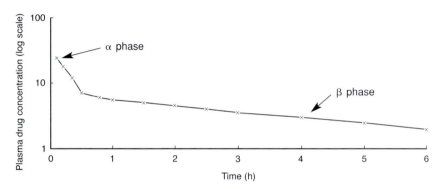

Figure 9. Plasma concentration of drug plotted against time on a logarithmic scale following an intravenous injection.

phase and elimination/metabolism (β) phase is more delineated. If the drug undergoes first-order elimination, as most do, then the β phase is a straight line on the semi-logarithmic plot as shown in Figure 9, above.

The equation describing the β phase line is:

$$C_t = C_0 e^{-Kt} \qquad (3)$$

where

C_t = plasma drug concentration at time t
C_0 = plasma drug concentration at time zero from extrapolation of the β phase line to the y axis
e = base for natural logarithms
K = first-order rate constant for the elimination (metabolism plus excretion) phase (in other tests this is often written as K_E)
t = time

By taking the natural logarithm (base e) of equation 3:

$$\log_e C_t = \log_e C_0 \ (- Kt) \tag{4}$$

As for any number x, $2.303 \log_{10} x = \log x$. Therefore, if equation 4 is converted from natural ($\log_e$) to common ($\log_{10}$) logarithms:

$$\log_{10} C_t = \frac{\log C_0 \ (-Kt)}{2.303} \tag{5}$$

The mathematical description of the β phase line from equation 4 is a straight line of slope $-K/2.303$.

K and C_0 can be obtained from the plot. This equation indicates that for a given time interval, the fractional change in concentration is fixed whatever time the interval starts and whatever the plasma concentration. This confirms the statement that for a drug which exhibits first-order (linear) kinetics, the elimination half-life is constant. Knowledge of $t^{1/2}$ or K allows calculation of the other as:

$$t^{1/2} = \frac{\log_e 2}{K} = \frac{0.693}{K} \tag{6}$$

($\log_e 2 = 0.693$)

Clearance is a more suitable measure of drug elimination than the elimination half-life or K, as it incorporates the volume of drug distribution. It is possible to calculate the total body clearance or individual routes of clearance, such as hepatic metabolism and renal excretion. Clearance, $t^{1/2}$ and V_d are mathematically interrelated:

$$t^{1/2} = \frac{\log_e 2}{K} = \frac{0.693}{K} \tag{7}$$

Clearance $= K \times V_d$

Substituting $0.693/t^{1/2}$ for K:

$$t^{1/2} = \frac{V_d \times 0.693}{\text{Clearance}} \tag{8}$$

Single oral dose

Most drugs are given via the oral route, a fact which complicates pharmacokinetics because the rate of absorption and bioavailability must also be considered.

In Figure 10, plasma drug concentration versus time has been plotted following a single oral dose: it only differs from that of an intravenous dose

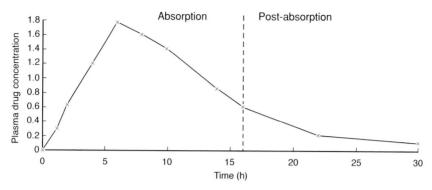

Figure 10. Drug concentration versus time plotted following a single oral dose.

during the drug absorption phase. Most oral tablets and capsules dissolve in the stomach and are absorbed by passive diffusion in the small intestine, which has a vast surface area available for drug absorption. Consequently, the rate of oral drug absorption is often related to gastric emptying; indeed, intestinal disease must be very severe before it affects drug absorption, since an immense 'reserve' surface area is available.

As the plasma drug concentration increases due to absorption, the rate of elimination also increases because both are usually first-order processes. At the time of peak plasma drug concentration (T_{max}), the rate of drug absorption = rate of drug elimination. The higher the dose administered, the higher the peak plasma concentration (C_{max}).

For a one-compartment model with a first-order absorption process with absorption rate constant K_A (analogous to first-order elimination rate constant K_E), the plasma concentration at any time, C_t, is given by:

$$C_t = \frac{K_A\, F A_0}{V_d\, (K_A - K_E)}\ (e^{-Kt} - e^{K_A t}) \tag{9}$$

where

F = bioavailability fraction
A_0 = the amount of drug administered
V_d = the apparent volume of distribution

NB: It is difficult (but fortunately rarely necessary) to determine K_A.

V_d cannot be determined by back extrapolation to time zero following an oral dose (cf. an intravenous bolus when $V_d = A_0/C_0$).

The $t^{1/2}$ corresponding to K_E can be obtained from the post-absorptive phase by plotting the log of plasma drug concentration against time and calculating the slope of the line.

Equation 9 introduces F, the bioavailability fraction. *Bioavailability is the amount of drug which reaches the systemic circulation.* When administered by mouth, some drugs undergo substantial pre-systemic metabolism in the gut and/or liver, and hence only a small percentage of the dose taken may reach the systemic circulation. Oral bioavailability should be calculated, if possible, with reference to plasma concentrations resulting from intravenous administration which gives a bioavailability of 100% (when the drug is injected directly into the systemic circulation). The area under the plasma concentration–time curve (AUC), calculated using the linear trapezoidal rule, represents the amount of drug in the systemic circulation and is used to estimate the bioavailability fraction *F*.

$$F = \frac{AUC_{oral}}{AUC_{i.v.}} \hspace{4cm} (10)$$

Low bioavailability may be due to incomplete absorption and/or gastro-intestinal/hepatic metabolism (the first-pass effect).

Multiple dosing

Most drugs are taken as multiple oral doses. If the total daily dose remains the same, mean C_{ss} will not be affected whether the drug is given once or four times daily, although this will affect the peak and trough plasma concentrations. If there is a close correlation between plasma concentration and effect, as with theophylline, excessively high peaks cause toxicity, and excessively low troughs cause loss of efficacy. Hence, oral theophylline is usually administered as a slow-release preparation; this has the convenience of twice-daily administration without the marked fluctuations in plasma concentrations that would result from twice daily administration of the same dose of a standard-release preparation. Sometimes it is not necessary to achieve a continuous finite plasma concentration, for example, as with the use of oral penicillin V in the management of bacterial tonsillitis.

For a drug with an elimination half-life of approximately 24 h and whose efficacy correlates with plasma concentration, a once-daily regimen would be suitable. Predictably, it would take approximately $5 \times t^{1}/_{2}$, i.e. 120 h, to reach the steady state (C_{ss}) plateau concentration. If it is clinically necessary to reach this plateau more rapidly, then as discussed previously, a loading dose will be required. Figure 11 shows plasma concentration–time curves for a drug with a $t^{1}/_{2}$ of 3 h given once daily (Figure 11(a)), and for a drug with a $t^{1}/_{2}$ of 24 h given once daily (Figure 11(b)) without a loading dose and (Figure 11(c)) with a loading dose.

If it is necessary to double the plateau concentration of Figure 11(b) to achieve a clinical effect, for example, for an antibacterial to eliminate an organism, this may be done by doubling the daily dose, either by giving that dose twice daily or by giving double the dose once daily, bearing in mind that

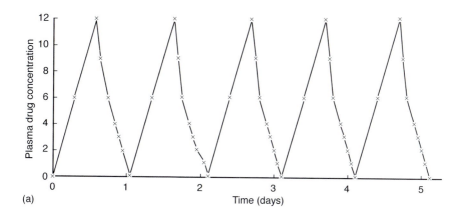

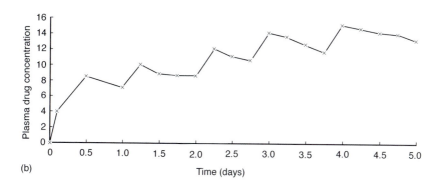

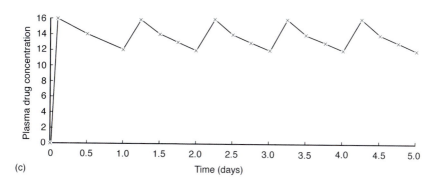

Figure 11. Plasma concentration–time curves for (a) a drug with $t\frac{1}{2}$ of 3 h given once daily, (b) a drug with a $t\frac{1}{2}$ of 24 h given once daily without a loading dose, and (c) a drug with a $t\frac{1}{2}$ of 24 h given once daily with a loading dose.

the latter option will result in a higher peak and lower trough concentrations than the former option.

Enterohepatic circulation

A confounding factor in the interpretation of pharmacokinetic data is entero-hepatic circulation: this occurs when a drug is eliminated in the bile and reabsorbed in the small intestine. If significant, this phenomenon can usually be identified as a second 'peak' in the plasma concentration–time profile following an intravenous bolus.

Effect of food

Food may alter oral bioavailability, C_{max}, T_{max} or have no effect. Most pharmacokinetic studies are performed on fasting healthy volunteers; however, patients cannot be asked to continually abstain from eating simply to take medications. Hence, it is essential to perform a study (usually a two-way, cross-over design) to examine the effect of food on the pharmacokinet-ics of an oral drug.

LINEAR AND NON-LINEAR PHARMACOKINETICS

In reviewing pharmacokinetic data from early drug studies in man, it is essen-tial to confirm whether or not a drug displays linearity as soon as possible, as this will have significant implications for the drug's management.

Linear pharmacokinetics

Most drugs are subject to first-order (linear) pharmacokinetics (i.e. the rate of drug elimination is directly proportional to the drug concentration). The consequences of linear kinetics are as follows:

1. The elimination $t^{1/2}$ is constant and independent of dose.
2. AUC is proportional to dose.
3. Composition of drug product(s) excreted is independent of dose.
4. Amount of drug excreted in urine is proportional to dose.
5. C_{ss} is proportional to dose and the elimination half-life.

Non-linear pharmacokinetics

The pharmacokinetic behaviour (absorption, distribution, metabolism and elimination) of some drugs is rate-limited. These processes can often be described by the Michaelis–Menten equation:

$$\frac{-dc}{dt} = \frac{V_m C}{K_m + C} \tag{11}$$

where

$\dfrac{-dc}{dt}$ = change in plasma concentration with time

V_m = theoretical maximum rate

K_m = the drug concentration at which the rate of the process is proceeding at half the maximum rate

C = the drug concentration

Figure 12 compares the log plasma concentration–time curves for drugs exhibiting linear and non-linear elimination kinetics during the post-absorption phase. Figure 13 illustrates the relationship of daily dose to C_{ss} for a drug exhibiting linear kinetics (e.g. diazepam) in comparison with a drug exhibiting saturation non-linear kinetics (e.g. phenytoin).

Non-linear kinetics are a disadvantage because the drug's kinetic behaviour is more prone to variation in a number of situations. The $t^{1/2}\beta$ is dependent

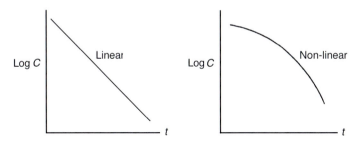

Figure 12. Linear and non-linear patterns of elimination curves (log drug concentration plotted against time).

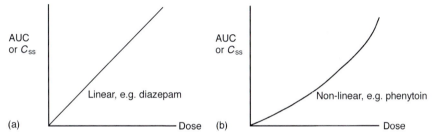

Figure 13. Effect of dose on area under concentration–time curve and on steady-state concentration: (a) linear and (b) non-linear kinetics.

on dose, and once the metabolism/excretion process is saturated, small incre-ments in dose may lead to disproportionately large increases in plasma concentration and subsequent toxicity. The dose/plasma concentration at which saturation occurs is often highly variable between individuals. Consequently, it is extremely difficult to predict the dose required to achieve a certain plasma concentration. In addition, there is unpredictable and delayed attainment of C_{ss}, and increased liability to competitive pharmacokinetic drug interactions. Minor changes in formulation are therefore more likely to lead to clinical (i.e. significant) bio-inequivalence.

In overdose, a number of drugs (e.g. paracetamol) saturate their normal metabolic pathways. At normal doses, phenytoin, alcohol and heparin are examples of drugs that exhibit non-linear kinetics.

Protein binding

Drugs bind to plasma and tissue proteins to a variable degree (for example, warfarin is 97% bound, whereas heparin is only <1% bound to plasma albumin). It is important to remember that only unbound 'free' drug is active and available for tissue penetration, metabolism and elimination. This is depicted in Figure 14.

Most drug assays measure total plasma drug concentration (bound and

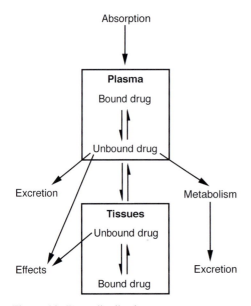

Figure 14. Drug distribution.

unbound drug) and are usually adequate. In certain circumstances (e.g. pregnancy, nephrotic syndrome and cirrhosis), protein-binding changes may alter the ratio of bound and unbound drug, and hence the drug's pharmacokinetics and pharmacodynamics, with potentially significant implications for drugs that are highly protein-bound.

POPULATION PHARMACOKINETICS

Since the initial studies of drugs in man usually involve limited numbers of healthy male subjects, the pharmacokinetic parameters of many drugs are calculated from a very homogeneous population. Although these data are often convenient to handle and of undoubted value, factors such as age, sex, race, genetic variations, body weight/surface area, renal function, disease and drug interactions may all influence a drug's pharmacokinetics. Patients tend not to be healthy young men within 10% of ideal body weight, and therefore to extrapolate pharmacokinetic data from these initial studies to a heterogeneous, general patient population can be misleading. One can design a study to investigate a single factor, such as renal function, by comparing a group of normal healthy subjects with a sex-matched group of patients with renal impairment. This type of study can determine the correlation, if any, of drug clearance with glomerular filtration rate and an appropriate dose adjustment if, for example, the drug is required for patients with impaired renal function. These studies are normally performed in hospital and often require a sequence of six to 12 blood samples from each patient. To examine a more varied population, a much more limited number of blood samples is obtained from a large group of patients taking the drug in Phase II or Phase III studies. The blood concentrations, time from dosing and all other factors are entered into a statistical program such as NONMEM that allows basic pharmacokinetic and random effect parameters to be estimated and thus elucidates some of the causes of population variation. This type of study allows the examination of many different factors in a large number of patients relatively inexpensively but has the disadvantage of confounding variables.

Adverse drug interactions

INTRODUCTION

The importance of rationally designed studies to investigate potential interactions in a drug development programme and the value of conducting *in-vivo* studies at an early phase are indicated in the Committee for Proprietary Medicinal Products (CPMP) 1997 publication *Note for Guidance on the Investigation of Drug Interactions*. In that document an interaction is defined as 'an alteration either in the pharmacodynamics and/or the pharmacokinet-

Table 4. Examples of serious drug interactions.

Drugs	Mechanism	Possible effect
Oral contraceptive and carbamazepine	Hepatic enzyme induction	Reduced contraceptive effects
Terfenadine and ketoconazole	Hepatic enzyme inhibition	Prolonged QT interval $\rightarrow$ cardiac arrhythmias
Cheese and phenelzine	Monoamine oxidase inhibition	Hypertensive crisis
ACE inhibitors and potassium-sparing diuretics	Hyperkalaemia	Cardiac arrhythmias
Lithium and thiazides	Reduced renal clearance of lithium	Convulsions

ics of a drug, caused by concomitant drug treatment, dietary factors or social habits such as tobacco or alcohol'.

BACKGROUND

Multiple drug use ('polypharmacy') is common and the potential for interactions almost infinite. While drugs are commonly prescribed concomitantly to increase efficacy (e.g. thiazides and beta-blockers to treat hypertension) or to reduce toxicity (e.g. a $5HT_3$ antagonist with cisplatin, the former reducing the emesis associated with cisplatin anticancer treatment), drug interactions may cause adverse effects (see Table 4).

One drug may reduce the beneficial effect of another drug; for example, NSAIDs will inhibit the diuretic effect of thiazides. Many interactions involving drugs with wide therapeutic margins are harmless. However, while some drugs are considered to be very safe when prescribed individually, their prescription in combination may have fatal consequences, as illustrated by the example of ventricular arrhythmias associated with concomitant administration of terfenadine (an antihistamine) and erythromycin (a macrolide antibiotic). Drugs with a narrow therapeutic index (e.g. anticoagulants) are of particular concern.

MECHANISMS

Adverse drug interactions may result from three mechanisms: pharmaceutical, pharmacodynamic and pharmacokinetic.

Pharmaceutical interactions

These may occur when two drugs (usually parenteral) are mixed or a drug is added to an infusion fluid. This may result in precipitation (e.g. thiopentone and suxamethonium, phenytoin and 5% dextrose) or inactivation (e.g. penicillin inactivated by hydrocortisone). In general, drugs should not be added to blood transfusions or blood products. Some drugs may also interact in the gut lumen, e.g. tetracycline with iron. Most of these interactions can be predicted from the physicochemical properties of the drugs and can be investigated *in vitro/ex vivo*.

Pharmacodynamic interactions

These are the most frequent interactions and usually result from the summation of effects of two drugs with similar pharmacodynamic actions or from the reduction of effect when two drugs have opposite pharmacodynamic actions. Pharmacodynamic interactions may often be predicted from the preclinical pharmacology and toxicology. Interactions may result from drugs acting at a common receptor, or from receptors and enzyme-controlled uptake processes causing a similar effect. One example of this type is hypnosedative drugs and ethanol, both of which will have a depressant effect on the central nervous system. Another example is aspirin and anticoagulants; not only may both drugs interfere with haemostasis by different mechanisms and increase the risk of bleeding, but aspirin may also precipitate gastric bleeding by inhibition of the biosynthesis of prostaglandin E_2 and direct gastric mucosal irritation.

Interactions may also result from indirect effects that alter physiological mechanisms and control loops. Hence, if a beta-blocker is prescribed for an insulin-dependent diabetic patient, there is a significant risk that in the event of hypoglycaemia, the symptoms (which are caused by adrenergic pathways) will be masked through beta-adrenergic blockade. Likewise, the rate of recovery from hypoglycaemia may be slowed because β_2 adrenoreceptors are also responsible for adrenaline-stimulated gluconeogenesis.

Pharmacokinetic interactions

Alterations in pharmacokinetics are of particular importance for those drugs with a narrow therapeutic index. Drug absorption, distribution due to changes in protein binding, metabolism and renal excretion must all be considered when determining which pharmacokinetic interactions are predictable and when investigating changes in blood concentration profiles in patients on concomitant therapy.

Absorption

Drugs which increase or inhibit the rate of gastric emptying are likely to affect

the rate rather than the completeness of absorption of most orally administered drugs. Intestinal P-glycoprotein, which acts as a transmembrane pump,
is potentially an important site for drug interactions; for example, digoxin
bioavailability is increased by concomitant administration of oral but not
intravenous talinolol (Westphal *et al.*, 2000). Some drugs may interfere with
enterohepatic circulation. It is postulated that this may be the cause of
occasional contraceptive failure in women simultaneously using oral contraceptives and some broad-spectrum antibiotics.

Distribution

Protein and tissue binding interactions, e.g. competition for albumin-binding
sites, are quite common *in vitro* but only rarely cause clinically relevant effects
in vivo because displacement of drug from binding sites results in increased
metabolism/elimination, leaving the concentration of unbound, free (i.e.
active) drug relatively constant. Some drugs may block specific transport
systems and prevent certain drugs from reaching their site of action; for
example, tricyclic antidepressants block uptake of adrenergic neurone-block-
ing drugs into presynaptic sympathetic nerve terminals, and hence a hypoten-
sive effect fails to materialise. The P-glycoprotein pump is responsible for
limiting the entry of some drugs into the CNS. Loperamide is an opioid used
to treat diarrhoea and rarely causes CNS effects. However, co-administration
with quinidine, a known inhibitor of P-glycoprotein, is associated with respiratory depression independent of changes in plasma concentration, indicating
increased CNS penetration (Sadeque *et al.*, 2000).

Metabolism

Altered drug metabolism is an important cause of adverse drug reactions.
Although drug-metabolising enzymes are present in many organs (e.g. gut
wall, lung and kidney), the liver is the major organ of drug metabolism. The
cytochrome P-450 (CYP450) enzyme system, which consists of many isoenzymes with a unique but sometimes overlapping range of drug substrates, is
the most important of the drug-metabolising enzyme systems responsible for
oxidation (Anon, 2000). Genetic polymorphisms exist for some of these isoenzymes and there are recognised and proven inhibitors and inducers for most
of them. For those isoenzymes such as CYP_{2D6}, which are genetically polymor-
phic, two phenotypically distinct populations can be identified (poor and
extensive metabolisers). Extensive metabolisers (over 90% of Caucasians) are
particularly susceptible to inhibitory drug interactions. Of the CYP450 isoenzymes, CYP_{3A4} is the most abundant and more than half of all drugs are
completely or partially metabolised by the enzyme (Anonymous, 1999). The
CYP450 system can also be affected by diet; for example, grapefruit juice
inhibits CYP_{3A4} (probably in the gut wall), and smoking induces CYP_{1A2} which

metabolises theophylline. The herbal remedy St John's Wort is a particularly broad-spectrum CYP450 enzyme inducer and its use has been implicated in the therapeutic failure of some anti-HIV regimens due to enhanced CYP450 drug metabolism and resultant low protease inhibitor plasma concentrations.

Excretion

Some drugs compete for transport mechanisms in the proximal tubules of the kidney. Competition for anion and cation transport and the effects of altering urine pH on excretion of weak acids and bases may be predictable and can be tested preclinically. If a clinically relevant interaction is possible, an *in-vivo* study should be performed in humans. Methotrexate excretion is inhibited by aspirin and NSAIDs and this may lead to bone marrow suppression. Digoxin levels are increased by concomitant amiodarone through a similar renal tubular mechanism.

EARLY PHASE DRUG INTERACTION STUDIES

Many pharmacokinetic and some pharmacodynamic interaction studies may be conducted in healthy subjects. While each new drug should be taken on a case-by-case basis, some pertinent principles for the selection of studies and design have been outlined (Posner and Rolan, 1998). In addition to preclinical review of the pharmacokinetic data to determine potential mechanisms and sites of interaction (e.g. P-glycoproteins, renal tubules and CYP450), the safety pharmacology studies, therapeutic index and the proposed indication and target population must be considered when determining potential clinically relevant interactions. It is often essential to conduct such studies before Phase II if the target population is likely to be receiving concomitant medication.

Most of these studies will be cross-over, with each subject acting as his/her own control. It is important to control potential confounding factors, such as diet, smoking, time of dosing, and posture. In view of the ubiquitous nature of the CYP450 enzyme system in drug metabolism, if there is evidence that the test drug may affect CYP450 activity, a common design is to give a 'cocktail' of CYP450 probe drugs while at steady state on the test compound. It may also be helpful to genotype the subjects, wherever possible, for CYP450 polymorphism at the time of the *in-vivo* interaction studies. For example, if the substrate is metabolised by CYP_{2D6} and if the investigation concerns a potential CYP_{2D6} inhibitor, then 'poor' metabolisers may show no interaction while 'extensive' metabolisers may be turned into 'poor' metabolisers by the enzyme inhibitor.

ADVERSE DRUG INTERACTIONS: CONCLUDING REMARKS

Adverse drug interactions are of increasing concern and must be taken into account in all drug development programmes. With improved understanding of the mechanism of many drug interactions and appropriate preclinical and early phase human interaction studies, many adverse drug interactions can be predicted and hence avoided by appropriate warnings to prescribers. However, the authors have no doubt that unexpected hazardous drug interactions will continue after a drug is licensed and they encourage doctors and pharmacists to report all suspected adverse drug interactions to the CSM. The CPMP's *Note for Guidance on the Investigation of Drug Interactions* is essential reading for those involved in drug development (Committee for Proprietary Medicinal Products, 1997).

REFERENCES

Adamson, H, Jacobs, A and Warrington, S (1998). Normal values for electrocardiogram intervals in young healthy subjects. *Int J Pharm Med* **12**, 289–291.

Anonymous (1999). The cytochrome P450 system and adverse drug reactions. *Adv Drug React Bull* 194.

Anonymous (2000). Why bother about cytochrome P450 enzymes? *Drug Ther Bull* **38**(12), 93–95.

Ayd, F (1972). Motivations and rewards for volunteering to be an experimental subject. *Clin Pharmacol Ther* **13**, 771–778.

Blackwell, B (1973). For the first time in man. *Clin Pharmacol Ther* **13**, 812–823.

Cardon, PV, Dommel, FW and Trumble RR (1976). Injuries to research subjects – a survey of investigators. *N Engl J Med* **295**, 650–654.

Cassileth, BR, Zupkis, RV, Sutton-Smith, K and March, V (1980). Informed consent – why are its goals imperfectly realised? *N Engl J Med* **302**, 896–900.

Committee for Proprietary Medicinal Products (1997). *Note for Guidance on the Investigation of Drug Interactions* (Issued as CPMP/EWP/560/95, effective June 1998).

Cudrin, JM (1969). Intelligence of volunteers as research subjects. *J Consult Clin Psychol* **33**, 501–503.

Dengler, HJ (1973). Early human trials: selection of investigators and subjects. In: *Clinical Pharmacological Evaluation in Drug Control*, WHO Regional Office for Europe, Geneva, pp. 41–42.

Dollery, CT and Davies, DS (1970). The conduct of initial drug studies in man. *Br Med Bull* **26**, 233–236.

Editorial (1984). How not to test drugs. *Nature* **307**, 490.

Eisenhauer, EA, O'Dwyer, PJ, Christian, M and Humphrey, JS (2000). Phase I clinical trial design in cancer drug development. *J Clin Oncol* **18**, 684–692.

Food and Drug Administration (1977). *General Considerations for the Clinical Evaluation of Drugs*. Document 77–3040 HEW, Washington, DC.

Frew, A and Holgate, ST (1995). Are bronchial challenge studies indicators of anti-asthmatic activity? In: Nimmo, WS and Tucker, GT (Eds), *Clinical Measurement in Drug Evaluation*, John Wiley, Chichester.

Froom, P, Ribak, H and Benbassat, J (1984). Significance of microhaematuria in young adults. *Br Med J* **288**, 20–22.

Hassar, M, Pocelinko, R, Weintraub, M *et al.* (1977). Free-living volunteer's motivations and attitudes towards pharmacologic studies in man. *Clin Pharmacol Ther* **21**, 515–519.

Huston, TP, Puffer, JC and Rodney, WM (1985). The athletic heart syndrome. *N Engl J Med* **313**, 24–32.

ICH Guideline (1994). *Topic E4: Dose–Response Information to Support Drug Registration*, International Federation of Pharmaceutical Manufacturers Associations, Geneva (Issued as CPMP/ICH/378/95).

ICH Guideline (1996). *Topic E6: Good Clinical Practice – Consolidated Guideline*, International Federation of Pharmaceutical Manufacturers Associations, Geneva. (Issued as CPMP/ICH/135/95).

Jagathesan, R, Lewis, LD and Mant TG (1995). A retrospective analysis of the prevalence of HIV seropositivity and its demographics in the normal healthy volunteer population of a Phase I clinical drug study unit (letter). *Br J Clin Pharmacol* **39**, 463–464.

James, IM (1976). Phase I trials. In: Good, CS (Ed), *Principles and Practice of Clinical Trials*, Churchill Livingstone, Edinburgh, pp. 17–22.

Joubert, P, Rivera-Calimlim, L and Lasagna, L (1975). The normal volunteer in clinical investigation: how rigid should selection criteria be? *Clin Pharmacol Ther* **17**, 253–257.

Kappas, A, Alvares, AP, Anderson, KE *et al.* (1978). Effect of charcoal broiled beef on antipyrine and theophylline metabolism. *Clin Pharmacol Ther* **23**, 445–450.

Lasagna, L and von Felsinger, JM (1954). The volunteer subject in research. *Science* **120**, 359–361.

Leopold, G, Burow, HM, Breitstadt, A and Nowak, H (1980). Modification of the bioavailability of drugs by external factors. In: Gladtke, E and Heimann, GG (Eds), *25 Years of Pharmacokinetics*, Fischer Verlag, Stuttgart.

Minton, N, Swift, R, Lawlor, C, Mant, T and Henry, J (1993). Ipecacuanha-induced emesis: a human model for testing antiemetic drug activity. *Clin Pharmacol Ther* **54**, 53–57.

Morrow, GR (1980). How readable are subject consent forms? *JAMA* **244**, 56–58.

Nakano, S, Ogawa, N and Kawazu, Y (1979). Influence of neuroticism on diazepam absorption. *Clin Pharmacol Ther* **25**, 239.

Orme, M, Harry, J, Routledge, P and Hobson, S (1989). Healthy volunteer studies in Great Britain: the results of a survey into 12 months activity in this field. *Br J Clin Pharmacol* **27**, 125–133.

Park, BB, Pirmohamed, M and Kitteringham, NR (1992). Idiosyncratic drug reactions. *Br J Clin Pharmacol* **34**, 377–395.

Posner, J and Rolan, P (1998). Clinical pharmacokinetics. In: Griffin, JP, O'Grady, J and Wells, FO (Eds), *The Textbook of Pharmaceutical Medicine*, Queens University, Belfast, pp. 119–122.

Quyyumi, AA, Wright, C and Fox, K (1983). Ambulatory electrocardiographic ST-segment changes in healthy volunteers. *Br Heart J* **50**, 460–464.

Reinberg, A and Smolensky, MH (1982). Circadian changes of drug disposition in man. *Clin Pharmacokinet* **7**, 401–420.

Ritter, JM, Lewis, LD and Mant TG (1999). *A Textbook of Clinical Pharmacology (4th edn)*, Arnold, London.

Rosenzweig, P, Brohier, S and Zipfel, A (1995). The placebo effect in healthy volunteers: influence of experimental conditions on physiological parameters during Phase I studies. *Br J Clin Pharmacol* **39**, 657–664.

Rosenzweig, P, Miget, N and Brohier, S (1999). Transaminase elevation on placebo during Phase I trials: prevalence and significance. *Br J Clin Pharmacol* **48**, 19–23.

Rotman, M and Triebwasser, JH (1975). A clinical and follow-up study of right and left bundle branch block. *Circulation* **51**, 477–484.

Royal College of Physicians (1986). *Research on Healthy Volunteers*, Royal College of Physicians, London.

Royal College of Physicians (1996). *Guidelines on the Practice of Ethics Committees in Medical Research Involving Human Subjects*, Royal College of Physicians, London.

Sadeque, AJ, Wandel, C, He, H, Shah, S and Wood, AJ (2000). Increased drug delivery to the brain by P-glycoprotein inhibition. *Clin Pharmacol Ther* **68**, 231–237.

Schoen, I and Brooks, SH (1970). Judgment based on 95 per cent confidence limits: a statistical dilemma involving multitest screening and proficiency testing of multiple specimens. *Am J Clin Pathol* **53**, 190–193.

Sibille, M, Deigat, N, Janin, A, Kirkesseli, S and Durand, VD (1998). Adverse events in Phase I studies: a report in 1015 healthy volunteers. *Eur J Clin Pharmacol* **54**, 13–20.

Silverman, K, Evans, SM, Strain, EC and Griffiths, RR (1992). Withdrawal syndrome after double-blind cessation of caffeine consumption. *N Engl J Med* **327**, 1109–1115.

Spealman, RD (1985). Environmental factors determining control of behavior by drugs. In: Seiden, LS and Balster, RL (Eds), *Behavioral Pharmacology: The Current Status*. Alan R. Liss Inc., New York, pp. 23–38.

Thomas, SHL (1992). Impedance cardiography using the Sramek–Bernstein method: accuracy and variability at rest and during exercise. *Br J Clin Pharmacol* **34**, 467–476.

Vaidya AB and Vaidya RA (1981). Initial human trials with an investigational new drug (Phase I and II): planning and management. *J Postgrad Med* **27**, 197–213.

Westphal, K, Weinbrenner, A, Giessmann, T *et al.* (2000). Oral bioavailability of digoxin is enhanced by talinolol: evidence for involvement of intestinal P-glycoprotein. *Clin Pharmacol Ther* **68**, 6–12.

Wheeldon, NM, McDevitt, DG and Lipworth, BJ (1992). Evaluation of *in-vivo* partial β_1/β_2 agonist activity: a dose-ranging study with carteolol. *Br J Clin Pharmacol* **33**, 411–416.

Zarafonetis, CJD, Riley, PA, Willis, PW *et al.* (1978). Clinically significant adverse effects in a Phase I testing program. *Clin Pharmacol Ther* **24**, 127–132.

FURTHER READING

Karalliedde, L and Henry, J (1998). *Handbook of Drug Interactions*, Arnold, London.

Rowland, M and Tozer, TN (1995). *Clinical Pharmacokinetics: Concepts and Applications (3rd edn)*, Lea & Febiger, Philadelphia.

Shargel, L and Yu, ABC (1999). *Applied Biopharmaceutics and Pharmacokinetics (4th edn)*, Prentice-Hall, New Jersey.

Stockley, IH (1991). *Drug Interactions*, Blackwell Scientific Publications, Oxford.

7

Phase IV studies

Brian D. Edwards, Hervé Laurent and Graham Wylie

INTRODUCTION

The nature of Phase IV studies has changed over the last 10 years because of increasing regulatory, commercial and pharmacoeconomic pressures to better define quality, safety and efficacy in relation to other (including non-pharmaceutical) treatments in the same therapeutic area.

This chapter will first discuss the driving forces that shape the design of Phase IV studies, identifying the objectives they must satisfy and the constraints with which they must comply. These driving forces are then categorised and sorted to explain their impact and to make them explicit, thus enabling the Phase IV protocol writer to create the most appropriate design. Other elements of the protocol writing process are discussed in the section '*Scientific method*', which attempts to summarise the essential value of scientific thinking in the design of any Phase IV study. The chapter then goes on to examine some of the more common designs of Phase IV clinical trials in detail, followed by a brief discussion of the issues of globalisation of clinical trial data post-authorisation, and the resulting logistical impact on study designs and operation.

DRIVING FORCES IN PHASE IV STUDIES

The major driving forces behind the development of Phase IV trials are commercial, academic, regulatory, efficacy and safety. This is a broad sweep of objectives, due to the catch-all approach of the Phase IV definition as 'any post-approval clinical study'. Figure 1 presents these major categories and offers a breakdown to a more detailed level.

Drilling down to the detailed driving forces, it becomes evident that there is some overlap between categories; consequently, final study designs tend to meet objectives from several categories. Tight mapping is undesirable, as this tends to constrain thinking and creativity. However, a balance must be sought

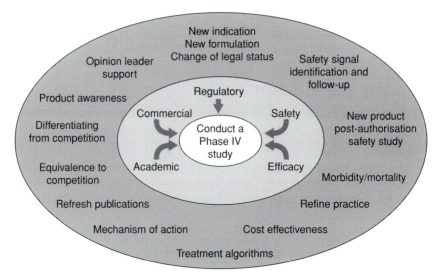

Figure 1. The range of Phase IV studies and how they interact with different driving forces.

between a broad set of objectives and the practicality or complexity of a study's final design. To achieve this balance, those designing the Phase IV study need to clarify the context in which it will be run. To help define context, certain questions are very helpful:

● What are the overall post-authorisation objectives of the full programme of work (of which this study is a part)?
● What objectives are being met elsewhere?
● What objectives remain for this study?
● What is the priority of objectives for this study?

CONSTRAINTS

Once the driving forces have been identified and the objectives defined, it is necessary to consider the major constraints. First and foremost are ethical considerations. Are the trial subjects being treated in accordance with the Declaration of Helsinki and subsequent amendments (*see Chapter 3*)? To answer such a question is not as straightforward as it may appear. Some patient groups are advocating the end to placebo controls or comparative arms, and the approach to this question varies significantly from country to country. This is in direct conflict with customary regulatory and scientific thinking, and can stretch the protocol writer's powers of innovation to their limit. Regulatory and ICH good clinical practice (GCP) requirements for post-authorisation studies are significant, although they are generally implemented at the low end of the permitted scale for monitoring. There are often strict budgetary constraints to reduce the overall cost of developing and marketing new products, especially where products have a small market potential. Lastly, the practicality of implementing the desired design may be limited by differences in medical practice and infrastructure between countries or even between regions within countries.

SCIENTIFIC METHOD

A logical approach to study design will minimise the risk of performing unnecessary trials and help to ensure that each trial has pragmatic and correctly balanced objectives that meet both internal and external needs. In maximising the chances of study success, scientific method is the final element to consider. The issues surrounding each product are unique, implying the need for a unique set of solutions. The drivers and constraints provide useful tools for clarifying study objectives and size, and for ensuring that appropriate expertise and experience are brought into play, but they must not replace creativity with a 'tick box' approach. The scientific design of the protocol is the key point at which to introduce this creative element. For the study to be accepted, it must gain the respect of the investigators and the wider medical community. It must be thoughtfully designed to properly address a serious question of interest to those health care professionals who will be using and paying for the drug. If these objectives are not met, ethics committees will not approve the study (the scientific merit of the questions studied is a critical element of ethical approval), the investigators will sign up and recruit slowly and inappropriately, and the data collected will be of poor quality. Since this is a potential waste of whatever resources are made available for the Phase IV work on a product, it is in the interest of the pharmaceutical company as a whole to ensure that this set of adverse circumstances does not materialise. The more credible the results from a study, the more useful they will be for marketing and sales, both directly through the company sales force, and indirectly through opinion leaders, publications and conferences. The cost and timing of the study need not be impacted by these design decisions.

For example, as discussed later, a product targeted at hypertension will invariably have to show equivalence with or superiority to other products in a head-to-head comparison in pre-registration studies in order to be granted a licence. Once approved, however, the context in which this product will be used is one of combining therapies to reach internationally agreed blood pressure targets. At this stage, it may be more helpful for primary care and other physicians to know that fewer therapies need to be used in combination to reach target blood pressure levels than with competitor products. This change in emphasis will move the study design away from replicating equivalence data toward a design where superiority may be demonstrable in terms of polypharmacy – a real issue in medical practice. This should make the study a more interesting and attractive one in which to participate and more likely to produce valuable, credible and reliable results, for no added cost. It is not possible here to detail how to be creative, but some areas of research do lend themselves well to the Phase IV environment. Indeed, certain types of information can only be provided by post-authorisation studies, for example:

- overall morbidity or mortality in very large samples of the patient population;
- the place for the product in complex treatment algorithms where many alternative therapies may be possible in countless combinations;
- overall cost-effectiveness in routine medical practice, without the intensive interventions of a pre-authorisation study;
- the incidence of rare suspected adverse reactions or specific benefits in patient sub-groups;
- compliance in routine medical practice (outside heavily structured clinical trials).

This is not an exhaustive list, but it may help to generate those sparks of creativity that can have a major impact on the success of a Phase IV protocol and of the product itself.

DEFINITION AND REGULATORY BASIS FOR PHASE IV STUDIES

The definition of what constitutes a Phase IV study can vary between companies and regulatory authorities. However, according to ICH Topic E8: *General Considerations for Clinical Trials*, Phase IV studies are all those (other than routine surveillance) performed after marketing approval and related to the approved indication (ICH Guideline, 1997). The EU pharmacovigilance guidelines define post-authorisation studies as those conducted within the conditions of the approved summary of product characteristics (SPC) or under normal conditions of use (EMEA, 1999). In relation to adverse reaction reporting and periodic safety update reports, reference to a post-authorisation study means any post-authorisation study of which the marketing authorisation holder is aware. A post-authorisation safety study (PASS) is any study conducted within the conditions of the approved SPC with the aim of identifying or quantifying a safety hazard related to the authorised medicinal product. Under the EU pharmacovigilance guidelines, any study where the number of patients to be included will add significantly to the existing safety data for the product, will be considered a PASS, provided that it complies with the criteria described in Section 5 of those guidelines. PASS is discussed further in *Chapter 13*.

Thus, Phase IV studies are not considered necessary for the granting of a marketing authorisation but they are often important for optimising the drug's use. They may be of any type but should have valid scientific objectives. Commonly conducted studies include additional drug–drug interaction studies, dose–response or safety studies, and studies designed to support use under the approved indication, e.g. mortality/morbidity studies and epidemiological studies. As a condition of the granting and maintenance of a marketing authorisation, companies may be required to perform certain post-authorisation studies at the particular request of the Committee for Proprietary Medicinal Products (CPMP). After initial approval, drug development may continue with studies of new or modified indications, new dosage regimens, new routes of administration or additional patient populations. If a new dose, formulation or combination is studied, additional human pharmacology studies may be indicated, necessitating a new development plan. As defined in Directive 91/507/EEC, Phase IV studies, except PASS, should comply with all the requirements of GCP.

In the UK, a code of practice for the clinical assessment of authorised medicinal products in general practice, known colloquially as the 'Phase IV Guidelines', was first published in April 1983. It was produced by a joint working party of the British Medical Association (BMA), the Royal College of General Practitioners (RCGP) and the Association of the British Pharmaceutical Industry (ABPI). Since then, the code of practice has been revised once, in May 1992, but this revision was limited to the section on ethical acceptance.

During 1992 the three bodies referred to above, together with the Committee on Safety of Medicines (CSM) and the Medicines Control Agency (MCA), formed a quintapartite working party to revise the guidelines for post-marketing surveillance studies. During the course of their deliberations it was felt that the guidance for Phase IV studies should be strengthened – to take account of the EC statement that its own guidance on GCP was intended to cover all four phases of clinical research, and to incorporate Phase IV studies in hospitals as well as in general practice.

After a product has been placed on the market, clinical trials exploring areas such as new indications, new methods of administration or new combinations are considered under the EU pharmacovigilance guidelines to be trials for new medicinal products and are not covered by the pharmacovigilance guidelines. In reality, however, a serious safety signal emerging from such studies is likely to have an adverse impact both with prescribers and with the regulatory authorities. Companies therefore need to consider the implications for the currently authorised SPC of such signals.

Apart from conducting further clinical trials, a product's efficacy can be demonstrated by arranging a systematic review or a pooled efficacy analysis, such as that conducted by Stein (1999) for six double-blind randomised trials performed with cerivastatin in primary hyperlipidaemia. An analysis of this type enhances the statistical power of pre-existing efficacy data, as well as better defining the adverse event profile. In a similar way, a meta-analysis of randomised controlled trials showed that intranasal corticosteroids produce significantly greater relief than oral antihistamines (Weiner *et al.*, 1998). Thus, multiple choices are available to a company for developing a product in Phase IV.

SEEDING STUDIES

Uncontrolled cohort studies that appear to be planned more for marketing advantage than for a specific scientific reason are known as 'seeding studies'. Their prime aim is to alter physician prescribing, and since this objective is nowhere mentioned in the protocol, such studies are held in very low esteem. The ABPI in the UK does not support the conduct of seeding studies that masquerade as Phase IV studies. The following features are suggestive of seeding studies:

- lack of control group;
- inadequate statistical power;
- involvement of a large number of doctors, each with a small number of patients;
- inappropriate use of sales representatives;
- vague safety aim, irrelevant or inappropriate outcomes;
- short-term studies with a drug intended for long-term use;
- paid for directly by the company's marketing department.

The change in attitude to seeding studies has been accompanied by a change in the regulations about how medicines are marketed, e.g. regarding the number of free samples that can be provided. However, a study is not necessarily invalidated simply because it is performed for marketing purposes. Companies are also finding other ways of raising awareness about their products, for example, through medical education programmes or by sponsoring a study to investigate the adequacy with which a disease is treated (e.g. the study of nursing practice in asthma conducted by Wesseldine *et al.*, 1999).

COMPARATIVE STUDIES: CLASSICAL PHASE IV RESEARCH

Studies designed to compare two or more active medications often form the basis of a classical Phase IV clinical trial programme. Numerous comparative studies have been conducted with antihypertensive drugs because the increasing choice available challenges companies to demonstrate efficacy and safety compared with market leaders.

Different chemical entities

It is difficult for physicians to choose between different treatments that may appear to have similar overall efficacy and safety and yet have different pharmacological modes of action. As an example of this situation, physical, social and psychological aspects of quality of life (QoL) were assessed in a multicentre, randomised, double-blind, parallel-group study comparing capto-pril, methyldopa and propranolol in 626 men with mild to moderate hyper-tension (Croog *et al.*, 1986). Hydrochlorothiazide was added if needed to control blood pressure. After a 24–week treatment period, all three groups had similar blood pressure control, although patients taking captopril alone or in combination appeared to tolerate therapy better, as indicated by a lower frequency of withdrawal due to adverse events, less sexual dysfunction, signif-icantly higher scores on measures of general well-being, and better scores for work performance, visual-motor functioning and measures of life satisfaction.

Antidepressants are another example of a crowded therapeutic class. In a randomised, allocation-concealed trial comparing fluoxetine with desipramine or imipramine, patients receiving fluoxetine were more likely to continue their original treatment although clinical and QoL outcomes were similar in all three groups (Simon *et al.*, 1999).

Medicines within the same pharmaceutical class

Studies can also be performed to compare drugs in the same pharmaceutical class: one such double-blind, parallel-group study assessed quality of life following treatment with atenolol, propranolol, captopril, and enalapril in 360 men with mild to moderate essential hypertension (Steiner *et al.*, 1990). After 4 weeks, atenolol, captopril and enalapril generally had equivalent effects on QoL as measured by psychometric questionnaires, whereas propranolol consis-tently showed worsening or less improvement. Numerous studies have addressed the differing risks and benefits of the calcium channel blockers: one double-blind multicentre study comparing nifedipine capsules with amlodipine showed better tolerability with amlodipine (Rees-Jones and Sweeney, 1994) whereas a double-blind randomised study comparing amlodipine with nifedip-ine retard showed a similar profile of adverse events (Lorimer *et al.*, 1994).

As with the results of any study, caution needs to be exercised when apply-ing conclusions to populations other than those studied (e.g. different ethnic groups). However, these examples illustrate how well-conducted and controlled studies can show differences between medicines in the same or a related class, thus helping prescribing physicians to make an appropriate choice.

Demonstration of efficacy in different patient groups

Many trials required for authorisation of a product are conducted in a selected subject group and do not include extremes of age or certain patient categories who might theoretically be at increased risk. Phase IV studies are often performed to demonstrate efficacy in these important patient groups, especially when the need for a product has been questioned. A good example in this context is the treatment of systolic hypertension in the elderly. The placebo-controlled Syst-Eur trial using nitrendipine (with added enalapril and thiazide as required) demonstrated a significant reduction in the risk of stroke (Staessen et al., 1997). Another example in a higher risk group was a study with enoxaparin, a low-molecular-weight heparin, in neurosurgical patients: a lower rate of venous thrombosis and an acceptable safety profile was demonstrated with enoxaparin plus compression stockings than with mechanical means alone (Agnelli et al., 1998).

To define efficacy more clearly in the post-authorisation phase, it is useful to see whether better end-points or harder clinical outcomes can be chosen than those used for authorisation. For instance, antihypertensive medicines are authorised based on the surrogate marker of a lower blood pressure. In order to establish a new product on the market, companies now often have to demonstrate that their product can produce clinically relevant results. Not only is a positive effect on congestive heart failure (CHF) an added bonus for an antihypertensive drug, underpinning its original indication, it is also an entirely new indication. The post-marketing development studies of angiotensin converting enzyme (ACE) inhibitors in the treatment of CHF illustrate how a group of antihypertensive products can be developed in the post-marketing phase to firmly establish their place in both the original and a new therapeutic area. The ACE inhibitor enalapril has been one of the most extensively evaluated in trials such as V-HeFT II (Veterans Administration Co-operative Vasodilator-Heart Failure Trial), CONSENSUS I (Cooperative North Scandinavian Enalapril Survival Study), and SOLVD (Studies of Left-Ventricular Dysfunction). In V-HeFT II the effect of enalapril was compared with that of hydralazine-isosorbide dinitrate in the treatment of chronic mild to moderate CHF. The study was a double-blind, double-dummy, parallel-group design in 804 patients and involved an external data monitoring board. It was concluded that mortality after 2 years was significantly lower in the ACE inhibitor arm of the study (Cohn et al., 1991). In CONSENSUS, the effect of enalapril on mortality in patients with severe CHF was compared with that of placebo. This was a randomised, double-blind, parallel-group study controlled by a steering committee and involving 253 patients. The study concluded that mortality was reduced at 6 and 12 months in the enalapril-treated group and it was terminated early on grounds of efficacy (CONSENSUS Trial Study Group, 1987). The first of the SOLVD studies to be published compared the effect of enalapril and placebo on survival in patients with reduced left-ventricular ejection fractions and mild to moderate CHF. This study followed a randomised, double-blind, parallel-group design and was under the control of a steering committee. The study concluded that the addition of enalapril to conventional therapy significantly reduced mortality in patients with chronic CHF and low ejection fractions (SOLVD Investigators, 1991).

NEW INDICATIONS, DOSAGE AND FORMULATIONS

New indications for a product can be developed in a number of different ways. They may be part of the initial planned development, be discovered in clinical use, or be postulated from the mode of action of the drug. These trials must comply with GCP, as in Phase III. Such studies are particularly important if the unlabelled use of a high-risk product is anticipated in an important therapeutic area. For example, variable benefits had emerged from the use of thrombolysis in acute ischaemic stroke, although uncertainties remained, particularly in terms of the timing of therapy. In the ECASS II study, patients with ischaemic stroke confirmed by computed tomography were randomised to alteplase or placebo in four blocks up to 3 hours and 3–6 hours after stroke onset (Hacke *et al.*, 1998). No statistical benefit could be demonstrated, although early treatment may have benefited some patients. This postulated benefit in a subgroup is being investigated further.

Important Phase IV development of a product may occur comparatively late in its life cycle, especially if new scientific data suggest a changing role for a group of products. This has been the case with beta-blockers in heart failure. It was previously taught that beta-blockers always aggravated heart failure. However, a growing body of experimental and clinical data accumulated to indicate their benefit in heart failure, although this might well depend on beta-selectivity. In the CIBIS II trial, patients with stable stage III or IV heart failure were randomised to bisoprolol or placebo and all-cause mortality and sudden deaths were reduced by such beta-blockade (CIBIS II Investigators and Committees, 1999). More recently, it was announced that a four-year study of carvedilol in heart failure was stopped a year early because the risk of death was substantially reduced.

Planned development and regulatory requirements

An example of planning would be the continuing development of an anticonvulsant drug post-authorisation. In the first instance, the drug would be tested as add-on therapy in adult patients with refractory epilepsy. Once sufficient data were available to substantiate its safety and efficacy in adults, studies might be set up to extend the indication for add-on therapy in children. It would also be important to examine the effect of the drug as monotherapy, first in patients in whom the new drug had been added to existing anticonvulsants prior to their withdrawal, and secondly in naive, newly diagnosed patients.

Increasingly the CPMP now expects companies to perform post-authorisation studies if they do not already have long-term data. This is particularly relevant for medicinal products designed for prolonged use (EudraLex, 1998a). For such products there should be safety data on at least 100 good quality cases of patients followed up for 1 year or more. Therapeutic areas that are most relevant in this context include chronic neurological disorders of the elderly (e.g. Alzheimer's disease and Parkinson's disease) and rheumatological disorders (e.g. osteoarthritis and rheumatoid arthritis). A randomised, blinded, placebo-controlled trial, for example, has shown that the selective oestrogen receptor modulator raloxifene reduces the three-year fracture risk in the spine in postmenopausal women with osteoporosis (Ettinger *et al.*, 1999). In a longer extension programme, Merck & Co. are performing two sequential double-blind extensions of their Phase III clinical trials to study the efficacy and safety of alendronate over 10 years in patients with osteoporosis.

Developing a product for self-medication

In the UK, once authorised, medicines are prescription-only medicines (POMs). However, if the indication is suitable for self-medication – or over the counter (OTC) sale – and the product itself is not a new chemical entity requiring more extended post-marketing experience, a company may consider it worthwhile to develop the product so that it can be switched from POM status to self-medication or pharmacy (P) status. Studies can be conducted to demonstrate that the product has an acceptable margin of safety during unsupervised use, including safety in overdose or following accidental misdiagnosis. These data can supplement those obtained through spontaneous reporting schemes. An even greater margin of safety is required for general sale list status because of the need to show that the hazard to health, the risk of misuse and the need to take special precautions in handling are all small. Certain categories of product, such as topical creams for minor skin complaints, are obvious candidates for planned development of this nature.

Discovery by chance

Around 1980, propranolol started to become a popular drug for the prophylaxis of migraine (Peatfield, 1984). This change in prescribing practice arose in response to a number of controlled clinical trials demonstrating that propranolol more than halved the number of migraine attacks, compared with previously, in about a third of patients and that another third derived some benefit. The doses required were much larger than those needed to achieve complete beta-blockade. The mode of action of propranolol in migraine prophylaxis remained far from clear because this property was not shared by all other beta-blockers. Thus, as has happened with other drugs, the therapeutic value of propranolol in this new indication was discovered purely by chance.

New dosage regimen

When phenytoin was first developed more than 50 years ago, and for many years thereafter, the drug was given three times a day. Subsequently, bioavailability studies demonstrated a long half-life sufficient to justify once-daily dosing, and this was later confirmed in clinical trials (O'Driscoll *et al.*, 1985). A company may also wish to investigate the value of intermittent therapy with a product compared with continuous therapy. A one-year randomised, double-blind, controlled trial, for example, has shown that, after remission has been induced, intermittent therapy with omeprazole or ranitidine is as effective as continuous therapy for controlling symptoms of gastro-oesophageal reflux disease (Bardhan *et al.*, 1999).

New formulations

New formulations of a drug may be developed for several reasons; for example, to enable a drug previously given several times a day to be administered once a day. Such formulations are variously known as slow-release, sustained-release, modified-release or long-acting, and examples abound of such products on the market, e.g. diclofenac (Voltarol Retard), theophylline (several forms), and diltiazem (Tildiem LA, Adizem-SR). In Europe there are guidelines defining 'the studies to be conducted in man which are specific to new extended release forms containing recognised active and safe medicinal substances so as to ensure a more prolonged action than the conventional pharmaceutical forms already marketed' (EudraLex, 1998b). In a double-blind, dose–response, cross-over study with each phase lasting 2 weeks, sustained-release diltiazem was shown to be comparable with the short-acting formulation in terms of efficacy and tolerability (Debrégeas and Duchier, 1997). Further examples of such studies are those performed with inhalation devices for pulmonary drug delivery. Pressurised metered-dose inhalers (MDIs) have been widely used to administer drugs for the treatment of asthma, e.g. β-agonists and inhaled corticosteroids. However, because of the hand–breath coordination required, some patients, particularly young children and the elderly, have difficulty in using MDIs. There is also a commitment to reduce the use of fluorocarbon propellants in such devices. Meades *et al.* (1992) evaluated the patient acceptability of a new dry powder inhaler (Diskhaler®) in 326 patients with asthma who were using MDIs or other inhalation devices. After 2 weeks of using the Diskhaler® to inhale salmeterol 50 μg twice daily, 97.8% of patients were assessed by the investigators as being able to use the device correctly. It was considered easy to use by 96.8% of patients and 49.8% preferred it to their previous inhaler device.

PRIMARY PREVENTION STUDIES

Primary prevention is an intervention to prevent a disease from becoming clinically manifest in the first place. Companies can specifically shape their product development to meet a public health agenda, such as reduction in deaths from coronary heart disease and stroke. The use of statins for this purpose was boosted by the West of Scotland coronary prevention study which established that treating hypercholesterolaemia with pravastatin 40 mg/day is an effective therapy to help achieve one of the primary goals of the UK National Health Service, namely the prevention of coronary heart disease (Shepherd et al., 1995). Treating high blood pressure helps to prevent stroke and is also a good example of a primary prevention target that can be evaluated in Phase IV (Staessen et al., 1997).

SECONDARY PREVENTION STUDIES

In secondary prevention, a more common indication than primary prevention, the intervention aims to reduce clinical recurrence of a disease. One of the most extensively studied areas of secondary prevention is that following myocardial infarction (Mehta and Eagle, 1998). Again the statins have an important role in secondary prevention, as shown by the reduction in ischaemic events occurring after atorvastatin 80 mg/day compared with placebo in patients referred for consideration of revascularisation (Pitt et al., 1999). In the AIRE (Acute Infarction Ramipril Efficacy) study, the effect of the ACE inhibitor ramipril and placebo on survival was assessed in a high-risk subset of 2006 patients with CHF following acute myocardial infarction (AIRE Study Investigators, 1993). A substantial reduction in premature death from all causes was found in the ramipril group; this was consistent across a range of subgroups and supported the concept of ACE inhibition for secondary prevention after myocardial infarction. It has also been suggested that hormone replacement therapy reduces cardiovascular events. However, such a benefit could not be demonstrated in a randomised double-blind, placebo-controlled trial of post-menopausal women with stable cardiovascular disease (Hulley et al., 1998). The balance of risks and benefits of a product for secondary and, in particular, for primary prevention has to be very favourable.

SIGNALS OF ADVERSE REACTIONS IN PHASE IV STUDIES

Many important pharmacovigilance signals, some of which have resulted in regulatory action, have originated in Phase IV trials, even though safety was not the primary purpose of the trial. One such important unexpected finding occurred in the Cardiac Arrhythmia Suppression Trial (CAST). The anti-arrhythmic agents flecainide, encainide and moracizine were compared with placebo to establish whether treatment of frequent ventricular premature beats or non-sustained ventricular tachycardia after myocardial infarction would reduce the risk of ventricular fibrillation. Surprisingly, increased mortality was detected in the treatment group in those patients with reduced left-ventricular fraction and subendocardial ischaemia due to a presumed pro-arrhythmic effect (Akiyama *et al.*, 1992).

Another Phase IV cardiovascular study to encounter problems concerned flosequinan, at one time authorised as a novel arteriovenous vasodilator therapy for cardiac failure. The PROFILE study examined the effects of flose-quinan compared with placebo in addition to conventional therapy. In 1993, an interim analysis at one year showed a statistically significant excess mortal-ity in patients receiving flosequinan 100 mg compared with placebo. With the 75 mg dose, there was an increase in patient hospitalisation and so the company concerned voluntarily withdrew the product (Moe *et al.*, 2000).

A pharmacovigilance signal can be generated even in a study not directly related to the current authorised indications for a product. In the MIDAS trial, 883 hypertensive patients were randomised to isradipine or hydrochlorothiazide. The objective of the trial was to measure the rate of progression of mean maximum intimal-medial thickness in carotid arteries over 3 years using quantitative B-mode ultrasound imaging. There was a higher incidence of major vascular events on isradipine and a significant increase in non-major vascular events and procedures (Borhani *et al.*, 1996). According to the editorial that appeared in the same journal issue, the signal from that trial helped to trigger a wide-ranging review of the risks and benefits of calcium channel blockers (Chobanian, 1996). If a company were to be faced with such a situation again, it should perform a risk/benefit analysis accord-ing to the EU pharmacovigilance guidelines (EMEA, 1999) and the Council for International Organizations of Medical Sciences (CIOMS) criteria (CIOMS Working Group IV, 1998) so that the relevance of such a signal for the regulatory status of the product could be evaluated. A safety signal gener-ated from a randomised controlled trial is one of the most robust forms of pharmacovigilance safety signal and, if supported by other evidence, is likely to have some impact on a current marketing authorisation. Thus, the CAST study led to a critical re-evaluation of the use of medicines as prophylaxis of ventricular arrhythmia as well as of other agents that prolong the QT inter-val in the ECG.

LARGE, SIMPLE, RANDOMISED PHASE IV STUDIES EVALUATING SAFETY

Randomised controlled Phase IV clinical trials do not have the problems of bias seen with cohort studies. However, if such trials are to be of value in identifying adverse reactions not seen in the pre-authorisation programme, the sample size needs to be very large, and this potentially makes such studies slow to conduct and very expensive. Also, to be meaningful, the entry criteria should not be restricted; in other words, the drug should be prescribed in accordance with the SPC (as described in section 5 of the EU pharmacovigilance guidelines) and yet the study should still reflect what happens in real life by analysing all patients who receive the product. As early as 1984, Yusuf *et al.* advocated large, simple, randomised clinical trials on widely used treatments for common conditions to study major end-points such as death. Reliable assessment of important differences would require trials where a substantial number of such end-points occur. Such trials would probably involve many thousands of patients, often more than 10 000, depending on the disease prognosis. Trial entry should be at the physician's discretion with minimal external monitoring and very few case record forms (CRFs). Telephone randomisation by a co-ordinating centre would permit immediate initial data capture without forms and ensure a reliable, precise list of every patient ever randomised, for example, by using an interactive voice response system (IVRS).

Typical examples were four open, prospective, uncontrolled safety studies performed using terbinafine in a total of 25 884 patients. As a result, the incidence of adverse events for terbinafine was more clearly defined and shown to be similar to the clinical trial profile. More importantly, serious adverse reactions were shown to be very rare, an important finding in view of the concern about potential hepatobiliary toxicity (Hall *et al.*, 1997).

As illustrated in the following three examples of studies designed to consider safety issues, other trial designs can also be used.

Hasford *et al.* (1991) conducted a multicentre, randomised trial to compare the incidence and severity of symptomatic hypotension on the first day of treatment with enalapril (*n* = 599) or prazosin (*n* = 583) in patients with CHF not adequately compensated with digitalis or diuretics. In the enalapril group, 0.5% and 4.7% experienced severe and moderate hypotension respectively, compared with 2.6% and 10.3% in the prazosin group (p < 0.000012).

Barrett *et al.* (1992) performed a randomised trial comparing the incidence of adverse events after administration of ionic, high-osmolality and non-ionic, low-osmolality radiocontrast agents during cardiac angiography. They found that treatment for adverse events was required in 29% of 737 patients who received ionic, high-osmolality agents and in 9% of 753 patients who received non-ionic, low-osmolality agents. Prolonged reactions, haemodynamic deterioration and symptoms also occurred more often in the high-osmolality group. Analysis showed that severe coronary disease and unstable angina were predictors of clinically important reactions, and the authors concluded that despite the increased cost, non-ionic contrast agents were to be preferred in patients with severe cardiac disease.

A third double-blind study, conducted in 25 180 patients in general practices, compared the safety of inhaled salmeterol, a long-acting β-agonist for regular use, with that of inhaled salbutamol (Castle *et al.*, 1993). Patients were randomised to salmeterol:salbutamol in a ratio of 2:1 and were treated for 16 weeks. There were no significant differences between the treatment groups in terms of serious adverse events, apart from the number of withdrawals due to asthma, which were fewer with salmeterol (2.91%) compared with salbutamol (3.79%) ($p = 0.0002$).

QUALITY OF LIFE AND PHARMACOECONOMIC STUDIES

There has been a growing emphasis on QoL and pharmacoeconomics (PE) associated with the use of different products. Companies are frequently required to justify their products for reimbursement agencies and to clear 'fourth hurdles' concerned with cost-effectiveness, such as the National Institute for Clinical Excellence (NICE) in the UK. In the past, many of the trials conducted to achieve these goals formed part of the Phase IV clinical trial programme.

Nowadays, however, QoL and PE measures are included in Phase III. In this context, one of the more popular tools used in clinical trials is the Short Form Health Status Measure or SF-36 (Ware, 1993). This instrument consists of 36 items covering nine dimensions. Patients find the SF-36 acceptable and it has levels of internal validity with good retest properties. However, no assessment is perfect and the SF-36 should form part of a portfolio of measures to assess many aspects of patient outcome. As an example of a Phase IV PE study, the cost-effectiveness of ondansetron and metoclopramide was compared in the prevention of acute emesis due to highly emetogenic chemotherapy (Cunningham *et al.*, 1993). Despite ondansetron costing over twice as much as metoclopramide, when overall efficacy and safety were taken into account, the two treatments were shown to be equally cost-effective in terms of the cost per successfully treated patient. QoL assessment and related issues are discussed further in *Chapter 14*.

A SUMMARY OF PRACTICAL DEVELOPMENTS IN PHASE IV CLINICAL TRIALS

The regulatory changes in clinical trials and pharmacovigilance have been accompanied by a number of practical changes. With the introduction of the EU Data Privacy Directive in 1998, companies must carefully consider whether they want patients in a post-authorisation safety study to provide consent to allow their personal data to be processed and stored.

To assist with general practitioner (GP) recruitment in the UK, site management organisations (SMOs) have been set up (*see Chapter 11*). SMOs can identify GP investigators through their own GP network, give access to out-of-hours providers and use innovative advertising techniques for attracting and selecting GPs. There have also been many developments in information technology to help promote the smooth running of trials, e.g. a dedicated extranet to ease data entry and enhance communication between investigator and sponsor/CRO, and hand-held data recording devices (e.g. PalmPilot™).

THE GLOBAL PERSPECTIVE

Although it is a gross oversimplification, in major pharmaceutical companies the spend on studies post-authorisation is generally greater than that on pre-authorisation. There are many reasons for this, the most important being that products are generally on the market for longer than they are in Phase II and III, and the product data need to be continually updated to keep pace with the speed of change in modern medicine and therapeutics.

Furthermore, the majority of studies undertaken are run nationally, not internationally. Overall, this means that a large percentage of all data is generated in national studies post-authorisation, and this fact presents specific challenges to companies attempting to collate and co-ordinate these data for safety, efficacy, commercial, academic and regulatory purposes. However, evidence abounds that if this huge volume of data cannot be rapidly accessed and combined, products suffer much more serious disruption in sales when issues arise.

Today, this risk is greater than ever before. Competitors and advocacy groups are challenging products in the courts regarding their labels or side-effects, sometimes even before they are launched. The media play a significant part in propagating claims and counter-claims, irrespective of their foundation in experience or data. The regulatory authorities may become involved at some stage with risk:benefit analyses or advisory board hearings, and the product may face withdrawal, label changes and more – all of which will have profound effects on sales and profitability. Companies find it difficult to defend their products against such activity or to determine the validity of concerns raised if they cannot easily and rapidly access their own data as a single entity. It does no service either to the medical profession or to patients if the company (which possesses the vast majority of available data on its own products) is unable to pinpoint scientific and objective responses to the issues raised.

For these reasons it is critical that Phase IV data are reliable, defendable and accessible. The data coding standards (e.g. the Medical Dictionary for Regulatory Activities, known as MedDRA) and the large patient data and safety data management systems available today make storage a simple matter compared with previously. Data management needs are often viewed as constraints on the Phase IV clinical trial programme. However, if the need for data access is recognised from the outset and if the logistics of data collection and storage are thoughtfully implemented, the constraints can be largely eliminated and this risk to product success can be significantly diminished.

CONCLUSION

Phase IV or post-authorisation studies cover a wide range of objectives and have changed over the last 10 years. Phase IV studies have now been accepted by many companies as a part of the drug development process. Although often conducted nationally, they should be part of a co-ordinated global programme to answer a series of overlapping questions. Apart from PASS, Phase IV studies should still comply with ICH GCP. However, the level and nature of safety monitoring may differ compared with pre-authorisation studies. In certain therapeutic areas, such as hypertension and chronic rheumatological disorders, there is increasing competition, a better understanding of the underlying pathophysiology, and growing academic and regulatory pressure to better demonstrate efficacy and safety. In other chronic diseases, such as diabetes mellitus or asthma, these trends may well develop as new chemical entities are authorised, causing companies to evaluate their products closely once marketed. Safety information in Phase IV studies in Europe is governed by the EU pharmacovigilance guidelines and such studies can be an important source of safety signals.

ACKNOWLEDGEMENTS

The authors wish to acknowledge Dr J.C.C. Talbot who wrote the corresponding chapter in the second edition of *Handbook of Clinical Research* (Lloyd and Raven, 1997). They also wish to thank Louisa Garvey for her excellent word processing skills.

KEY REGULATORY DOCUMENTS

The following documents can be downloaded from the EMEA website http://www.eudra.org/emea.html:

- CPMP/ICH/291/96: ICH Topic E8: *Note for Guidance on General Considerations for Clinical Trials.*
- CPMP/PhVWP/108/99: *Pharmacovigilance Guidelines.*
- CPMP/EWP/553/95: *Note for Guidance on Medicinal Products in the Treatment of Alzheimer's Disease.*
- CPMP/EWP/556/95: *Points to Consider on Clinical Investigation of Slow-acting Anti-rheumatic Medicinal Products in Rheumatoid Arthritis.*
- CPMP/EWP/563/95: *Note for Guidance on Clinical Investigation of Medicinal Products in the Treatment of Parkinson's Disease.*
- CPMP/EWP/784/97: *Points to Consider on Clinical Investigation of Medicinal Products in the Treatment of Osteoarthritis.*
- CPMP/EWP/238/95: *Note for Guidance on Clinical Investigation of Medicinal Products in the Treatment of Hypertension.*
- CPMP/180/95: *Guideline for PMS Studies for Metered Dose Inhalers with New Propellants.*

REFERENCES

Acute Infarction Ramipril Efficacy (AIRE) Study Investigators (1993). Effect of ramipril on mortality and morbidity of survivors of acute myocardial infarction with clinical evidence of heart failure. *Lancet* **342**, 821–828.

Agnelli, G, Piovella F, Buoncristiani, P *et al.* (1998). Enoxaparin plus compression stockings compared with compression stockings alone in the prevention of venous thromboembolism after elective neurosurgery. *N Engl J Med* **339**, 80–85.

Akiyama, T, Pawitan, Y, Campbell, WB *et al.* (1992). Effects of advancing age on the efficacy and side effects of antiarrhythmic drugs in post-myocardial infarction in patients with ventricular arrhythmias. *J Am Geriatr Soc* **40**, 666–672.

Bardhan, KD, Müller-Lissner, S, Bignard, MA *et al.* (1999). Symptomatic gastro-oesophageal reflux disease: double blind controlled study of intermittent treatment with omeprazole or ranitidine. *Br Med J* **318**, 502–507.

Barrett, BJ, Parfrey, PS, Vavasour, HM *et al.* (1992). A comparison of nonionic, low-osmolality radiocontrast agents with ionic, high-osmolality agents during cardiac catheterization. *N Engl J Med* **326**, 431–436.

Borhani, NO, Mercuri, M, Borhani, PA *et al.* (1996). Final outcome results of the Multicenter Isradipine Diuretic Atherosclerosis Study (MIDAS). *JAMA* **276**, 785–791.

Castle, W, Fuller, R, Hall, J and Palmer, J (1993). Serevent nationwide surveillance study: comparison of salmeterol with salbutamol in asthmatic patients who require regular bronchodilator treatment. *Br Med J* **306**, 1034–1037.

Chobanian, AV (1996). Calcium channel blockers. Lessons learned from MIDAS and other clinical trials. *JAMA* **276**, 829–830.

CIBIS II Investigators and Committees (1999). The Cardiac Insufficiency Bisoprolol Study II (CIBIS II): a randomised trial. *Lancet* **353**, 9–13.

CIOMS Working Group IV (1998). *Benefit-Risk Balance for Marketed Drugs: Evaluating Safety Signals*, CIOMS, Geneva.

Cohn, JN, Johnson, G, Ziesche, S *et al.* (1991). A comparison of enalapril with hydralazine-isosorbide dinitrate in the treatment of chronic congestive heart failure. *N Engl J Med* **325**, 303–310.

CONSENSUS Trial Study Group (1987). Effects of enalapril on mortality in severe congestive heart failure. Results of the Cooperative North Scandinavian Enalapril Survival Study (CONSENSUS). *N Engl J Med* **316**, 1429–1435.

Croog, SH, Levine, S, Testa MA *et al.* (1986). The effects of antihypertensive therapy on the quality of life. *N Engl J Med* **314**, 1657–1664.

Cunningham, D, Gore, M, Davidson, N *et al.* (1993). The real costs of emesis – an economic analysis of ondansetron vs metoclopramide in controlling emesis in patients receiving chemotherapy for cancer. *Eur J Cancer* **29A**, 303–306.

Debrégeas, B and Duchier, J (1997). Efficacy and tolerability of once-daily sustained-release and conventional diltiazem in patients with stable angina pectoris. *Clin Drug Invest* **13**, 59–65.

EMEA (1999). *Pharmacovigilance Guidelines*, European Agency for the Evaluation of Medicinal Products, London (Issued as CPMP/PhVWP/108/99).

Ettinger, B, Black, DM, Mitlak, BH *et al.* for the Multiple Outcomes of Raloxifene Evaluation (MORE) Investigators (1999). Reduction of vertebral fracture risk in postmenopausal women with osteoporosis treated with raloxifene: results from a 3-year randomized clinical trial. *JAMA* **282**, 637–645.

EudraLex (1998a). *The Rules Governing Medicinal Products in the European Union. Volume 3C: Medicinal Products for Human Use – Clinical Investigation of Medicinal Products for Long-Term Use*, European Commission, Brussels.

EudraLex (1998b). *The Rules Governing Medicinal Products in the European Union. Volume 3C: Medicinal Products for Human Use – Clinical Testing of Prolonged Action Forms with Special Reference to Extended Release Forms*, European Commission, Brussels.

Hacke, W, Kaste, M, Fieschi, C *et al.* (1998). Randomised double-blind placebo-controlled trial of thrombolytic therapy with intravenous alteplase in acute ischaemic stroke (ECASS II). *Lancet* **352**, 1245–1251.

Hall, M, Monka, C, Krupp, P and O'Sullivan, D (1997). Safety of oral terbinafine: results of a postmarketing surveillance study in 25,884 patients. *Arch Dermatol* **133**, 1213–1219.

Hasford, J, Bussmann, WD, Delius, W *et al.* (1991). First dose hypotension with enalapril and prazosin in congestive heart failure. *Int J Cardiol* **31**, 287–293.

Hulley, S, Grady, D, Bush, T *et al.* (1998). Randomized trial of estrogen plus progestin for secondary prevention of coronary heart disease in postmenopausal women. *JAMA* **280**, 606–613.

ICH Guideline (1997). *Topic E8: General Considerations for Clinical Trials*, International Federation of Pharmaceutical Manufacturers Associations, Geneva (Issued as CPMP/ICH/291/96).

Lloyd, J and Raven A (1997). *Handbook of Clinical Research (2nd edn)*, Churchill Communications Europe, London.

Lorimer, AR, Anderson, JA, Laher, MS *et al.* (1994). Double-blind comparison of amlodipine and nifedipine retard in the treatment of mild to moderate hypertension. *J Hum Hypertens* **8**, 65–68.

Meades, C, Churcher, KM and Palmer, JBD (1992). An evaluation of the ease of handling the Diskhaler dry powder inhaler by asthmatic patients. *Eur J Clin Res* **3**, 43–50.

Mehta, RH and Eagle, KA (1998). Secondary prevention in myocardial infarction. *Br Med J* **316**, 838–842.

Moe, GW, Rouleau, JL, Charbonneau, L *et al.* (2000). Neurohormonal activation in severe heart failure: relations to patient death and the effect of treatment with flosequinan. *Am Heart J* **139**, 587–595.

O'Driscoll, K, Ghaldiali, E, Crawford, P and Chadwick, D (1985). A comparison of single daily dose and divided dose of phenytoin in epileptic outpatients. *Acta Therapeutica* **11**, 375–385.

Peatfield, R (1984). How to treat migraine. *Br J Hosp Med* **31**, 142–144.

Pitt, B, Waters, D, Brown, WV *et al.* (1999). Aggressive lipid-lowering therapy compared with angioplasty in stable coronary artery disease. *N Engl J Med* **341**, 70–76.

Rees-Jones, D and Sweeney, M (1994). A comparative study of amlodipine and nifedipine in treatment of stable angina pectoris in general practice. *Br J Cardiol* **1**, 229–233.

Shepherd, J, Cobbe, SM, Ford, I *et al.* (1995). Prevention of coronary heart disease with pravastatin in men with hypercholesterolemia. *N Engl J Med* **333**, 1301–1307.

Simon, GE, Heiligenstein, J, Revicki, D *et al.* (1999). Long-term outcomes of initial antidepressant drug choice in a 'real world' randomized trial. *Arch Fam Med* **8**, 319–325.

SOLVD Investigators (1991). Effects of enalapril on survival in patients with reduced left-ventricular ejection fractions and congestive heart failure. *N Engl J Med* **325**, 293–302.

Staessen, JA, Fagard, R, Thijs, L *et al.* (1997). Randomised double-blind comparison of placebo and active treatment for older patients with isolated systolic hypertension. *Lancet* **350**, 757–764.

Stein, E (1999). A pooled efficacy analysis of cerivastatin in the treatment of primary hyperlipidemia. *Clin Drug Invest* **18**, 433–444.

Steiner, SS, Friedhoff, AJ, Wilson, BL, Wecker, JR and Santo JP (1990). Antihypertensive therapy and quality of life: a comparison of atenolol, captopril, enalapril and propranolol. *J Hum Hypertens* **4**, 217–225.

Ware, JE (1993). Measuring patients' views: the optimum outcome measure. *Br Med J* **306**, 1429–1430.

Weiner, JM, Abramson, MJ and Puy, RM (1998). Intranasal corticosteroids versus oral H1 receptor antagonists in allergic rhinitis: systematic review of randomised controlled trials. *Br Med J* **317**, 1624–1629.

Wesseldine, LJ, McCarthy, P and Silverman, M (1999). Structured discharge procedure for children admitted to hospital with acute asthma: a randomised controlled trial of nursing practice. *Arch Dis Child* **80**, 110–114.

Yusuf, S, Collins, R and Peto, R (1984). Why do we need some large, simple randomized trials? *Stat Med* **3**, 409–422.

8

The clinical trial protocol

Nina Downes

INTRODUCTION

A thought for every protocol writer: 'Under carefully controlled conditions humans do what they damn well please.' (Harvard's Law of Human Behaviour).

When faced with the task of writing a clinical study protocol, it is as well to bear Harvard's Law in mind. One of the greatest challenges for the protocol writer is to predict and make allowances for the real-world behaviour of the myriad different individuals who will be involved in the clinical trial with the expectation that they will behave 'according to the protocol'. This chapter will attempt to give some practical guidance on how to tackle the job of writing a protocol. It will cover the main decisions to be made, along with the scientific and practical considerations to be taken into account when making those decisions, and will offer advice on how to defeat Harvard's Law, if possible.

The average clinical trial protocol may be a 100–page text and writing such a document is no mean feat. It is not simply a question of beginning at page 1 and going forward from there; protocol writing requires careful thought and a structured plan of action. Because everyone works differently, there is no single infallible formula for the task of protocol writing; however, irrespective of individual approach, it is essential first to step back and think about the plan.

DEFINITION AND PURPOSE OF THE PROTOCOL

Section 1.44 of the International Conference on Harmonisation (ICH) good clinical practice (GCP) guideline defines the protocol as: 'A document that describes the objective(s), design, methodology, statistical considerations, and organisation of a trial. The protocol usually also gives the background and rationale for the trial ...' (ICH Guideline, 1996). According to the guideline, the term 'protocol' also encompasses any protocol amendments; furthermore, the background and rationale for the clinical trial may be described in other trial-related documentation, e.g. the investigator's brochure, provided that this is referenced in the protocol.

The protocol is, in short, the reference document that describes *why* the trial is being conducted, *how* it should be executed and *what* is to be done in *any* eventuality. The protocol, therefore, is used by many different people involved in the trial and it must set out clearly all the information that is required to conduct the trial. The degree of detail contained in the protocol is a matter of judgement but guidance may be found in the sponsor company's standard operating procedures (SOPs), with which the protocol writer must comply. A sensible rule of thumb for the writer is to include the right amount of detail necessary for the reader of each section to be able to understand exactly what is required to conduct the study. For example, the description of blood pressure measurement will be far more detailed in a protocol for a hypertension study where this is the primary efficacy measure than in a protocol for another disease area where blood pressure is assessed as part of the general safety check.

The protocol users will include all study site staff (investigators, study site co-ordinators, research nurses, pharmacists and dispensing staff, laboratory staff, and members of other departments who are to perform any special procedures, e.g. electrocardiography (ECG), radiography, endoscopy, etc.), as well as study monitors, the clinical trial supplies department, data managers, statisticians, report writers, auditors, regulatory inspectors and ethics committees. This catalogue of potential users emphasises the need for the trial-related information in the protocol to be comprehensive.

The protocol must specifically inform study site staff about how the study treatments will be assigned, how the subjects are to be treated, and what assessments are to be performed when, with what equipment and by whom. It will describe how the study medication will be packed and when it will be dispensed, returned and tracked. It will also specify whether special storage facilities are required. Details relating to the obtaining of biological samples will be defined, together with the allocation of responsibilities for their analysis. The protocol will stipulate the action to be taken if an adverse event occurs, particularly if the situation constitutes an emergency.

In addition, the protocol will describe how the data collected in the study will be analysed. This will be relevant not only to the data managers and statisticians who will be responsible for data handling and analysis, but also to the ethics committees and regulatory authorities.

The end product of the clinical study is usually a clinical study report and this may or may not be included in a marketing authorisation application (MAA). The protocol will form part of the clinical study report (ICH Guideline, 1995); it is therefore important that the protocol writer should consider the requirements for this final report. Even at the protocol writing stage there should be a clear idea of the data to be collected, the analyses to be performed, and the shape of the data tables.

WRITING A PROTOCOL

Writing a protocol is a time-consuming exercise, but the effort is well spent if the result is a good sound document. As a prelude to writing, some research will be useful to answer the following questions:

- Why is the protocol needed?
- Where does the study fit into the clinical development plan for the product?
- Is the study required for a regulatory submission?
- What question must the study be designed to answer?

Answers to these questions will usually be provided by staff from the sponsor company involved in developing the drug. Advice should be sought from the regulatory affairs department for all studies intended for inclusion in an MAA, and the marketing department should have input, especially for later phase studies that will be used when marketing the product. It is common practice for the marketing and regulatory departments to be involved from the beginning in developing the clinical development plan for the product.

The marketing department will usually discuss and define the maximum and minimum labelling and summary of product characteristics (SPC) require-ments for a product; a clinical development plan detailing the studies aimed at achieving the best possible labelling will require input from the regulatory and other departments. The clinical development plan should map out those studies required to demonstrate the efficacy and safety of the proposed dose(s) in the proposed formulations in the chosen patient population. ICH Topic E8 (*General Considerations for Clinical Trials*) provides further details and guidance regarding the purpose and content of clinical development plans (ICH Guideline, 1997).

The protocol writer will also require input on the disease area in question, common treatments for the disease and methods used to assess the disease in clinical studies. This can be obtained from a number of sources, e.g. the medical literature (both textbook and on-line search), sponsor company medical advisors, investigators, pharmacists, etc. If the proposed study is destined for an MAA and there has been a precedent approval of a similar product, this type of information may be generally available. For example, under the Freedom of Information law in the USA, the Food and Drug Administration (FDA) provides such information on New Drug Applications (NDAs). Similarly, the European Agency for the Evaluation of Medicinal

Products (EMEA) publishes information on the basis of approvals in Europe via the European Public Assessment Report (EPAR). Posters at symposia, congresses and medical meetings can also be a useful source of this information because they often describe details of study design, patient population selected, assessments used and their timings.

If the study is to be multinational or global, cultural differences in the treatment of the target disease in different countries need to be understood by the protocol writer. A protocol for a disease area characterised by cultural differences in disease management will usually be a compromise. Depending on the extent of these cultural differences, it may not even be possible to design a compromise protocol; in such cases the best way forward may be to conduct more than one study.

The judgement call as to whether to proceed with a compromise protocol is a difficult one and is not usually made by the protocol writer alone. The situation should be discussed with a variety of disciplines within the sponsor company (e.g. regulatory affairs, medical advisors, marketing department, etc.). In such circumstances it is also common practice to consult an expert panel or steering committee of investigators/opinion leaders from the countries where the study is to be performed and the product is to be registered. In the USA, prior to conducting any study, a pre-investigational new drug (IND) meeting is usually held to discuss study designs. In Europe too it is becoming increasingly common for the sponsor company to meet with one or more of the regulatory authorities to obtain some guidance on their requirements. This exercise may result in similar opinions or, less helpfully, in opinions that differ from country to country.

A decision to undertake many separate studies is not ideal in terms of time and financial resource but sometimes there can be no alternative. Conversely, a decision to conduct one compromise study presents challenges of a different nature, e.g. finding investigators who are willing to be sufficiently flexible to work with the protocol. It is the task of the protocol writer to make the compromise as acceptable as possible, given the existing range of cultural and practical differences.

Knowledge of the preclinical and clinical development of the drug is also required and a good source for this information is the investigator's brochure. If no clinical studies have been conducted previously, it will be necessary to produce an investigator's brochure in addition to the protocol. The required contents for an investigator's brochure are listed in Section 7 of the ICH GCP guideline (ICH Guideline, 1996).

Once all this knowledge has been assembled, but before starting to write the protocol, it is essential that the study design and possible subject numbers be discussed with a statistician. Writing the protocol is a futile exercise if it is subsequently discovered that the sample size is so large that the study is not affordable within the budget provided or that subject numbers are impossible to achieve.

THE SKELETON PROTOCOL: THE MAIN DECISIONS TO BE MADE

There are many different approaches to writing a protocol but sketching out a 'skeleton protocol' that outlines the main decisions or 'bones' is a good starting point. The exact details can be fleshed out later. The first step in developing the skeleton is to map out a study schedule as the main decisions are made; this can then be used for expanding into the larger protocol document. The study schedule (see Table 1) should not only show the visit timings, study phases (e.g. screening, run-in, dose titration, wash-out, treatment, follow-on, etc.) and assessments, but also include relevant notes on how specific assessments are to be performed. It is also useful at this stage to note key inclusion/exclusion criteria and/or eligibility requirements for progression from one study phase to the next.

Table 1. Example of a study schedule.

	Visit 1 (day –7) wash-out	Visit 2 (day 0) baseline	Visit 3 (day 7)	Visit 4 (day 14)	Follow-up (30 days after end of treatment)
Informed consent	×				
Inclusion/exclusion	×	×			
Medical history	×				
Primary diagnosis	×				
Concurrent diagnoses	×	×	×	×	×
Concomitant medication	×	×	×	×	×
Clinical assessment	×	×	×	×	×
Randomisation		×			
Dispense treatment	×	×			
Overall clinical assessment: Investigator			×	×ᵃ	×
Subject			×	×	×
Assessment of relapse					×
Acceptability of treatment			×	×	
On-treatment adverse events			×	×	×
Collecting of used/unused trial medication			×	×	

The exact layout of the final protocol document is usually governed by sponsor company SOPs, and electronic shell or template protocols are generally available. These make life very much easier for the protocol writer because they will contain wording for standard sections that are included in every protocol (e.g. for handling adverse events). However, these sections must be checked each time to confirm that the wording is relevant to the protocol being developed.

The contents of a clinical trial protocol are listed in detail in Section 6 of the ICH GCP guideline (ICH Guideline, 1996); hence, only thoughts relevant to the main considerations for the skeleton outline will be elaborated here.

Objectives and end-points

The objective (or aim) of a trial is the question (preferably only one) that the trial is seeking to answer. This could be either efficacy or safety, although in efficacy trials, safety is always considered as a second objective. It is invariably tempting to try to answer too many questions in a single protocol, with the attendant risk of answering none properly. It is good advice to keep things simple and to have one primary objective. Clarity of thought is required. Suggestions from opinion leaders to measure the fashionable 'thing of the moment' should be considered cautiously in the light of the objective of the study and the overall development of the product, as stated in the clinical development plan. Additional satellite studies, which are not part of the main protocol, may be a practical solution in such cases.

It is important to get the primary objective right, i.e. the question that the study is designed to answer: it must be well-defined with a well-founded rationale that is logically explained in the introduction to the protocol. The primary objective will dictate the primary end-point measurement upon which the statistical sample size is calculated. Careful formulation of this objective will also help to convince ethics committees that the question needs to be answered and that it is being addressed by the trial in an ethical way with the best interests and safety of the subjects in mind.

As with the primary objective, the primary end-point measurement (sometimes called the primary outcome measure or primary variable) requires careful thought. The term 'end-point' implies not only that this must be the actual defined measurement or assessment but also that there is a time point of clinical interest. For example, in a hypertension study, a reasonable objective would be 'to compare the efficacy of drug A with that of drug B in the treatment of hypertension'. Suitable end-points for comparing the effect of the two treatments would be either:

● the percentage of subjects who achieve a target diastolic blood pressure (e.g. 90 mmHg) at the end of treatment (e.g. at 12 weeks); or
● the change from baseline in diastolic blood pressure at the end of treatment (e.g. at 12 weeks).

If at all possible, an end-point should be something that is unequivocal to measure; this is known as a *hard* end-point. Hard end-points are objective measurements that are not dependent on the opinion of the observer.

Common examples of hard end-points are death, blood pressure, laboratory values, etc. However, while some disease areas readily lend themselves to such hard end-points, many do not.

Disease areas in which the main clinical manifestation necessitates measurement of subjective symptoms such as pain, discomfort or irritation, present the protocol writer with a different challenge. In such cases, there may be a surrogate marker of the disease that could be used, but care must be taken to ensure that the surrogate marker accurately correlates with disease levels and symptoms and that it is an accurate predictor of clinical outcome. An example of a surrogate marker may be a laboratory value that changes as disease activity changes. Alternatively, scoring systems can be used in an attempt to quantify symptoms. Scoring systems have been developed and validated in many different disease areas and are regularly employed as research tools. It is preferable to select a recognised and validated scoring system and it is well worth searching the literature and consulting experts to decide on the most appropriate instrument. If the disease area does not have a recognised and validated symptom scoring system, one can be developed in consultation with a panel of clinical and regulatory experts.

Certain diseases are characterised by subjective symptoms (e.g. itching, pain or irritation) that can only be scored by the subject, and by related symptoms (e.g. redness) that can be assessed by the investigator. While it is tempting to use only the investigator score, the acceptability of this approach depends on the relative importance of the symptom scored by the investigator. For example, while the investigator can assess redness of the eyes in allergic conjunctivitis, the most sensitive measure of the disease is the itching that can only be assessed by the subject. A score of clinical effectiveness as judged by the investigator and the subject is often included as an additional measurement.

Ultimately, the protocol writer has to justify the choice of primary end-point, and clarity of thought is required to ensure that this choice is as objective as possible.

Choice of study design

Many different designs are used in clinical studies (*see Chapter 5*). The design chosen depends on why the trial is being conducted (e.g. for an MAA or for market support), the phase of the study and the study end-point (subjective or objective).

There are two main types of design, comparative or non-comparative. Non-comparative designs are used when safety and tolerability data are required. Human pharmacology studies (Phase I) used to collect safety and tolerability data are often non-comparative. Some therapeutic confirmatory studies (Phase III) are also non-comparative if long-term safety data are required, e.g. in chronic diseases such as rheumatoid arthritis where the treatment will be used continuously or intermittently over a number of years. Comparative designs are used when comparing treatments. The two most commonly used comparative designs are:

- *Cross-over:* each subject receives one study treatment and then crosses over to receive the other treatment. In this design, responses are compared within each subject.
- *Parallel-group:* each subject receives only one of the study treatments for a predetermined period. In this design, responses are compared between groups of subjects.

The cross-over design appears to be a very attractive option at first sight because it offers certain advantages: each subject receives all treatments to be compared and this minimises individual subject variability and results in smaller subject numbers. By contrast, in a parallel-group trial, because each subject receives only one of the treatments and comparisons are made between groups of subjects, individual subject variability must be taken into account and larger subject numbers are required. The disadvantage of the cross-over design is that it can only be used for efficacy trials if an adequate wash-out period can be included so as to avoid the effect of the first treatment being carried over to the second. For this to be possible, the disease in question must be stable and the wash-out period must be sufficiently long to ensure that baseline status is the same at the start of both treatments. This design is not appropriate in diseases where it would not be ethical to withhold treatment, if the subject's safety would be at risk during wash-out, or if the wash-out period would need to be too long to be practical. The cross-over design is often used in later phase studies, destined for marketing use, where the aim of the study is to assess subject acceptability of the treatments being compared; since all subjects receive all treatments, a comparative measure is provided for acceptability of use.

Parallel-group designs are usually the design of choice for most therapeutic exploratory (Phase II) and therapeutic confirmatory (Phase III) studies intended for regulatory submissions, a context in which an objective scientific assessment of the relative efficacy and safety of two or more treatments is required. Subjects enter the trial and are randomised to one of the treatments to be compared and the between-treatment group responses are analysed. These trials are often conducted in a single- or double-blind fashion, especially where there is a subjective primary end-point. If two treatments are to be compared, this is referred to as a two-arm, parallel-group study; a comparison of three treatments will be a three-arm, parallel-group study, and so on.

Choice of comparator

For comparative studies it is important to select the right comparator (e.g. placebo, standard treatment or no treatment). In the early phases of drug development a placebo is used as the comparator, where possible, to assess whether a drug really works. In life-threatening diseases, however, comparison with placebo is only possible when the study treatment (or placebo) are added to existing therapy. Some regulatory authorities, including the FDA, request placebo-controlled trials in order to prove efficacy; this is meaningful for comparison purposes with treatments already licensed. Patient populations, or responses to previously licensed treatment, can change over the years and the FDA argues that comparison with a placebo eliminates this possible bias. Two placebo-controlled trials showing similar results are generally required to prove that the results have not been generated by chance. Most European regulatory authorities require comparison against the standard or 'gold standard' treatment. In practice, therefore, a series of studies is required and most MAAs include comparisons with both placebo and standard treatments. ICH Topic E10: *Choice of Control Group in Clinical Trials* provides guidance on choosing a comparator for clinical studies (ICH Guideline, 1999).

As the drug approaches the market place, other comparative trials may be conducted for marketing purposes in different countries against less well-known treatments.

Bias and how to avoid it

Studies should be designed to avoid bias, if possible. For example, if investigators know which treatment is which, they may be tempted to give the new treatment either to subjects who have failed on previous therapy or to those they think will do well. This phenomenon is known as selection or allocation bias and it can be avoided by using randomisation, a process based on the strict allocation of subjects to treatment groups by chance. In its most simple form, randomisation of subjects to two treatment groups could be performed depending on whether an odd or even number is drawn on cutting a pack of cards or whether a tossed coin comes up heads or tails. However, in the sophisticated setting of clinical trials, randomisation is performed using computer-generated random number tables that are used to produce blocks of treatment numbers balanced to contain equal numbers of each treatment being studied. Hence, the next subject to be randomised is assigned the next subject number in the block. Block size must be sufficiently large to prevent investigators from identifying treatments, and yet sufficiently small so that faster recruiting sites can be (re-)supplied easily and quickly. Block size is related to the number of treatment arms in a parallel-group study and to the minimum recruitment target at each site. For example, if two treatments are to be compared, block size must be in multiples of two (i.e. four, six or eight, etc.) and will usually bear some relationship to the minimum number of subjects expected at each site (e.g. where 24 subjects per site are needed, then a block size of eight would appear sensible).

Observer bias is said to be present if the investigator knows which treatment a study subject is taking: in these circumstances, subjects taking a new treatment might be scored more optimistically (or pessimistically). To eliminate observer bias, studies are conducted blind, i.e. the treatments are identical in appearance so that the observer does not know which subject is taking which treatment. Where only the observer is blind to the treatment, the study is said to be single-blind. In theory, to remove observer bias, only the observer needs to be blinded. However, subjects often give clues to the observer about what they are taking; consequently, many studies are conducted in a double-blind fashion (i.e. the treatments are identical in appearance so that neither the observer nor the subject can distinguish one treatment from another). This approach is successful provided that the treatments are identical in terms of appearance, smell, taste, texture, formulation and dosage regimen. However, it becomes problematic when one or more of these characteristics are different. One solution then is to use a special form of double-blinding known as the double dummy technique. For example, let us suppose that a capsule taken twice daily is to be compared with a tablet taken four times daily. Dummy (placebo) capsules and tablets will have to be made and subjects will then take either active capsules twice daily plus dummy tablets four times daily or dummy capsules twice daily plus active tablets four times daily to retain the blind nature of the study.

Stratification is another technique sometimes used in comparative studies in order to avoid bias. It is employed in circumstances where a particular factor is thought to affect subject response and ordinary randomisation does not ensure even allocation of subjects with this factor to each treatment group. This imbalance of subjects between the randomised treatment groups could then bias the trial results. Stratification takes place before randomisation to ensure that subjects with this factor are distributed equally between the treatment groups and that treatment allocation is equally balanced. For example, if males and females are thought to respond differently to treatment, separate randomisation lists would be generated for each sex substratum so that allocation to treatment is balanced within each substratum. Subjects would then be stratified (assigned) to a male substratum or a female substratum.

Subject selection criteria

The selection or eligibility criteria define the population to be studied. They define which subjects are to be included and which excluded. A balance always has to be struck between a well-defined study population on the one hand, and the presence of so many exclusion criteria on the other that recruitment becomes difficult. In early studies, e.g. human pharmacology (Phase I) and therapeutic exploratory (Phase II) studies, eligibility criteria are very well defined in order to tightly control the subject population, thus allowing the effect of the drug to be studied closely. However, as the drug development programme progresses to therapeutic confirmatory studies (Phase III) and therapeutic use studies (Phase IV), it becomes increasingly important for the study populations to reflect the wider population of patients who will ultimately be treated. To extrapolate results from a trial conducted in an extremely tightly defined population to the general patient population can be of questionable validity. The protocol writer must bear the study phase in mind and aim for a balance between scientific integrity and final application.

In addition to defining the inclusion criteria, sponsor SOPs often detail certain standard exclusions, e.g. concomitant therapy (possibly affecting the course of the disease or leading to drug interactions) and contra-indicated therapy. The SOPs will also cover the issues of informed consent and how to deal with women of childbearing potential, pregnant women, nursing mothers or subjects who cannot comply with a protocol (e.g. alcoholics or drug users).

Methodology/assessments

A broad outline of the assessments for efficacy and safety will suffice for the skeleton protocol. However, the final protocol must include a full description of the methodology, recording equipment, its calibration and use.

The protocol user must be provided with accurate and detailed instructions for all measurement procedures to ensure that all observations are performed in a standard manner. This is particularly important where there will be two or more participating centres. Blood pressure, for example, can be measured in a variety of ways: by taking the mean or the median of three readings, or by taking readings until two are within a certain margin of each other. It can also be measured using a conventional sphygmomanometer or a special random zero sphygmomanometer to exclude observer bias. Whichever technique or instrument is chosen, the same observer and the same sphygmomanometer should be used in order to minimise variation in the measurements. This must be stated in the protocol to ensure standardisation.

If laboratory assessments are required, details of relevant tests and sample collection procedures must be included in the protocol. Rather than performing all the automated tests on offer, it is advisable to consider only the relevant ones. Otherwise there is a risk of finding a value by chance outside the normal reference range for a clinically irrelevant parameter; this will then need to be explained in the clinical study report. In a multicentre study, use of a central laboratory makes data handling and analysis easier because there is only one set of reference ranges. However, the stability of the blood/serum sample over the period required for courier transport often dictates whether or not a central laboratory is practical from a logistical point of view. Bacteriological and other samples can also be transported if appropriate media are used. The laboratory should be consulted for its expert advice.

In the case of adverse events, precise instructions must specify by whom, to whom and within what time frame serious adverse events (SAEs) should be reported. The adverse event section is typically a sponsor company standard that is included in the protocol template or in the sponsor company SOPs. It is usually based on ICH Topic E2A: *Clinical Safety Data Management: Definitions and Standards for Expedited Reporting* (ICH Guideline, 1994) and ICH Topic E6: *Good Clinical Practice – Consolidated Guideline* (ICH Guideline, 1996). The ICH guidelines do, however, allow the protocol writer to detail certain exceptions from immediate reporting to the authorities for SAEs in disease areas where they will predictably be numerous. For example, deaths in oncology studies are expected and are frequently listed as not requiring immediate reporting.

The source data to be included in the source documentation, such as the patient notes, should be listed in the protocol. Source data that are expected to be recorded directly into the case record form (CRF) should also be described. Items expected to be recorded only on the CRF are usually data from rating scales or study-specific scoring systems that are not usually found in patient notes because they are primarily research tools. Patient notes must always contain the results of any measurements or observations that may affect any future care the subject may receive, especially from a safety point of view. Thus, details such as the fact that a subject has consented to participate in a clinical trial, the name of the trial (usually including details of the treatments being studied), and the randomisation or subject number, together with all adverse events, must be recorded in the patient notes.

Statistical considerations

The protocol writer should always seek statistical advice (whether from inside a sponsor company or from an external consultant). Statisticians will be able to provide a wealth of information about the appropriate design of the trial, the pros and cons of the proposed comparator, not to mention the calculation of sample size and the production of the statistical analysis sections.

The number of subjects required (sample size) should be calculated using the primary variable or end-point at the time of interest. As discussed above, it is helpful if this end-point is as objective as possible (e.g. complete cure, survival, etc.). Statisticians should also be consulted about subject numbers at the skeleton protocol stage because it is pointless to proceed with the task of writing a full protocol if subject numbers turn out to be so large that they are not practical from the viewpoint of either recruitment or funding. There are several different ways of calculating sample size, depending on whether the trial is designed to show superiority against placebo or another treatment, or to show equivalence or non-inferiority against the standard treatment. In order to calculate sample size for a trial that aims to show that one treatment is superior to another, the statistician usually requires a measure of the variability (standard deviation) in the proposed primary variable and a definition of the clinically relevant difference that is to be detected. This information is often available from previous trials or publications of similar studies. However, if the trial is being conducted in a situation where there is no precedent, clinical advice must be sought. In order to check the accuracy of the estimate of variation used to calculate the original sample size, a formal calculation of the variability should be planned once some of the baseline assessments have been completed. In some protocols a series of calculations is performed, based on different standard deviations, and the sample size is initially selected on a 'best guess' basis and later adjusted once some real data become available. To ensure that the number planned for enrolment will still yield the calculated number of subjects completing the study, allowance must be made for subjects who simply drop out. Although there is no hard and fast rule for defining this overage, precedent may again be helpful. In general, however, the longer the study, and the more compli-cated and/or unpleasant the assessments and procedures, the higher the attrition rate, especially in studies in less serious disease areas.

In a multicentre study it is important to have sufficient numbers of subjects at each site so that the numbers allocated to each treatment group are adequately balanced and similar populations are ensured. The statistician will wish to specify expected subject numbers per site. In practice, however, some sites recruit more subjects than others and the protocol will often specify a maximum number to be recruited per site. From the outset, sites should only be selected if the study monitor feels that they have a good chance of recruit-ing the numbers required.

The statistician will write the statistical analysis section in the protocol and will specify the statistical tests to be applied at the end of the study. The statistical analysis section will also describe the patient populations to be analysed and will usually include a description of the response criteria. This description of the response criteria will define the variables to be compared and the time points at which these comparisons will be made for all variables (primary and secondary).

Ethical considerations

The protocol should state the rationale for conducting the study. The basis for the study should be ethical from the subjects' point of view and should be statistically sound to enable the primary objective or question to be answered adequately and unequivocally. To place subjects at risk from a treatment that is unproven and potentially dangerous is clearly not ethical. The ICH GCP guideline (section 6.2.3) requires that the study rationale should include a summary of the known and potential risks and benefits of the treatment under investigation. The protocol writer must take a 'helicopter' view when assess-ing the ethics of the study:

- Has every possible precaution been taken to ensure the safety of the subject?

- Are the assessments really necessary, especially those that involve some risk to the subject (e.g. invasive measurements)?
- Is the comparator (especially if it is placebo) ethical to use or is the subject being deprived of current proven effective treatment?

Guidance on ethical issues, including a discussion of the Declaration of Helsinki, is provided in *Chapter 3.*

Informed consent procedures in the subject groups concerned, particularly in special groups such as children, women of childbearing potential, and mentally ill or incapacitated subjects, should be considered thoughtfully. The protocol must also address the important ethical issues of confidentiality, compensation and indemnity, audit and finance as far as these affect the interests of the subject.

Organisation, practicalities and logistics

For the study to be successful, it must win the commitment of all participants. One way of ensuring this commitment is to actively involve all participants in the development of the protocol, with the protocol writer usually acting as co-ordinator and final editor. It is relatively easy to achieve this within sponsor company departments and with site staff in a single-centre study. However, in larger multicentre studies, it is difficult to involve all sites and/or personnel, and some creative compromise may be required. For example, it may be helpful to appoint a principal investigator from each participating country, or to form a steering committee/expert panel.

Above all, it should be possible to conduct the trial from a practical point of view. For example, there is no point in organising a study in a hospital setting when the patients with the disease being studied are treated only in primary care. There are many other practical issues to consider; for example, the cultural acceptability and practicality of study assessments in the clinics in the countries where the study is to be performed. Questions of practicability and feasibility should never be far from the protocol writer's thoughts.

ADMINISTRATIVE SECTIONS

Once these main decisions have been made in the skeleton protocol, the first draft of the protocol proper can be written by elaborating on each of the aspects discussed above and adding administrative details, as set out in the sponsor company SOPs and the ICH GCP guideline. These administrative details will include assigning a protocol number, and adding the names of sponsor company personnel (including the sponsor's medical expert) and the addresses of other institutions that will be participating in the study (e.g. the central laboratory). These aspects are well defined in Section 6 of the ICH

GCP guideline (ICH Guideline, 1996) and will not be repeated here. Standard sponsor wording for many of these sections (e.g. publication policy, quality assurance, financing and insurance, etc.) will be contained in the protocol template or in the sponsor SOPs, but these sources must be checked to ensure that the wording is appropriate for the protocol in hand.

PROTOCOL REVIEW AND SIGN-OFF

Once the first draft of the protocol has been written, it should be circulated for critical review and comment to all those who have had input. The protocol will typically be refined through several drafts before it is finalised. At this stage the protocol writer, often in consultation with a small core team, acts as editor of all comments received.

The protocol will then usually undergo review by a committee of individuals as specified in the sponsor company SOPs, and a final protocol will result. In many cases the individuals involved at this stage are heads of departments who have not had previous input; they are therefore able to be highly objective about the protocol. The review procedure will define the steps for initial review and dealing with modifications requested, the remit of the reviewers and a time frame for review. There is usually a final sign-off procedure before the protocol is given the 'green light'. The review process can be long and involved because the reviewers have often not been party to previous discussions about the protocol. However, a well-written protocol will help to reduce the time taken to achieve sign-off.

PROTOCOL AMENDMENTS

It is worth taking time over the protocol to get it as right as possible first time so that amendments are kept to a minimum. However, because the real world is unpredictable and situations can change during the lifetime of a clinical trial, protocol amendments often become necessary. The procedures for dealing with and tracking amendments are customarily defined in sponsor company SOPs. However, from a general point of view, there must be a procedure for review and sign-off, and ethics committee approval will need to be sought before implementing the protocol amendment (unless there is an immediate hazard to the subject).

AND FINALLY...

Writing a protocol is a very important task – get it right and the clinical trial is off to a good start. However, it is merely the starting point: Harvard's Law and its close relative, Murphy's Law ('If anything can go wrong, it will.'), are always just around the corner to challenge us all!

REFERENCES

ICH Guideline (1994). *Topic E2A: Clinical Safety Data Management; Definitions and Standards for Expedited Reporting*, International Federation of Pharmaceutical Manufacturers Associations, Geneva (Issued as CPMP/ICH/377/95).

ICH Guideline (1995). *Topic E3: Structure and Content of Clinical Study Reports*, International Federation of Pharmaceutical Manufacturers Associations, Geneva (Issued as CPMP/ICH/137/95).

ICH Guideline (1996). *Topic E6: Good Clinical Practice – Consolidated Guideline*, International Federation of Pharmaceutical Manufacturers Associations, Geneva (Issued as CPMP/ICH/135/95).

ICH Guideline (1997). *Topic E8: General Considerations for Clinical Trials*, International Federation of Pharmaceutical Manufacturers Associations, Geneva (Issued as CPMP/ICH/291/96).

ICH Guideline (1999). *Topic E10: Choice of Control Group in Clinical Trials*, International Federation of Pharmaceutical Manufacturers Associations, Geneva (Reached Step 4 in July 2000).

9

Case record form design

Pauline Pentelow and Karen Grover

INTRODUCTION

The case record form (CRF) came into being as a way of regularising the collection of clinical trial data. Before CRFs, clinical trial data were collected from a variety of sources, with all the attendant problems for standardisation and threats to accuracy. The now traditional paper-based CRF has been a very important tool for the clinical trial team. However, the advent of electronic data capture, permitting data to be entered directly into the database, confronts the CRF designer with fresh challenges. This chapter will describe the overall CRF design process; highlight those aspects of design that are significant for the success of the CRF; and consider the effect of electronic data capture on CRF design for the future.

DEFINITION AND PURPOSE OF THE CRF

The CRF is the document used to record the data on which the eventual analysis and reporting of the clinical trial will be based. Although the study protocol provides the detailed methodology for running the trial, the CRF is the main day-to-day tool that enables the correct information to be captured at the right time. CRF design must therefore reflect the two principal uses of the document in the trial, the *collection* and the *extraction* of data. The CRF is significant to the investigator (or research nurse) who will complete it; to the monitor who will review it to ensure accuracy and consistency; and to the data manager who will use it to construct and fill the database.

From the *investigator's* perspective, the CRF should be clear, unambiguous, and easy to follow and complete. Because the investigator will often be seeing subjects as part of a busy clinic day and will not have the opportunity to refer back to the protocol and other documentation, the CRF should contain comprehensive instruction and guidance. It should also enable the investigator to ascertain the subject's eligibility to continue in the trial at any given point.

The *monitor* will review the completed CRF against the protocol requirements in order to validate and clarify entries. The CRF should therefore be designed to minimise uncertainties and to facilitate entry verification, for instance cross-checks between related data.

The final recipient of the CRF is the *data manager*, who will use it first to design the database and then as the source of the data to fill the database. By encouraging clear and unambiguous responses, minimising the amount of free text and guiding the investigator to make the correct entries in the right places, the CRF designer contributes to the creation of a clean database with a minimum need for query resolution between the investigator, monitor and data manager.

REGULATORY REQUIREMENTS

All the elements of a clinical trial, including the CRF, must comply with good clinical practice (GCP), follow the guidelines of the International Conference on Harmonisation (ICH) and adhere to the specific requirements of the regulatory authorities that will review the clinical study report as part of the overall regulatory submission.

The ICH GCP guideline (section 8.2.2) indicates that the CRF should form part of the protocol, implying that the protocol should not be finalised until the CRF is completed. Because this advice is often ignored, there is potential for the CRF and the protocol to contain discrepancies as each proceeds separately through the editorial process. The discipline of constructing the CRF can highlight problems in the protocol and assist in its correction. On the other hand, constructing the CRF from an early draft of the protocol can be fraught with danger if the refining process for both documents is not coordinated.

The various ICH and GCP guidelines and regulations have little to say about CRF design *per se*; the requirements are conventionally covered in standard operating procedures (SOPs) and other in-house documentation. However, because the CRF is a critical document in the conduct of the trial, and may in some cases be regarded as source data, its completion should be according to GCP requirements. Thus, the CRF should contain guidance to the investigator to help ensure such compliance.

THE DESIGN AND REVIEW PROCESS

Because of the significance of the CRF in the successful completion of the clinical trial, and the importance of its design to the different contributors to that endeavour, a team-based approach to CRF design and review is highly recommended. Ideally, this team would, as a minimum, include:

- CRF designer
- medical advisor
- clinical monitor (also representing the investigators)
- data entry leader
- data manager
- statistician.

Working from initial versions produced by the CRF designer, the experts in this team can make a significant contribution to ensuring that the final CRF meets its objectives.

CRF design starts with the protocol. From this document, the designer will initially generate a skeleton plan showing the visits and each associated assessment. The assessments are then reviewed to determine which are visit-specific and which are 'global'. Using this information the designer can map out the number of pages required and what will appear on each page. Implicit in this process is the need for the CRF designer to have the latest copy of the protocol (ideally, although rarely, the final version) and to be informed immediately of any change to the study design.

Where possible, standard pages will be used and adapted to maintain conformity with other studies. New pages, designed specifically for the study, will follow standard formats. The designer next distils the requirements of the protocol into clear, simple and unambiguous questions and creates appropriate areas for data to be recorded, using the design pointers that will be discussed later. The designer will also translate the requirements of the protocol into a series of instructions for the investigator, as a guide through the various assessments required at each visit and as a reminder of actions that must be taken. Once completed, this first version should undergo quality control review by an independent person to check the CRF against the protocol as well as for internal consistency.

The first version is then sent for review by the study team, either by issuing a copy for each member, or by circulating a single copy around the team. The latter is the better option since changes are not duplicated and amendments suggested by one team member may stimulate thought in others. When the review cycle is complete, a team meeting should be scheduled to discuss the suggested changes and review their overall implications. This meeting will also serve to inform the designer as to which changes are essential and which are not.

The CRF designer will then generate the second version, again for review by the team. At this stage, unless the protocol has changed, any changes should be minor and a meeting for overall review will not be necessary.

In parallel with this activity, the designer will select the printer who will be briefed about the number of CRFs required, the design characteristics, the type and weight of paper and card required, and the deadline for distribution.

Receipt of comments on the second version will stimulate production of the final version. After quality assurance review to check that all required changes have been made, the final version is sent to the project leader for approval. To prevent a continual stream of adjustments to the design, it is best to limit approval authority to one member of the team. The approved artwork can then be sent to the printer, who should generate a proof copy of the CRF which will be as close to the finished article as possible in terms of binding, materials and format. Approval to print should come from the project leader, based on a final review of the proof.

The importance of the CRF in the trial means that each step in its generation should be carefully documented. Copies of each version, annotations, review meeting decisions, quality control/quality assurance checks, and approval documentation form part of the raw data for the trial and should be retained and archived in a GCP-compliant facility.

PURPOSE OF THE INFORMATION TO BE COLLECTED

The two main purposes of the data collected on the CRF are to answer the hypothesis formulated in the study protocol, and to provide relevant safety data relating to the study drug. The protocol will have been carefully written and reviewed in order that the right questions are asked to obtain the information required. The purpose of the CRF is to ensure the precise collection, collation, analysis and reporting of these data. The accuracy of the data is of paramount importance. Any discrepancy between the data required by the protocol and those collected on the CRF will undermine confidence in the findings of the study.

It is sometimes tempting when conducting the trial to collect secondary information that may be of 'academic' interest but is not strictly required by the protocol. Not only may this be unethical, it also makes the CRF lengthy and unnecessarily complicated. For all parties using the CRF, its most desirable characteristics are brevity and simplicity. The collection of unnecessary data can also result in delays at the end of the data management process because of time spent 'cleaning' data that are not germane to the study.

To avoid these pitfalls, the designer should ensure that the CRF:

- requests the *precise* information required by the protocol;
- requests *only* the information required by the protocol;
- requests the information in such a way that completion is simple, relatively quick, and as unambiguous as possible, and that all assessments are straightforward to complete;
- presents the information clearly, in a logical sequence, and with as uniform a style as possible to facilitate its interpretation by data entry staff;

- presents the information clearly to enable the investigator to review the subject's continuing eligibility;
- phrases the questions and orders the assessment sequence so as to minimise the number of queries arising; and
- has been accepted and is 'owned' by all members of the study team.

IDENTIFYING AND ENSURING THE INTEGRITY OF THE CRF

For security reasons, each CRF book, and each page within the CRF, must be uniquely identifiable to the centre conducting the trial, to the trial itself, and to the subject whose data it contains. Because the subject must not be identifiable by name, a unique system of codes is needed, usually consisting of the subject's initials and identification number within the trial.

Each page of the CRF will usually contain the following information:

- unique patient identification (e.g. subject number, CRF number and subject initials);
- name of the sponsoring pharmaceutical company responsible for the trial;
- identification of the trial itself (e.g. a unique trial code name or number);
- number or code identifying the centre in which the subject has been recruited;
- visit number for each assessment;
- study day/assessment reference;
- page number (ideally expressed as 'page n of nn'); and
- an indication of the eventual distribution of copies in cases where the CRF is printed on 2- or 3-part no-carbon-required (NCR) paper.

These identifying items ensure that any loose CRF pages can always be confidently assigned to the correct study, centre, subject and assessment. They also provide the data manager with the means to check that all CRF pages for a given subject have been received, or to establish which are missing.

LAYOUT STYLE

General principles of good design should be applied to the CRF. Its pages should be easy to read and understand, and they should lead the person completing the form from one assessment to the next in an orderly and logical fashion. The CRF should look good; it is an advertisement for the sponsor and its quality and appearance send a strong signal to its users. A document that is attractive and easy to use indicates the importance that the sponsor attaches to the study and encourages careful and accurate completion. A wordy and complicated CRF will be viewed as a burden by the investigator, and is an invitation to error or misinterpretation. Furthermore, investigators running a busy clinic will be completing the CRF in an environment that is less than ideal for the purpose. The document should thus be simple and clear, with directions where necessary to aid completion of the required assessments.

The layout of the form, text style and phrasing of questions can all play an important part in ensuring that quality information is collected. The following considerations will help the designer to create a CRF that will encourage accurate completion.

Formatting and sequencing pages for multiple assessments

Wherever possible, multiple assessments at a visit should appear in the CRF in the sequence they are performed. When multiple assessments are repeated at subsequent visits, they should appear in the same format and sequence for each visit. This will not only help the investigator to develop a 'visit routine', but will also assist database building in data management, and therefore data entry.

Encouraging investigator comments in the right place

Used sensibly, white space is conducive to completing the CRF and can be used to guide the investigator from one assessment to another. However, too much white space will encourage note-writing and this is unhelpful for the data manager. To discourage note-writing, a global comments page can be provided, on which the investigator can make any necessary remarks and indicate the page number to which the comment refers. The availability of this global comments page can be referenced on every other page of the CRF.

Choosing a readable font

Font styles can influence the 'readability' of the CRF. A serif font (e.g. Times New Roman) is ideal for text articles, where the reader's eye moves from left to right and reading is often achieved by scanning. A simpler sans serif font (e.g. Helvetica or Arial) has a much cleaner appearance on a form and encourages a more detailed review of the content.

Choosing the appropriate point size

Text that is too small or is cramped into a small area does not encourage the reader to take notice. If text is to be read, it needs to be readable; it must be of a reasonable size, well spaced and well ordered. Footnotes are often used in CRFs, but they will go unnoticed or be ignored if the text is not easily readable. Text smaller than 10 point is too small for easy reading, even by someone with perfect vision, and text larger than 12 point is too large and

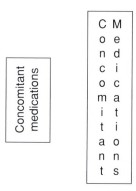

Figure 1. Which is easier to read?

may appear to be a section heading. Text used for questions or completion instructions should ideally be 12 point, with 10 point being reserved for minor instructions, e.g. (dd/mm/yyyy) for date format prompts.

Dealing with rotated text

If text needs to be turned 90 degrees, e.g. for tab edges or column headers, the text should be turned as complete words, and not printed as individual letters stacked on top of each other (see Figure 1).

Dealing with hyphenation

Hyphenation may be an efficient way of fitting more text on a page, but it carries the simultaneous disadvantage of making text harder to read. If hyphenation must be used, care should be taken. Hyphens placed too close to the beginning or end of a word may render it almost unreadable. There is also a danger that hyphenating a word may have unintended results, as illustrated by the example of 'the-rapist'.

UNIFORMITY

Uniformity of layout is very important for a CRF. When a particular drug is being tested in various trials, it is advisable to develop project standards that can be used across all trials. All will be helped if similar information is presented in a standard way across a series of trials. The designer does not have to start from 'square one' on every CRF; the investigator becomes accustomed to the format and therefore makes fewer errors; and the data manager can economise on database design.

Four types of data are collected in most trials:

- *Baseline data:* inclusion and exclusion criteria, demographics, medical history, baseline laboratory data, vital signs and physical examination, and previous medications.
- *Efficacy data:* assessments that are specific to the objective of the study (assuming that it includes an efficacy evaluation).
- *Safety data:* ongoing records of vital signs, physical examination, laboratory data, and adverse events.
- *Compliance data:* test medication accounting, concurrent medications, withdrawal/end-of-study records.

Several of these sets of data could be collected on global, standard forms. Thus, demographics, medical history, laboratory data, vital signs, physical examination, previous medications, concurrent medications, adverse events, and withdrawal/end-of-study records could each become standard CRF modules that would require minimal or no modification from study to study or from product to product.

INSTRUCTIONS FOR COMPLETION

Every CRF should provide precise but sufficient information for the investigator to carry out the visit assessments, enter any additionally required information (adverse events, concomitant medication), review subject eligibility and ensure the subject's continuing compliance with the study protocol.

A flow chart or table of contents at the beginning of the CRF book, perhaps on the inside front cover where it is constantly visible, will be a ready reference point for the investigator and will define the precise requirements for the entire trial and at each visit or assessment point. It could also indicate the time between visits, and thus assist with scheduling the next appointment.

A general instruction page should also appear in the CRF, again where it is easily accessible or constantly visible, such as on a wraparound writing shield. This should give guidance to the investigator on how to complete the CRF and how to deal with corrections to entries made in error. Date and time formats should also be explained here, and information provided on how to deal with unknown or missing data. Because the study may be global, but using a CRF in English, the designer should always bear in mind that English may not be the first language of the investigator. In such cases, graphics are very useful to illustrate what is required.

It may also be beneficial to include a smaller flow chart or list of assessments to be carried out at the beginning of each visit; this could be placed on the reverse of tabbed dividers between visits. Such prompts are particularly useful for assessments that are not necessarily recorded on the visit pages, but on global pages; they will remind investigators to ask the relevant questions and to take appropriate actions.

Further prompts and instructions should also appear throughout the CRF, e.g. reminders to prompt subjects for information on adverse events, or to ensure that laboratory reports, ECG traces, etc., are placed in the correct wallet or sent to the correct destination. Instructions should also highlight any departures from routine practice, e.g. requests for a specific set of laboratory analyses rather than the standard battery.

Some individual assessments may warrant their own instruction page. This may be the case where numeric codes are used to indicate the route of administration of concomitant medications, or the action to be taken following an adverse event. Instructions on how to record dosages and frequencies are helpful, as is a reminder listing prohibited medications opposite the concomitant medications page.

Data management queries commonly arise when inter-related information appears on two or more pages of the CRF. Prompts placed alongside the first of a series of inter-related entries will minimise internal inconsistencies in the data. For example, if an adverse event is treated by medication, a corresponding entry should appear on the concomitant medication page.

AVOIDING TRANSCRIPTION PROBLEMS

Badly designed or poorly phrased questions will lead to misunderstandings, incorrect entries, and problems for the data manager. Since database lock is a rate-limiting step in the production of the report, and hence time to registration, it is imperative that the CRF is designed to avoid delays from large numbers of queries being generated close to this time. Many potential transcription problems can be eliminated by improving the design of the form. Simple enhancements are outlined below.

Number lines

Lines should be numbered where similar information is required repeatedly, for example, on adverse events or concomitant medications pages. If each line is given a number, it is apparent to the investigator that it demands a unique entry. This ensures that the corresponding fields in the database also contain unique data. The numbering of each entry line should be sequential over continuation pages. The database will be sequentially numbered, and if the CRF pages match those numbers, transcription problems can be avoided.

Example of required format

Provide an example of the format of text entry required, perhaps on the first line of the page.

Think about how the data will be entered on to the database

If more than one identical assessment is to be taken twice on one day, it is easier for data entry purposes if each observation is listed on a separate line, rather than on one line running across the page. This is because in the database, the date must be associated with each observation. Figure 2 illustrates a CRF page designed to collect the date, and then two observations of time and temperature across the page. Data entry personnel have to enter the date, time 1 and temperature 1, and then refer back to re-enter the date and pick out time 2 and temperature 2, missing out those already entered.

Date (DDMMYYYY)	Time 1 (HH:MM)	Temperature (¡C)	Time 2 (HH:MM)	Temperature (¡C)
	:	.	:	.
	:	.	:	.

Figure 2. CRF page designed to collect the date, and then two observations of time and temperature across the page. A simple, easier to complete format is illustrated in Figure 3.

It would be more appropriate to design a CRF page with each observation of time and temperature on a different line (see Figure 3). To minimise the repetitive completion of date fields, instructions could be given to complete the date only when it changes; alternatively, the cell can be shaded to indicate that the date is definitely the same. Exactly the same information is conveyed, but the page is much easier not only for the investigator to complete, but also for data entry personnel to read and transcribe on to the database.

Date (DDMMYYYY)	Time (HH:MM)	Temperature (°C)
	:	.
	:	.
	:	.
	:	.

Figure 3. CRF page showing a preferred format with each observation of time and temperature on a different line.

Include units of measurement on the form

For example, the investigator should be in no doubt whether height is required in centimetres only or in metres and centimetres. This can be achieved by ensuring that the units of measurement are specified and that the boxes provided for entry are appropriate to the units, including position of the decimal point, as shown in Figure 4.

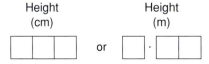

Figure 4. Data entry boxes on the CRF showing the required units and the position of the decimal point, where appropriate.

Guide the quality of text entries

The interpretation of hand-written entries, especially if they are medical terms, microbial species or medications, can be a nightmare for data entry and data management personnel. This is especially true if the study is multinational because different nations have their own ways of forming letters. It is significantly easier to interpret block capitals than script. Instructing that text entries should be in block capitals and giving an example entry is the best way to prevent illegible text entries. Providing the appropriate amount of space is also very important, but may be difficult to judge; the clinical and medical monitors can advise on this aspect. Too much space encourages the investigator to wax lyrical; too little space results in abbreviations or cryptic comments overflowing their allotted space.

Minimise graphical data

Even something as apparently simple as a linear visual analogue scale can cause problems for data management. The linear scale may be cut by a straight line, which is easy to interpret; by a tick, a circle or a squiggle cutting the line at more than one point; or the respondent may have used a cross that misses the line altogether. If there is no alternative to graphical data, e.g. to depict the site of a lesion, the CRF designer should work with the data manager to establish how the data will be coded for the database. The graphic can then be designed to reflect this coding. However, alternatives to such data collection methods should be sought wherever possible.

QUESTION FORMATS

If a clinical trial is to be successful, it is vital that CRF questions are formulated so as to be understood and to yield an answer in the correct format. All questions should be worded to eliminate confusion and to ensure that their answer cannot change (for example, the CRF should elicit the date of birth of the subject, not his/her age). Questions should never be in the form of a double negative and, wherever possible, should require a positive, not a negative response. The question: 'Is the patient unable to swallow tablets?' could easily prompt the wrong answer. Rephrasing the question to: 'Does the patient have difficulty swallowing tablets?' yields the same information, i.e. Yes (the patient is unable to swallow tablets) or No (the patient is not unable to swallow tablets), but there is much greater confidence that the answer is right.

It is easier, quicker and usually more accurate if the investigator can tick a box instead of writing something in it. For example, if 0 = No and 1 = Yes, the form will be easier to complete (and less likely to be wrong) if the investigator is asked to tick one of two discretely coded boxes rather than having to write the code number in the box. Also, if 0 = No and 1 = Yes, care must be taken to ensure that this usage is continued throughout and does not change to 1 = Yes and 2 = No in mid-CRF.

By the same token, in a series of Yes/No options, the boxes should appear in two columns. All Yes boxes should appear in one column, and all No boxes in the other, so that the investigator is less likely to tick the wrong box inadvertently. The sequence of Yes and No columns should not change either part way through a list of questions or through the CRF as a whole.

Forms must state clearly whether more than one box may be ticked. An end-of-study form, for example, might ask the investigator to tick the box that matches the reason for withdrawal. The database will be constructed on the expectation that only one box will be ticked. However, unless instructed otherwise, the investigator may tick the boxes for 'Adverse event' *and* 'Protocol violation' if an adverse event was treated by a prohibited medication.

It must also be clear whether a response to a Yes/No option will exclude or necessitate withdrawal of the subject from the trial. It may be useful to adopt a particular style for such questions, e.g. shading or emboldening all the 'right' or all the 'wrong' answers, so that the investigator can see at a glance the result of any line of questioning. For inclusion/exclusion questions, it is therefore advisable to make Yes the 'right' answer to all inclusion criteria, and No the 'right' answer to all exclusion criteria.

Questions requiring free text answers are to be discouraged wherever possible. It is never safe to encourage free text, as the amount of information cannot be regulated, and the answers may be ambiguous or, in extreme cases, self-contradictory.

If a question necessitates comparison with baseline or other data, e.g. for changes in severity of symptoms, the location of the reference data should be indicated on the CRF. In such cases, it is advisable to work closely with the medical monitor, the statistician and the data manager to ensure that adequate guidance is given on how to specify the degree of change. It would be unwise to base such assessments on subjective judgement; wherever possible, a grading scheme employing an unambiguous scale should be used.

The layout of questions and their corresponding answer boxes can greatly affect the ease of CRF completion. There are several ways to align more than one row of questions, as shown in Figure 5. Example (a) is untidy, difficult to complete, and time-consuming for data entry personnel who will have to search for the information. Example (b) is much clearer for data entry

(a)
Married? ☐ Yes ☐ No
Aged between 18 and 45 years inclusive? ☐ Yes ☐ No
Received any other investigational drug within 30 days? ☐ Yes ☐ No

(b)

Married?	☐ Yes	☐ No
Aged between 18 and 45 years inclusive?	☐ Yes	☐ No
Received any other investigational drug within 30 days?	☐ Yes	☐ No

(c)

Married?	☐ Yes	☐ No
Aged between 18 and 45 years inclusive?	☐ Yes	☐ No
Received any other investigational drug within 30 days?	☐ Yes	☐ No

(d)

Married?	☐ Yes	☐ No
Aged between 18 and 45 years inclusive?	☐ Yes	☐ No
Received any other investigational drug within 30 days?	☐ Yes	☐ No

Figure 5. Four examples illustrating how ease of CRF completion is affected by different alignments of rows of questions and corresponding response boxes. Version (d) is the clearest and easiest to use.

purposes, but it could be difficult for the investigator to differentiate between lines if a longer list of questions was presented. This problem is overcome in example (c) to some degree, but example (d) probably offers the clearest layout for both the investigator and the data manager.

SECTIONS FOR COMPLETION BY THE SUBJECT

Some parts of the CRF, such as questionnaires and diary cards, are intended for completion by the subject, rather than by the investigator. The CRF designer should recognise that the typical subject may have a limited vocabulary and little medical knowledge. Because subjects in a clinical trial may also be quite ill and in pain, extra care should be taken with the wording of questions designed for subject completion and with the layout of these portions of the CRF. The following points in particular should be borne in mind:

- Most people over the age of 40 cannot read text of point size less than 10 without assistance (such as spectacles).
- Medical jargon should be banned. All text should be as simple as possible so as to be understood by anyone.
- Full examples of each entry required should be given. For example, particular problems can arise over the recording of time, as some people are not familiar with the concept of a 24-hour clock.
- An attractive, easy-to-use format will encourage subjects to continue to use the diary card.
- Prompting by listing potential symptoms may cause these to 'appear'.
- Text entry should be minimised.
- It is better to have several diary cards, each covering a short period (no more than 2 to 4 weeks) than to have one card covering an extended period. The loss of one of several diary cards in the former arrangement is clearly less disastrous.
- The diary card itself should be robust.

PRINTING REQUIREMENTS

The production of artwork for a commercial printer to reproduce must satisfy a number of essential requirements:

- The dimensions of any artwork supplied to the printer must be appropriate to standard paper sizes.
- Allowance must be made for a binding margin to ensure that binding holes are not drilled through text.
- If coloured graphics are to be generated, colour-separated copy is required.

- If artwork is supplied to the printer as an electronic file, the printer must have access to the same program (type and version) and templates that have been used for the design. Most commercial printers use Apple Macintosh as the industry standard, and the CRF design programs used most commonly are unfortunately not compatible with the standard. Thus, where compatibility issues cannot be resolved, it may be necessary to supply the printer with camera-ready copy.
- 'Crop marks' on the copy show the printer the exact position of the artwork. They also allow for the finished job to be trimmed to the specific size required.

It is essential that the printer should receive absolutely clear and precise instructions on printing and assembling the CRF. These specifications are very detailed and include the weight of paper for each individual page, the colours of NCR sets, ink colours, logo formats, type of binding, position of wallets, etc. The printer will need as much advance notice as possible concerning number of CRFs to be printed, the weight of paper to be used, and any special or unusual requirements. Many printers will not carry large amounts of stock and will have to order paper and card specially. An unusual requirement will probably be difficult to source, as the materials will be in short supply. Failure to notify the printer well in advance will have an adverse impact on CRF production timelines.

Before final print approval is given, the printer should supply a proof copy of the CRF for review by the data manager and the clinical trial manager. If the proof copy stage is omitted, the first time anyone sees the finished CRF will be when it arrives at the centres, and this is not a good time to discover mistakes.

It is best to form a working relationship with a small and trusted group of printers who are expert in CRF printing, appreciate the time constraints and understand the cost of any delay. By seeking competitive quotations within this group and, from time to time, outside it, the CRF designer can ensure that the printer provides good value for money.

THE ELECTRONIC CRF

The management of clinical trial data using paper-based CRFs, although long accepted as the industry standard, is not highly efficient in terms of data recording and subsequent data processing. The paper-based system is dependent on legible data recording supported by manual and computer-assisted data integrity checks performed by monitoring and data management staff.

As information technology has advanced, various attempts have been made to improve the data collection and data management process. The initial focus was on scanning technology to 'read in' the paper CRF. This resulted in some improvement in data management but data collection was still dependent on pen and paper. However, the advent of secure electronic data transfer systems and acceptance of the 'electronic signature' has made it possible to enter data directly into the database from a remote location. This development has generated great interest because it would limit transcription errors and reduce the time taken to lock the database at the end of the study.

Since good laboratory practice (GLP) preceded good clinical practice (GCP) in defining magnetic computer media as source data, it is not surprising that the first element of the traditional CRF to be replaced was the manual recording of laboratory data (haematology, biochemistry and urinalysis). Analytical instruments and laboratory computer systems are typically able to present results as an electronic computer file. Laboratory results now tend to be sent directly to data management in an electronic format for direct inclusion in the trial database. This development has reduced the need for these data to be transcribed on to the paper CRF.

Although other clinical data can now also be generated electronically, e.g. ECG traces, ambulatory blood pressure measurements, spirometry results, etc., the majority of clinical trial data are still collected on paper CRFs. The next stage of CRF development, therefore, is to make an electronic version that replaces paper as the interface between the investigator and the database.

While many systems and methods are currently proposed as being appropriate for collecting data via an electronic representation of the CRF (e-CRF), the advent of the Internet and mobile telecommunications capability is felt to offer the most appropriate technology base to build electronic data collection systems for clinical trials.

The merits of the e-CRF

The merits of collecting data electronically can be summarised as follows. Data can be checked at the time of entry against appropriate field validation criteria, thus providing assurance that correct data have been entered. The inclusion of traditional monitoring and data management validation checks in the e-CRF should also reduce the number and frequency of data query forms. The e-CRF can aid compliance by cross-checking key data. Instructions for completing the e-CRF can be presented on screen and as validation help messages. Moreover, the acceptance of an appropriate electronic signature by regulatory authorities means that e-CRF data can be 'electronically signed' by the investigator. Finally, if the data are being entered directly to a centralised database, monitoring staff and data management personnel will be able to review data more quickly and easily.

e-CRF issues still to be addressed

A number of issues still need to be addressed before electronic collection of data becomes fully accepted:

- Currently, it takes much longer to design and deploy e-CRFs, together with the supporting database and information technology (IT) infrastructure, compared with the design, printing and distribution of the traditional paper CRF. Since the availability of the CRF is one of the key elements in study initiation, the time to set-up needs to be reduced considerably.
- The e-CRF, unlike the paper CRF, will have technical problems. There must be adequate support to ensure continuity of data collection whenever access to the e-CRF system is unavailable. Sending patients home from a scheduled visit 'because the Internet is down' is unlikely to prove a popular option.
- The concept of incorporating validation checks into the e-CRF has considerable merit, but if these checks slow down the data collection process significantly, the result will probably be unacceptable and unworkable for research staff.
- If electronic checks are to be considered foolproof, it is of paramount importance that many 'dummy runs' are undertaken before the e-CRF is released.

e-CRF and paper CRF: similarities and differences

Paper CRFs may be designed by monitors, data managers and CRF design specialists, or the design may be contracted out to a specialist CRF design company. The design of the e-CRF still incorporates the traditional CRF skills but also needs technical IT support to design the data entry screens, to provide electronic data collection scheduling, validation checks and database interaction, and to maintain overall system security. The electronic checks will typically involve computer programs or scripts that are written specifically to check or validate data before they are written to the trial database.

Similarities

Wherever possible, the e-CRF should be similar in design to its paper counterpart since the layout and data collection flow are designed to reflect the traditional data collection sequence and procedures. If significant design changes are implemented, then SOPs, monitoring plans and guidelines will have to be amended accordingly.

The e-CRF should be designed to have a format similar to the traditional CRF and should include many of the design features illustrated in earlier sections of this chapter. This will assist the transition from the paper to the electronic version for research staff who are unfamiliar with electronic data collection methods.

The header information is still critical in the e-CRF, and electronic checks should be included here. This information is essential to identify the subject-specific data record for the corresponding e-CRF page and visit when it is stored in the trial database. It is used to check that the subject initials, centre number, visit date and subject number are of the correct data type and format and reflect what is anticipated. Where a series of data 'pages' are collected during a visit, this header information should automatically be carried over to all pages for that subject visit.

Where tick boxes are used in the e-CRF, validation can be set so that only one box can be ticked. Date fields can be checked to ensure that they are in the correct format and fall within expected ranges, e.g. date of birth can be used to automatically verify the subject's age and this can be checked against the age inclusion/exclusion criteria for the trial. Numeric data fields can be checked against appropriate reference ranges and values falling outside these limits can be flagged or noted for confirmation.

Differences

The e-CRF pages for collecting adverse events, concomitant medication and other across-visit observations need to be designed differently. The form should be designed to retrieve previous observations and records that require a relevant status update for that visit (see Figure 6).

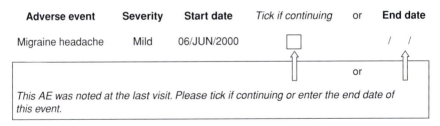

Figure 6. Example of a form that retrieves previous observations and records to permit relevant status update.

Drop-down selection menus can be used for coded fields. An associated option would be to have lists of standard terms or comments held within the database that can be referenced and used as part of the e-CRF design. There might also be options to incorporate special computer-generated components into the e-CRF design, e.g. date selection where standard elements are available (see Figure 7).

Thus, while many of the traditional CRF design skills will still be appropriate for the design of e-CRFs, there will also be a need for in-depth understanding of the computer-enabled e-CRF design components that must be developed and deployed to enhance the data collection process. The most probable solution will be to include a database programmer in the CRF design team to advise on technical design and functional elements.

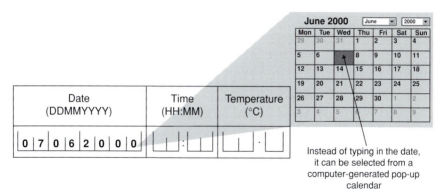

Figure 7. Date selection from a computer-generated pop-up calendar.

All the traditional monitoring and data management scheduling, checking and validation elements will need to be incorporated into e-CRF design. This will necessitate enhanced planning and co-ordination early in the life of the study to allow completion of additional up-front work before trial initiation.

The development of the e-CRF will continue as technological advances present more reliable and flexible design and data collection opportunities. The cultural change, training and support associated with the e-CRF environment will remain the most challenging aspect of moving from paper to electronic records.

CONCLUSION

Good CRF design has a critical influence on the success of a clinical study. By asking the right questions in the right way, and by providing appropriate space for data to be entered correctly, the designer ensures that the CRF accurately captures the data generated in the study. By allowing the data to be presented in a clear format, the CRF designer aids the data manager in designing the database and in transferring the data into it. Because of the crucial nature of the document, it is essential that the various experts involved in the trial, in particular the CRF's main users, are represented in the design process.

The move to e-CRFs will require few if any changes in the application of basic CRF design concepts. However, the increased complexity of the e-CRF, with its potential for in-built validation and parallel database development, means that the e-CRF designer will have to be involved at an early stage of study planning and that the e-CRF design team will include at least one more expert, a database programmer.

ACKNOWLEDGEMENTS

The authors are grateful to Chris Wilkinson for his input and assistance with the section on printing requirements.

FURTHER READING

Bohaychuk, W, Ball, G and Sotirov, K (1999). CRF design and planned data capture. *Applied Clinical Trials* **8**, 64–74.

Code of Federal Regulations (1997). 21 CFR Part 11: Electronic records; electronic signatures. *Federal Register* **62**, 13 429–13 466.

ICH Guideline (1996). *Topic E6: Good Clinical Practice – Consolidated Guideline,* International Federation of Pharmaceutical Manufacturers Associations, Geneva (Issued as CPMP/ICH/135/95).

10

Clinical trial supplies

Paul O'Connor and Linda Hakes

INTRODUCTION

Once the decision has been to taken to conduct a clinical trial and the form it will take has been chosen, the manufacture of the clinical trial supplies must be considered. The key to the success of this part of the process is timely and appropriate communication across the whole study team; this will reduce errors and improve overall understanding of the responsibilities within each role. It is not essential for a study monitor or an investigator to have training in the elements of good manufacturing practice (GMP), but they should understand that the preparation of clinical trial supplies has many potential pitfalls.

No clinical trial can proceed without the materials to be tested, the clinical trial supplies, and therefore it is essential to begin planning these in parallel with the study protocol. The provision of clinical trial supplies is usually organised by a special group, often within the product development department, and it is prudent to discuss a proposed trial with this group at an early stage so that any potential difficulties can be identified and resolved.

Until the last few years, the manufacture and supply of clinical trial supplies were outside all pharmaceutical legislation, and although responsible organisations took great care to ensure the quality of supplies, there was no guidance or regulation from external authorities. This has changed and clinical trial supplies are expected to be manufactured in accordance with GMP conditions and to comply with basic legal labelling requirements. The European Commission has revised the rules governing GMP in regard to medicinal products for human and veterinary use (*see Further Reading* at the end of this chapter), with Annex 13 of these rules dealing specifically with the manufacture of investigational medicinal products.

Very few regulatory bodies have had an active inspection programme covering clinical trial supplies units. However, regulatory inspectors in the past have entered the clinical trial supplies area of a pharmaceutical company as part of a US Food and Drug Administration (FDA) pre-approval inspection and Medicines Control Agency (MCA) 'specials licence' inspection. More recently, the MCA has carried out voluntary inspections of clinical trial supplies manufacturing areas with a view to assessing compliance with current GMP. However, the recent European Clinical Trials Directive has initiated the requirement for Member States to actively inspect clinical trial supplies manufacturing facilities and analytical laboratories and to issue a report. Indeed, sites outside the EC may be inspected at the request of a Member State.

One effect of the growth in regulatory interest has been an increase in the detail of documentation required for the entire clinical trial supplies process and a consequent extension of the lead time needed between placing an order and receiving the supplies. A clinical trial can be invalidated by poorly prepared supplies or by an inability to produce adequate documentation of the history of those supplies. It should be expected that, when assessing a marketing authorisation application (MAA) for a product following the completion of clinical trials, the regulatory body will scrutinise these data closely. Meticulous patience in this respect is a good investment.

The impact of this lead time on the study can be reduced if preparations start sufficiently early. Good communication and co-operation between the medical and clinical trial supplies groups will yield dividends in terms of prompt start-up, well-designed patient packs, and management of expiry dates of supplies while they are 'out in the field'.

PLACING AN ORDER FOR CLINICAL TRIAL SUPPLIES

In most companies, an order for clinical trial supplies must be placed by the study manager or by the physician responsible for the study. Practice and procedures may vary from company to company. In some cases the supplies will be prepared locally and in others they will be sent from a foreign affiliate or from an external contract manufacturer. In almost every case, however, the information required will be similar, although format and timing may vary. As a general rule, it is never too early to discuss clinical trial requirements with the supplies group. The following details and documents will almost certainly be needed at some stage, and it is better to err on the side of too much information rather than too little:

- name and strength of product(s), including placebo and comparator (if any);
- dosage form (tablet, capsule, etc.);
- number of subjects;
- dose and duration of treatment;

- study design (double-blind, cross-over, etc.);
- location of study;
- starting date of study;
- estimated completion date (important for shelf-life of products);
- availability of regulatory and ethical approval;
- pack size (one–week, one–month supplies) and overage (if any);
- name of person responsible for the study;
- address for dispatch of supplies; and
- copy of the study protocol.

MANUFACTURE OF CLINICAL TRIAL SUPPLIES

The manufacturing process and its consequences vary depending on the development stage of the product. Phase I supplies, for example, are often manufactured for a particular study and used within a short time period because very few stability data are available and these studies are of short duration. At the other end of the development timetable, Phase III and Phase IV supplies generally closely resemble the marketed product, are manufactured in large batches and are held in stock against future orders.

The formulation and manufacturing process often changes during the development of a product, and this has implications for the conduct of clinical trials. A product may enter Phase I as a simple solution or suspension, evolve into a capsule for Phase II, become compressed into a tablet in Phase III, and acquire a film coat for the market. Such changes are acceptable, even necessary, in order to produce a dosage form that is suitable for the market and for large-scale manufacture, but the changes must be supported by appropriate data, particularly relating to bioequivalence. In some cases, when the drug is readily soluble, dissolution data may be sufficient to demonstrate that two products are equivalent, but in most instances, bioavailability data will be required. It may be possible to demonstrate this in animals, but often data from human subjects will be needed. Careful planning and close co-operation between formulators and clinicians will avoid the expense of unnecessary bioequivalence studies. Sometimes the data can be collected as part of an ongoing clinical study, but there must be good *in-vitro* evidence for equivalence before a new dosage form is introduced into a study. Serious clinical effects can result if the new product is significantly more or less bioavailable than the original.

More subtle changes may be less easy to detect and can lead to problems when additional supplies are ordered. It is not uncommon for two visually identical capsules to contain the same drug in the same dose but in a different formulation. Changes may become necessary in order to manufacture the product on large-scale equipment at high speed; for example, it may be necessary to increase the lubricant content for tablet punching. Stability issues may also necessitate alteration of the formulation. Requests for additional supplies for an ongoing study should therefore be very specific to ensure that the correct formulation is provided. Some companies use formulation numbers or codes which should be referenced in any order. Others rely on cross-referencing to previous supplies for a particular study, and thus the reference number of the previous supply should be quoted on any new orders.

As stated earlier, it is expected that clinical trial supplies will be manufactured according to GMP. This ensures that cross-contamination is avoided and that there is full traceability of all ingredients as well as of the finished product. Stability studies will be performed to ensure that the product remains within specification during its shelf-life under the recommended storage conditions. These stability studies have implications for the packaging of clinical trial supplies (see below).

BLINDING OF CLINICAL TRIAL SUPPLIES

Since most clinical studies are conducted under double-blind conditions, it is desirable that the treatments should be identical in appearance. This is usually relatively easy to achieve for the manufacturer's own product and matching placebo. For example, identical capsule shells can be filled with different doses of the test drug or placebo. Alternatively, it is often possible to produce tablets of identical size but containing different doses of drug. There are pitfalls to this approach, however, which may preclude such a neat solution. For example, drug substances which are coloured may result in tablets of different hue, according to dose, due to the various other constituents such as lactose or starch used to generate tablets of similar size. More seriously from a therapeutic standpoint, differences in bioavailability may result from inevitable differences in formulation in the attempt to achieve identical dosage forms.

A greater difficulty arises when a comparator drug is needed to match the test drug. Several options are available but all take time and have potentially serious disadvantages. The first option, if the comparator product is off-patent, may be to purchase bulk drug substance and formulate a product to match the one under test. This requires a full formulation development effort, culminating in a bioequivalence study with a commercial brand of the drug in question. Analytical data and stability methods will be needed, and the total development time is unlikely to be less than 12 months. This is an expensive and time-consuming option.

A second approach, often regarded as a short-cut, is to purchase the commercial brand of the required drug, crush or grind the tablets/capsules, sieve to remove fragments of capsule shell or coating material, and then fill into capsules of the company's choice. On occasion, the ground material may even be compressed into tablets. This approach can be successful, but the pitfalls are large and deep:

- stability data will be needed on the reprocessed product;
- bioequivalence with the original product will need to be demonstrated;
- modified-release products cannot be treated in this way because the grinding/crushing will disrupt the mechanism controlling release of the drug;
- the original manufacturer may challenge the validity of the data on the reprocessed product.

A less dramatic option, which is quicker and cheaper if the comparator product is of a suitable size, is to 'blind' it by placing it intact inside an opaque capsule shell, perhaps with some inert filler such as starch or lactose to prevent rattling. In these circumstances, bioequivalence data are unlikely to be necessary although disintegration/dissolution testing should be performed. Similarly, stability is unlikely to be seriously affected unless the product is moisture-sensitive. Tests should be performed to confirm the stability of the blinded product, although it may be possible to start the study on the basis of short-term stability data, provided that longer-term tests are conducted concurrently.

If the product is too large to fit inside a capsule shell (not uncommon), the apparently simple solution of breaking the tablet in half should be viewed with caution. Such action may, perhaps surprisingly, have a significant effect on the bioavailability of the product. This is almost inevitable if it is a controlled-release formulation. In addition, care must be taken to ensure that both halves of the *same* tablet go into one capsule shell. Tablets seldom break into two identical halves and therefore failure to keep matching halves together could lead to serious variation in the administered dose. It should be noted further that inserting a half tablet into a capsule shell is not usually a satisfactory method of achieving a lower dose. All dosage units supplied for use in a clinical trial must meet pharmacopoeial standards for dose uniformity. As these apply to the whole tablet only, it will be highly unusual for broken tablets to satisfy these requirements. Finally, although this technique is very simple, it is also very labour-intensive because the capsules often have to be filled by hand. The manufacture of 20 000 capsules, each containing a single tablet or capsule, is likely to require great dedication by the clinical trial supplies staff.

Other techniques that have been used to blind solid dosage forms for clinical trial supplies have included press-coating of tablets, film-coating and use of cachets. All suffer from disadvantages related mainly to the need for stability data, bioequivalence data, or both. The only way to avoid this is to adopt a double-dummy design and ask the originator of the comparator product to supply matching active product and placebo. This has the advantage of shifting the responsibility to someone else, but the counterbalance is that the control of the process has also moved to another organisation. Although most companies would not deliberately delay supplying clinical trial products to another, such an activity is unlikely to be high on their list of priorities. Consequently, if they have a conflict of resources, manufacture or shipment is likely to be postponed in favour of their own trials.

In order to satisfy GMP and good clinical practice (GCP) requirements, as well as regulatory commitments to an investigational new drug (IND) application or clinical trial exemption (CTX), it is necessary to have certificates of analysis from the supplying company to confirm that the products comply with the specification and that the active product is identical, except in appearance, to the commercial product. As the product does not originate in-house, it may also be reassuring for the receiving company to have a simple identity test to confirm that active and placebo have not been confused.

Blinding of dosage forms other than tablets and capsules can be even more difficult. Oral liquids usually have a distinctive taste and/or smell, which the manufacturer attempts to mask with flavouring agents. It is seldom possible to achieve an identical match with a placebo or comparator product and so a compromise must be accepted. The usual approach is to match the tastes as closely as possible and to ensure that no product is significantly 'nicer' or 'nastier' than the other to keep subjects from identifying the test product. To achieve this, the placebo can be given the taste characteristics of the active product (e.g. bitterness) by using appropriate flavouring agents.

Injections are relatively simple to blind if they are water-white solutions, but if the drug is naturally coloured, ethical considerations preclude the inclusion of a colouring agent in the placebo or comparator product, even if a colour match were possible by such means.

It is also possible for inhalers to be blinded. This is a specialist technique carried out by some contract manufacturers. The difficulty arises in effectively dismantling the units, removing the active product and replacing it with an inactive powder, such as lactose, prior to re-assembly.

Medical devices, such as intra-vaginal devices and insulin pens, are now much more commonly used in the context of clinical research activities. Attempting to blind such products is difficult and provides a significant challenge to the imagination of the study designers.

It should be remembered that blinding refers only to the physical and organoleptic characteristics of the product, and that the blind may be broken very quickly when the subject starts to use the product. For example, some drugs produce very specific side-effects or have a distinctive physiological effect, such as colouring the urine. It is impossible to match such effects in the placebo or comparator products.

Although double-blind studies are probably the 'ideal', single-blind studies can be very effective, especially when the investigator (or assessor) is blinded. Use of this type of study should be considered in the early phases of development when it may be difficult to justify expending great effort on achieving well-matched clinical trial supplies.

OBTAINING COMPARATORS

If it is decided that comparator products will be sought from another company, it is helpful to follow some simple guidelines. In this specific context, the need for good communication becomes very clear indeed. The monitor or physician responsible for the study must liaise closely with the clinical trial supplies group in order to determine exactly the requirements of both companies. Most companies are willing to supply products for clinical trial use to another company and all require similar information to assess the request. In this process it will be necessary to:

- Calculate the quantity of product required for the study. This must include analytical samples, retention samples, overage to allow for subjects who drop out, packaging losses, and variable dosages or intervals between subject visits.
- Send a copy of the protocol, or at least a draft, to the company being approached to supply the comparator.
- Request details of any analytical tests that may need to be performed (identity, assay if more than one strength).
- Request a reference standard of the active ingredient for identity test purposes.
- Request certificates of analysis and a statement to confirm that the formulation is the one required (usually the commercial formulation).
- Request details of recommended packaging materials or confirmation that the product will be stable in the packaging proposed for the study.
- Recognise that the other company will expect sight of the results of the study before publication.
- Recognise that the other company will expect to be notified of any adverse events that could be attributed to its product.

It is always best to contact the supplying company by telephone first to determine if such a request is likely to be considered and whether there will be a charge for the supplies. This is also the ideal opportunity to find out the probable lead time for the supplies. In practice, it can take up to 3 months to obtain medical approval and 6–9 months for the supplies to be made and delivered. The request for supplies may be submitted by either the medical or the clinical trial supplies group, but both should discuss the request to ensure that it is accurate and has included all the relevant details.

If the comparator is to be supplied from another country, it will be necessary to ensure that importation of the product is legal and that it may be used in the countries of choice for the clinical study. If it is sourced from outside the EC, analytical testing on importation is a requirement of the regulatory bodies. Following tests in the country of entry, however, further testing is not necessary if the product is subsequently to be sent to other EC countries. Advice should be sought from the regulatory departments in both companies.

It is not unheard of for a company to purchase a comparator product on the open market and then repackage it to suit the demands of the clinical trial. This is often the case if the new drug is challenging the market leader. The other company may not be willing to supply its expensively researched and manufactured drug to a company intent on ousting it from its market position with a new, alternative treatment. By the same token, the company conducting the trial may wish to preserve a certain degree of confidentiality regarding the therapeutic areas in which it is interested. On repackaging the materials, this type of approach faces the same stability challenges that have already been discussed.

PACKAGING

The presentation of clinical trial supplies can play a crucial role in creating a professional image, influencing subject compliance and ensuring the integrity and quality of the product. Packaging is therefore an important factor for consideration and should be discussed with the clinical trial supplies group at an early stage to avoid confusion later.

The existence or absence of stability data is often the deciding factor when selecting a particular type of packaging for a clinical trial. If something special is needed, this requirement should be identified in good time so that the studies necessary to support the use of the pack can be initiated. Most companies prefer to use only one or two types of packaging in order to simplify the support work needed. These are usually a bottle-type pack and a blister pack. It is important to remember that if stability data in the actual pack of choice are not available, it is highly unlikely that the pack can be used.

There are many types of blister material, all with different characteristics, of which the most significant are probably moisture permeability and cost. As a general rule (although it is an oversimplification), the better the moisture barrier, the higher the cost. An increasingly important factor is the environmental impact of the material, and cost may be related more to ease of recycling than to packaging performance.

Blister packs have the advantage of offering protection to each individual dosage unit. There is no danger of spilling the rest when one is removed from the pack, and no risk that the remaining contents will become contaminated. Such packs can also provide a reminder to the subject to take a dose through the use of 'calendar' type printing on the blister card to act as an *aide mémoire* and thus improve compliance. However, subjects who lack manual dexterity may find blister packs difficult to use and in some countries (e.g. the USA) this presentation is unusual and consequently may not be appropriate. Indeed, if blister packs are used in the USA, the FDA now prefers them to be child-resistant. Manufacturers have found this issue difficult to resolve. The disadvantage of such packs is that they are more complicated to produce, often require external contracting, and can be relatively bulky.

Bottles, by contrast, are quick and cheap to prepare and are relatively compact. However, they can be abused by subjects who may leave the cap off (especially if it is child-resistant, as preferred for bottles in the USA) or spill the contents.

The decision on an appropriate pack design for a particular study should be made as a result of discussion between the medical and pharmaceutical experts, taking into account the needs of the trial subjects, the characteristics of the product, the preferences of the investigator/pharmacist and staff, and the accountability checking which may need to be done by the study monitor. Common sense can be a good asset in such decisions; for example, a child-resistant bottle will not be the most suitable packaging for a trial involving a new treatment for arthritis.

A particular packaging problem arises in relation to comparator products. Even if a study is single-blind (i.e. there is no manipulation of the comparator to make it identical to the test product), the packaging will probably need to be identical for all components. There is the risk therefore that a competitor product will be distributed for use in the clinical trial in packaging different from that in which it is marketed. This means that stability studies will be needed to support the use of this packaging and therefore analytical methods will need to be obtained or developed. Adequate time must be allowed for this in the preparation stages of the study. The European Community guide to GMP demands that, on completion of such tests, the sponsor should not issue an expiry date in the new packaging that is any later than that in the original packaging. Alternatively, in the absence of suitable stability data, expiry must not exceed 25% of the remaining shelf-life of the product or 6 months, whichever is shorter.

Injectable products present a special challenge since it is impossible to pack a competitor product into ampoules or vials matching one's own 'house' style. It is also highly unlikely that the other company will be willing to make supplies in ampoules or vials that differ significantly from their own. Alternative approaches therefore must be adopted. This may involve formulating the comparator in-house, with all the attendant development costs, or designing secondary packaging so that all products are in identical cartons. If the product is administered by a different individual from the one performing the clinical assessment (e.g. nurse v. physician), the blindness of the study may be maintained. This technique is known as the double-observer method.

The need for drug accountability under GCP has led to the development of sophisticated packaging to facilitate the reconciliation of returned supplies. This is often costly, and the value of expending so much time and effort should be questioned. Once a pack has been handed to a subject, accountability becomes almost meaningless since there is no guarantee that the subject has taken all the units extracted from the pack. The main purpose of account-ability is to be sure that supplies were used for the declared clinical study; the exercise therefore relates to the bulk supplies and the distribution of subject packs. Counting of tablets returned by subjects is of dubious value although apparently advocated by some regulatory authorities. Whatever level of accountability is selected for a particular study, the checking of supplies at the investigator site is the responsibility of the study monitor. At the conclusion of the study, it is usually most efficient if the monitor and another individual (often the pharmacist at the hospital) check and record the quantity of the supplies remaining. It is not generally appropriate to return them to the clini-cal trial supplies group, and it is often possible to arrange destruction locally, after the documentation process. If this is not convenient but is nonetheless required, it may be helpful to use an external contractor in these circum-stances. If the supplies are destroyed, it must be in accordance with local health, safety and environmental requirements, and a certificate of destruc-tion must be retained in the study files.

Another aspect to have received lively attention is the assessment of subject compliance. This has driven the development of novel packs with the aim of improving or monitoring compliance. Most of these devices are expensive and use modern microelectronics to provide the reminding or monitoring function. Devices have been developed which give an audible signal, record the time of opening the bottle, or release the container lid at specific times. Careful consideration should be given to the objectives of the study before deciding to use such devices because they are not typical of the type of pack used by the average patient. There is a risk that compliance will be different from that achieved when the product is used in routine medical practice.

A recent addition to the clinical trials 'toolbox' has been the development of interactive voice response systems (IVRS). These sophisticated information technology systems bring the world's telephone networks and advanced computing technologies together in a single easy-to-use data collection and reporting system. Subjects can dial in and use the numbers on their telephone keypads to answer pre-recorded questions covering everything from compli-ance to adverse reactions. The information can be automatically forwarded to the investigator and onwards to the sponsor, thereby giving up-to-the-minute information on the trial.

LABELLING

The labelling of clinical trial supplies can be a source of major discussion and/or confusion between the clinical trial supplies staff and those running the study. This is because it has often been impossible to label clinical trial supplies strictly in accordance with the regulations for labelling pharmaceuti-cal products and, until recently, there have been relatively few regulations specifically covering clinical trial supplies. However, for supplies in Europe, useful guidance is given in Annex 13 of the European Community guide to GMP (*see Further Reading*).

It is always advisable to contact the registration/regulatory group within the company, preferably at the appropriate affiliate office, to confirm any regulatory requirements for labelling. However, it must be made clear that the question relates to clinical trial supplies and not to commercial products. A degree of flexibility may be needed in interpreting the requirements in order to satisfy both the law and the needs of the clinical trial. In order to avoid possible conflict with local labelling policies within hospitals, the pharmacy at the study site should be consulted whenever possible.

In general, labels should carry the following information:

- name of the sponsor;
- pharmaceutical dosage form;
- route of administration;
- reference to the study or protocol number (allowing identification of the trial site and investigator);
- the name and address of the supplying organisation;
- a means of identifying the product and its batch number (usually a combination of the study number and the subject number);
- directions for the trial subject (where appropriate);
- a statement that the product is 'For clinical trial use only';
- storage conditions;
- the period of use (expiry or re-test date);
- the words 'Keep out of reach of children', except where the product is for use only in hospital.

Annex 13 of the GMP guide allows some leeway in the labelling of product packaging, depending on the information given on the outer packaging.

Some countries have special labelling requirements or require specific wording to be included on the label. Most of this information will be available from the clinical trial supplies group, which can advise on sensible, legal label design. The European Clinical Trials Directive also specifies that at least the outer packaging must have labelling in the national language of the country where the trial is to be conducted. It makes good sense to have all labels in the native language of the subject and therefore, in multinational studies, translations will be needed. The compact and concise nature of the language used on pharmaceutical labels requires special skill, and translations must be sought from native speakers of the language(s) in question.

The need for greater efficiency in clinical trial supplies manufacture has led to the use of multilingual labels and booklet labels. These are apparently unpopular with some authorities, and acceptance may depend on whether 'their' country's language is on the front of the booklet or is most prominent on the multilingual label.

The need to be able to break the code of a blinded study in an emergency has stretched the imagination of clinical trial supplies groups and label manufacturers. Several options have been developed and many may be of value in some circumstances. The most obvious and simple means of providing code-break information is to print an emergency 24–hour telephone number on the label. However, this can lead to problems if trial subjects attempt to use it to gain extra information about the study and the drugs being used.

A more sophisticated solution is the use of labels with a special pouch containing the identity of the medication in the pack. The pouches work in the same way as salary envelopes, and must be torn open to reveal the information. Thus there is no risk that subjects or investigators will cheat by breaking the code covertly. Another simple option is the use of scratch-off panels on the label.

IVRS can also be used as an unblinding tool. It is password-protected to eliminate accidental unblinding of the trial and its use can instantly notify the sponsor and initiate immediate follow-up.

Ultraviolet (UV) ink to mark packs with an identifier has also been used to a limited extent. These inks can be read only under UV light and therefore the information is invisible under normal circumstances. It should be recognised, however, that there is a small risk that the pack may be exposed to UV light unexpectedly (e.g. in a discothèque), causing the code to be broken inadvertently. Such inks can be used to good effect during the packing operation if packing of the product is performed separately from labelling. The unlabelled packs can be marked with this 'invisible' ink and then checked at the labelling stage to confirm that the correct packs have been used. The label may then be affixed over the ink since it has fulfilled its purpose. However, the use of these inks is uncommon and cannot be used as a substitute for good traceability through the manufacturing documentation.

Special labels can also be used to document the supply of medication to the subject. If subjects receive medication at more than one visit, it is important to assess that all their supplies relate to the same randomisation and that an individual who starts on drug A does not mistakenly receive drug B halfway through the trial. If the supplies are prepared with multiple-part labels, a 'flag' can be detached from the pack at the time of dispensing and attached to the case record form. This label will provide confirmation that the correct subject number or kit number was dispensed.

DOCUMENTATION

In order to comply with GMP and GCP requirements and to provide total traceability within the company concerning the preparation and fate of clinical trial supply materials, it is essential to fully and accurately document the preparation, packaging and labelling of the supplies for any particular study. Good version control of documents is imperative because instructions may change as the development of the product progresses.

Documentation may take a variety of forms but must specify all the relevant details and must contain the signatures of all the individuals who performed specific tasks. In order to make it easier to identify these individuals in the future, by which time they may have left the company, it is useful to maintain a signature log of all those who sign such documents, in any capacity. This should include the person's full name (printed), their usual signature and usual initials.

Documents for manufacturing operations should be written in the form of instructions that are easy to follow and be such that the individual performing the operation can sign against the instruction to indicate its completion. The documents must include the unit and batch formula of the product and the batch numbers of all the ingredients used. In some cases it will be necessary to record in-process readings such as time, temperature, pH, etc. Reconciliation should occur at the end of the manufacture, packaging and labelling operations, and abnormal discrepancies must be investigated. Packaging documentation should specify the name of the product, the type of packaging components used, and the number or quantity of product in each pack. A sample of the label applied to the packs should be attached to the packaging documentation and this should be approved by an appropriate, responsible person to confirm that all labelling requirements have been met and that the instructions on the label are accurate. It is expected that intense quality control (QC) checks will be performed during the labelling operation. Self-inspection or independent audit of the whole manufacturing process is integral to the quality assurance (QA) system.

All documentation should be reviewed by an independent person, at least before the product is released for use. This independent person should be unconnected with the actual manufacturing or packaging process, and in many companies will be a member of the QA/QC department. The European Clinical Trials Directive demands that a Qualified Person of appropriate experience and qualifications (as specified in Directive 75/319/EEC) should carry out a review of batch documents as well as quality control of batch manufacture.

Ideally, the documents should be reviewed (and signed) before the manufacturing/packaging process starts, and again on completion when all the signatures and in-process readings will be in place. For an external contract manufacturing/packaging operation, initial sign-off by the contract giver is an essential part of the process because seemingly straightforward requirements are often interpreted quite differently from what was intended.

Documentation should also record the location of the operation and the identification of any equipment used. This helps to trace cross-contamination, if it is found at any stage, and to ensure that if equipment is found to be faulty, all those materials processed using it can be traced. It is helpful to have logs to record equipment and room usage to avoid the need to search through individual batch records in the event of a problem.

Stock cards (or an equivalent computer system) should be maintained for each batch of product, drug substance and excipient used in clinical trial supplies, and dispatch records should show the details of each shipment, including product(s), quantity, destination, date and time of dispatch, and method of dispatch. Written confirmation of receipt should be retained with these records.

The European Community guide to GMP expects all batch-related documents to be retained by the manufacturer/packager for at least 2 years following the conclusion or discontinuation of the trial to which they pertain. It should also be noted that following manufacture, there is a requirement in Europe for samples of blinded investigational medicinal products to be retained.

EXPIRY DATING

All pharmaceutical products have a limited shelf-life, and it is usual for commercially marketed products to be marked with an expiry date on the label, in accordance with the product licence. Expiry dating of repackaged comparators has been described earlier. During a drug's development, however, supplies may be provided for use in a clinical trial before extensive stability data have been gathered. This limits the shelf-life that can be claimed for the product, although the shelf-life may be extended as more data become available. This poses a dilemma: should the supplies be marked with a relatively short expiry date, in accordance with current information, even though they may be suitable for use for a much longer period? Or should no expiry date be declared and reliance placed instead on recalling the supplies when they are no longer suitable for use?

The decision on how to resolve this problem must lie with each individual company and will depend to a large extent on the systems used for tracking supplies and on the resources available for updating the expiry date, if necessary. The advantage of an expiry date on the subject pack is that it is fail-safe. The subject will be alerted to the fact that the product may not be suitable for use and will either contact the investigator or, if the supplies have been lurking at the back of the medicine cabinet for some time, will dispose of them. If no date is present, there is nothing to warn the subject or to serve as a reminder that the product is getting old.

Updating clinical trial supplies that have had an extension to their expiry date is a difficult task and requires either the return of all supplies to the company for relabelling (an expensive exercise) or the provision of new labels to be attached to the packs at the investigator site. This activity is usually coordinated and controlled by the study monitor, but in some circumstances it may be advisable for a member of the clinical trial supplies group to visit the investigator site and supervise relabelling. The operation should always be checked by a second person. It is important that the addition of the new label with date and batch number does not cover the original batch number, although the old expiry date may be covered. The use of additional labels should be described in the trial documentation and in the batch records.

DISPATCH OF SUPPLIES

Clinical trial supplies are very valuable, not necessarily because of their intrinsic monetary worth, which is usually difficult to estimate at this stage, but because they are often in short supply. In Phase I/II it may take several months to produce enough drug substance to make more clinical trial product and so losses in transit must be avoided at all costs. Distribution of supplies to investigator sites should be covered by documented procedures and must be handled through reputable and reliable carriers. Signed documentation of all transactions should be retained so that the history of the supplies can be traced through a complete paper trail. Receipt of supplies should be acknowledged and non-delivery investigated promptly. Most carriers now perform computer tracking of deliveries and so the location of a shipment at a particular point in time should be easy to determine. If it is necessary to move supplies between investigator sites, company procedures must be followed and the details carefully recorded. It is often advisable to contact the clinical trial supplies unit for advice because labelling requirements may vary between sites.

Special storage requirements should be clearly marked on the outside of all shipping cartons, and investigators should be notified in advance so that suitable arrangements for correct storage can be made. It should be remembered that most pharmacies or investigator sites have limited storage capacity, and it may be helpful to send the supplies for a large study in several smaller shipments at appropriate intervals. If refrigerated storage is necessary and transportation is not directly under the company's control, it may be advisable to use temperature-sensitive strips in the shipment to monitor the conditions to which the goods are exposed. If a box is off-loaded from an aircraft in the tropics, the recommended storage conditions can be exceeded quite quickly, but without monitoring strips this might never be detected. Similar problems can occur at the other end of the temperature range during northern winters when products may be subjected to sub-zero temperatures, which can be equally damaging to sensitive products such as vaccines and aerosols. It may be necessary to carry out a 'dummy delivery' to the investigator site using the chosen packaging with a temperature recorder inside to give assurance as to the suitability of the chosen transportation arrangements.

For international shipments, great care must be taken with the documentation to ensure that delays are not encountered in customs. It has been known for all the containers of a double-blind study to be opened by over-zealous customs officials who did not understand the word 'placebo'. Care in preparing the documentation should minimise such risks although it is unlikely that they can be eliminated completely. For this reason, tamper-evident packaging is highly desirable. It is also helpful to attach a packing note to the outside of shipping cartons to assist identification by customs officials or at the receiving warehouse. A contact name and telephone number of the originator can also help to explain the shipment.

Within Europe, international tariff numbers are used to identify products by category, and use of the correct number will greatly facilitate a shipment's passage through customs. Shipping documentation also needs to state the value of a shipment, but it is usually difficult to assign a realistic value to clinical trial supplies. The true monetary value is seldom known during the early stages of development, and since the product cannot be sold because it is unlicensed, the question of the commercial value of the shipment does not arise. Most companies have a policy for assigning a value for customs purposes, and the clinical trial supplies group will work in conjunction with the finance or export department to ensure that the correct value is declared.

Another consideration when transporting clinical trial supplies is the potentially hazardous nature of some materials. It is unlikely that most tablets or capsules would present a serious hazard if spilt in transit, but liquids may be corrosive and broken glass is a hazard in itself. International regulations concerning the shipment of hazardous goods must be observed.

It is important to recognise the special requirements for transportation of supplies originating outside Europe. The importation of clinical trial supplies from outside Europe for use within is allowed, provided that a Qualified Person has reviewed the batch documentation and its quality control and has been satisfied that the supplies have been manufactured according to the principles of GMP. It is expected that this will include full analytical testing.

DISPOSAL OF CLINICAL TRIAL SUPPLIES

At the end of a clinical study surplus drug supplies may remain with the investigator or supplies may be returned from subjects who have participated in the study. These supplies must be accounted for and destroyed in an appropriate manner. It is expected by the regulatory authorities that returns should be destroyed only after trial completion and compilation of the final report. All drug products that have been dispensed to subjects must be destroyed if unused. It is not possible to guarantee the quality of these returns and so they cannot be used for other subjects or studies. Unopened packs stored in a controlled manner at the investigator site may be re-usable if absolutely necessary, but the preferred option is to destroy them. The savings to be made by re-using supplies seldom outweigh the hazards of sorting out blinded supplies. Re-use is generally only acceptable for studies involving very expensive products or when subjects are running short and further supplies are unobtainable. Open-label supplies are easier to use elsewhere, but the quality of the product must be assured. If there is any doubt, destruction is the safest option. However, there may be restrictions concerning the retention of all surplus materials until the study has been analysed and reported. Regulatory affairs departments can provide advice on this aspect.

Destruction of unwanted supplies must be documented and should be performed either by returning the supplies to the company, often to the clinical trial supplies unit, or by arranging destruction locally and obtaining certification of the fact. Incineration is generally recommended but this should comply with all the appropriate legislation, particularly that relating to environmental issues. If there is any doubt about the appropriate method of destruction, environmental health or waste disposal officers at the local authority should be consulted.

CONCLUSION

The conduct of clinical trials is one of the most expensive aspects of the development of new medicinal products. It is important, therefore, that the studies should produce high-quality data in the shortest possible time. More companies are trying to use single, larger, complicated trials in an attempt to gain the greatest amount of information about a product and thus reduce the lead time to market. A key element in ensuring this goal is the close cooperation between those responsible for the clinical aspects of the study and those responsible for the provision of the clinical trial supplies. As stated at the start of this chapter, communication is everything. Clinical trial supplies units can provide valuable support and advice: this will help ensure that supplies are obtained on time and packaged in a way that is convenient for the subject and the investigator. Only by such co-operation can new products be developed efficiently for the benefit of patients.

FURTHER READING

Directive 75/319/EEC (1975). Council directive on the approximation of provisions laid down by law, regulation or administrative action relating to medicinal products.
EudraLex (1998a). *The Rules Governing Medicinal Products in the European Union. Volume 4: Good Manufacturing Practice – Medicinal Products for Human and Veterinary Use*, European Commission, Brussels.

EudraLex (1998b). *The Rules Governing Medicinal Products in the European Union. Volume 4, Annex 13: Manufacture of Investigational Medicinal Products*, European Commission, Brussels.

European Parliament and Council Directive (2000). Common Position adopted by the Council with a view to the adoption of a Directive of the European Parliament and of the Council on the approximation of the laws, regulations and administrative provisions of the Member States relating to the implementation of good clinical practice in the conduct of clinical trials on medicinal products for human use. (Procedure number: COD 1997/0197. Common Position document date: 20 July 2000.)

Food and Drug Administration (1991). *Guidelines on the Preparation of Investigational New Drug Products (Human and Animal)*, FDA, Washington.

HMSO (1968). *The Medicines Act 1968*, Her Majesty's Stationery Office, London.

Howieson, G and Scaiff, C (2000). Child resistant packaging. *Clin Res Focus* **11**, 4–6.

Medicines Control Agency (1997). *Rules and Guidance for Pharmaceutical Manufacturers and Distributors 1997* (also known as the *Orange Guide*), The Stationery Office, London. (The UK version of EudraLex Volume 4, containing all the Annexes and defining the roles and responsibilities of the Qualified Person.)

11

Investigator selection

Shirley Wildey

INTRODUCTION

The aim of this chapter is to introduce clinical research personnel to the importance of selecting the right investigator and team for a clinical trial in order that the trial is conducted within agreed timelines and to the highest standards. Time spent on obtaining meaningful feasibility information and giving due consideration to the site selection process will be rewarded when the study is recruited on time with few drop-outs.

IDENTIFICATION OF INVESTIGATORS

Traditional methods

The important consideration when selecting investigators is to identify and recruit those who are competent and motivated to conduct the trial according to the protocol, within the agreed timelines and in compliance with good clinical practice (GCP) guidelines. Tried and tested over many years, the *traditional sources* for identifying potential investigators include company databases, marketing colleagues, literature searches and personal recommendation.

Company databases

Many companies have developed their own databases listing investigators by geographical region, therapeutic interest, clinical trial experience, research facilities and contact details. For many companies, this has become a global database that provides an opportunity to select investigators for international studies from a single source. It is important to take account of local data protection laws when storing personal data electronically, but this issue can be resolved by obtaining the investigators' signed agreement to their data being stored for the use of the company and its affiliates only. In some cases, these databases are linked to an investigator website, allowing investigators to enter data directly to the database and to accept responsibility for the update of that information.

Provided that the database is kept up to date, it can contain a wealth of information regarding the performance of the investigator in previous studies for the company. In some cases, the database can be linked to a clinical trial management package to provide important performance metrics. These may include an indication of number of data queries raised at the site, number of protocol violations, enrolment data, and start-up times, i.e. the amount of time from study initiation to first subject enrolled. The database will also alert clinical monitors if there are any ongoing studies at the site (for their own or other companies) that could cause conflict problems, both with regard to clinical trial populations and to prioritisation of workload.

Marketing colleagues

Marketing and sales colleagues will be able to provide lists of 'good prescribers' for a particular therapeutic area. These lists can be used to send a mailshot to doctors to sound out their interest in taking part in a clinical trial. Such doctors may not be experienced investigators but they may have an interest in the drug. It is useful to be able to train and nurture inexperienced but enthusiastic investigators because they often become the better trialists. Sales and marketing departments will always be able to recommend opinion leaders. For some drug development programmes, it is common to have external consultants and opinion leaders assigned to provide information and advice and to lend a prestigious name to subsequent publications. These experts may be able to suggest other possible investigators with a particular interest in a study or to provide a network of contacts to recommend new investigators.

Literature searches

Literature searches of published works in journals or on commercially available databases may locate key centres or doctors with relevant research interests and be an indicator of successful completion of previous clinical trials. The editorial board listed on the inside cover of a journal will indicate eminent experts in a given disease area. Medical directories in most countries list information on specialties, location and personnel involved in health services, with some details of individual interests. Previously archived studies may also reveal information about potential new investigators. Lists of attendees and speakers at conferences and congresses may prove helpful for mailings about the study to generate interest from doctors. Likewise, attendance by clinical research staff from the sponsor at such meetings is a productive way of making contacts with potential investigators.

Recommendations

Current investigators already selected for a study may provide a number of personal recommendations on others who may be interested in the study, and a network of contacts can be developed in this way. Some investigators may suggest colleagues within the same institution or other doctors with whom they have previously collaborated on other studies. Tracking the career of a junior doctor who has been a good co-investigator on a study may provide a first-rate principal investigator of the future.

With regard to investigators who have worked on previous company studies, it is helpful to discuss the overall performance of their sites with the monitors involved in those studies. A monitor's evaluation of an investigator's study conduct can be the most effective guide to identifying good investigators. There is no better way to identify potential investigators than personal recommendation.

Alternative strategies

As the health care industry has progressed over recent years to providing more information in the public domain, *alternative 'web-enabled' strategies* for identifying investigators have evolved in parallel with the more traditional approaches listed above.

Surfing the Net

In the USA it is common to advertise studies to physicians on the Internet and this practice is growing in Europe. A number of sites have been set up to target physicians and give lists of studies in which interested doctors can participate. This is an excellent method of attracting motivated investigators who have a population of patients not previously used in clinical trials, and it offers an option to move away from the professional trialist.

Data mining from commercial databases

A number of commercial databases are available that analyse prescription data collected across countries or regions. From prescription information, it is possible to drill down and identify investigators with a high volume of potential patients, enabling those to be targeted who have a high throughput of patients with the condition to be treated. Data mining may also provide an opening for contacting doctors who have the required patients but who have not yet had an opportunity to participate in clinical trials.

Using investigator networks

Instead of selecting individual investigators, a Site Management Organisation (SMO) or an investigator network may be used. These are commercial, profit-making organisations that provide groups of investigators or sites, and offer a centralised site management function with a focus on quality and efficiency of trial conduct.

SITE MANAGEMENT ORGANISATIONS

This section will describe the different models of SMOs and similar clinical investigator networks, and will consider their benefits and their suitability for undertaking clinical studies.

The SMO market place in Europe is relatively new and is expanding rapidly, currently accounting for a market share of 5% in clinical trial Phases II to IV (Getz, 1999a). The market place is not clearly defined and offers a mixture of models and practices, e.g. owned-site, network and hybrid. The type of model describes how the SMO operates in terms of identification, screening and recruitment of potential subjects. There are two basic varieties:

- The *owned-site* or *research site* model has its own centres where subjects are seen for study visits. The investigators may be employees of the SMO or contractors and will be supported by research nurses and administrative staff. In this model, it is possible to exert good management control of SMO sites. Subjects are recruited using a variety of approaches, e.g. database searching of referring practices and direct patient advertising. This model is particularly suitable for chronic stable diseases, e.g. osteoporosis, migraine, and hypertension but less so for acute diseases.
- The *network* model uses community physicians or general practitioners (GPs) as investigators, but again usually with the strong support of research nurses. The study visits are conducted at the GP surgery, with subjects recruited largely from the GP practice. This type of SMO has a regional co-ordination structure, offers site training/support, and quality assurance (QA) systems are in place. Subjects are recruited through database searches and following direct consultations with their doctor. In general, direct patient advertising is less effective in this model. The network model is particularly suitable for acute diseases, e.g. infections, and paediatric studies.

Other *hybrid* organisations exist alongside these two broad SMO models (Getz, 1999b). They combine aspects of both and are set up according to country-specific health care systems, culture and politics.

Most SMOs work in primary care and operate within a single country in Europe but the trend is for them to become multinational. Increasingly, some SMOs have also established links with secondary care, either for subcontracted services or as an additional source of potential subjects. A small number of SMOs work exclusively in secondary care.

Many SMOs originally specialised in a single therapeutic area, e.g. women's health. Almost all have grown beyond their origins and are now multispecialty operations. Generally, it is essential to consider SMOs, whether they focus on primary or secondary care, as capable of running studies in most therapeutic areas. In other words, a primary care SMO has the potential to run clinical trials in any disease area where subjects are actively managed by their GP.

SMOs can provide rapid start-up of studies across a network of sites. The protocol approval process is expedited because SMOs have developed relationships with and understand the requirements of ethics committees. They offer a single point of reference for all regulatory documentation. Importantly, they produce good feasibility for subject recruitment and routinely use a variety of recruitment strategies.

SMOs are a 'one-stop shop', offering a simplified process for negotiating contracts and investigator budgets. Instead of several financial agreements with all sites, the sponsor has a single contract with the SMO, which negotiates separately with its group of investigators.

SMOs will have their own standard operating procedures (SOPs) to describe their working practices and they provide efficient study management, with a project manager as the main communication contact. Their advantage over individual investigator sites is that they can be judged more easily on performance and quality and should be able to provide historical evidence of performance from previous similar studies, e.g. regarding data query rates and enrolment targets.

SELECTION CRITERIA

Now that the methods of searching for potential investigators have been identified, the selection criteria for the study will need to be defined so that a profile of investigator and site requirements can be built up.

Study phase

The study phase will dictate if the clinical trial should be conducted in a specialised clinical pharmacology unit or would be more suited to general practice.

Geographical location

The scope of the study will define whether sites need to be found in a single country, across several European countries or globally. Influence may be brought to bear by the marketing department to place the study in those countries where there is a priority for the product's current or future sales. The incidence of the disease indication in a particular country needs to be considered, with special reference to the local strategy for treating patients with that disease. For example, diabetic patients are well controlled in most countries in Western Europe due to the nature of the health care system there. This is different from the situation in Eastern European countries where the diabetic patient population is less well controlled. This influences site selection because potentially fewer sites could be required in Eastern than in Western Europe to achieve the same number of subjects.

Primary or secondary care

The patient management strategy within a country will determine whether the clinical trial population to be studied is found in primary care or in hospitals.

Patient population

The investigator should confirm that sufficient patients are to be found at the site for potential recruitment into the study. As a rule of thumb, because investigators are often over-optimistic about potential subjects and may be unaware of how they fit the eligibility criteria, recruitment numbers suggested by the investigators themselves should be halved. Realistic patient availability needs to be assessed by thorough feasibility checks at the site: historical recruitment should be reviewed and any factors that may influence patient suitability must be addressed.

Timelines

The timelines of the study can affect whether an investigator can reasonably take part and make an adequate contribution to the study. The starting date may fall at a time when the investigator is on holiday or away at a conference and no medical cover is available. There may be a conflict with another study starting at the site. All such factors need to be taken into account when selecting a site. Clear definition of the study timelines will enable the investigator to ensure that there are no conflicts in undertaking to participate in the study. If the recruitment period is to be shortened, the investigators need to understand the implications for their sites, themselves and their staffing levels.

Facilities and resources

Any specific type of equipment that will be needed at a site, e.g. specialised photographic equipment for an alopecia study, must be defined at the selection stage in order to check site suitability. If the equipment is to be provided to the site, there needs to be adequate space to store and use it.

Similarly, the investigator must have sufficient staffing levels to provide the clinical and administrative support required for the study to be conducted to the stipulated timelines. Investigators frequently underestimate the amount of work generated by a clinical trial and consider that their regular support team can cope with yet another study. Resources at sites may be constrained for many reasons, including competing studies, restricted timelines, anticipated high recruitment, or a high screening rate from advertising for patients. Such issues need to be discussed in depth with the investigator, and contingency plans must be drawn up for providing additional resources to the site, where necessary.

Regulatory constraints

Strong regulatory constraints may affect the ability of some sites and some countries to carry out the study. The length of time required for regulatory and ethics committee approval, both regionally and nationally, must be taken into account prior to investigator selection. If a study is seasonal, e.g. in seasonal allergic rhinitis, the approval time for the study may prohibit the involvement of certain countries if the resultant start date does not coincide with the start of the disease 'season'.

Financial arrangements

Although there are more important selection criteria, financial remuneration will inevitably be a deciding factor for the investigator. It is important to identify and exclude those investigators who are only interested in their own financial gain and who will participate in a study but may not produce the quality of data required within the stipulated timelines. Equally, fees need to be set at a level sufficient to reward investigators for their expertise and therapeutic specialism, and to encourage them to take part.

FEASIBILITY

To achieve the specified numbers of evaluable subjects, the selection of sites is critical to the success of the study. A good feasibility survey must be undertaken at an early stage in the selection process to ensure that a study can be conducted in the country or at the site of choice. The survey will gather and analyse data on the availability of potential subjects fulfilling the inclusion and exclusion criteria, realistic recruitment rates within stated timelines, current and comparator treatments, competitor studies, and regulatory and ethical issues. The initial feasibility survey may also check investigators for proven experience in trials in a particular indication. The questions asked must provide sufficiently well-founded responses to permit a decision on which countries and sites are to be used.

Good feasibility will make an immeasurable difference to a study. The monitor will feel confident about the site's capabilities and there should be fewer drop-outs and fewer site replacements due to poor or no recruitment. The feasibility survey should complete those parts of the selection process that can be performed by telephone, fax and e-mail prior to visiting the site for a site selection visit.

SITE SELECTION VISITS

Although some investigators may have been involved in the feasibility survey, not all investigators will have been approached about the study beforehand. Initial contact with these other investigators is usually by letter, outlining the rationale for the study, the type of product and its stage of development, a brief description of the study design, the type of study population and measurements involved, the approximate time schedule, other products to be used in the study, and any particular treatment to be used. Investigators need to be provided with sufficient information to decide whether they consider it worth proceeding to the site selection meeting.

It is essential to remember that collaboration on a clinical trial may last for several years and that establishing a good relationship with the investigator from the outset is of paramount importance to the success of the liaison. A telephone call to the site will confirm the correct form of address, not only with the investigator's correct title but including key qualifications.

Once an investigator has expressed interest, a confidentiality agreement, a summary protocol and other relevant information will be sent, and arrangements made for the site selection visit. Prior to the visit, a letter should be sent to the potential investigator, confirming the arrangements for the meeting, including an agenda for the discussion and indicating whether any other members of staff need to be present. It is also courteous to suggest the approximate duration of the visit to allow the investigator and site staff to book sufficient time in their diaries.

For optimum results, the meeting should be a two-way process in which the monitor needs to impart information to and obtain information from the investigator so that the latter's suitability can be assessed. Therefore, good verbal and non-verbal communication is vital to encourage the sharing of information rather than a one-sided presentation to the investigator.

Monitors must meticulously prepare for this first visit by familiarising themselves thoroughly with the preclinical and clinical development of the trial product and by re-reading the protocol to ensure that they feel confident about discussing it. It could be advantageous to provide a short summary of the investigator's brochure. The monitor should know the investigator's background and be *au fait* with the investigator's research interests, recent publications and any other facts that might lend a broader perspective by which to judge suitability. Such preparation will also help in developing a professional relationship, as the investigator will feel flattered at the interest shown.

The monitor must be absolutely clear on any aspects of the study that are not open to negotiation and on any study features that must be complied with by the site. It is important that these non-negotiables are emphasised during the site selection visit and that the investigator clearly understands their importance. Frequently, there can be pressure to recruit investigators too quickly, with the result that they are accepted as participants despite reservations about their commitment to the study schedule, for example, or to the number of subjects required.

The agenda for the site selection visit should cover the following points:

- Introduction to the study drug, including pharmacology (animal and human), toxicology, clinical development and regulatory status. The 10–minute summary of the investigator's brochure is useful at this point.
- Protocol review, focusing on eligibility criteria, randomisation/treatment allocation, safety and efficacy, adverse event reporting, required equipment and procedures, enrolment periods, treatment periods and follow-up visits.
- Discussion of subject recruitment issues, including estimates of the number of potential subjects who would be eligible for the study based on retrospective data over a specified time period. The investigator should be able to provide documented evidence, e.g. a database listing or clinic lists, where possible. The timelines should be discussed in detail, as should the obligations of the investigator to recruit the required number of subjects within those timelines. The meeting should establish how subjects are to be identified for participation in the study, e.g. from advertising, referrals from colleagues, etc. Similarly, the recruitment strategy needs to be defined in terms of whether the site will recruit in cohorts of subjects or in a steady flow.
- Case record forms (CRFs) and their completion.
- The qualifications of the investigator and support staff should be reviewed, together with the investigator's experience with similar studies and other clinical trials, particularly to identify any areas of potential conflict. The amount of resource available at the site must also be confirmed in case contingencies need to be developed to provide extra resource in order to carry out the study at the site. The responsibilities of the ancillary staff, e.g. pharmacist or dietitian, will also be identified and agreed at the site selection visit.
- The facilities at the site must be assessed as to their suitability for the study. This assessment should check the availability of special equipment and procedures for calibration and inspection, according to the manufacturer's schedules. Central/local laboratory requirements must also be reviewed at this stage.

- GCP and regulatory issues must be covered, including the informed consent process, investigator responsibilities with regard to GCP, insurance and indemnification issues, and regulatory approval.
- The name and address of the central/regional independent ethics committee (IEC) must be identified, and details of the approval process, including submission dates, must be discussed. The impact of ethics committee approval on the start date of the study will be clearly emphasised.
- The monitoring process must be explained, including frequency of visits, site contacts, availability of space, and source data verification (SDV) procedures.
- Arrangements for the study drug must be checked, including storage, handling and accountability. These aspects may be discussed with the appropriate site personnel, e.g. the hospital pharmacist.
- In reviewing the financial aspects, it is important to be clear whether the payment is a flat fee per subject or if there is some flexibility to negotiate with individual sites.

It is unlikely that all issues will be resolved at this initial meeting and a note should be made of any points outstanding that need to be dealt with, either before or at the study initiation meeting (*see Chapter 12*).

Following the selection visit, the monitor needs to consider critically the information collected in order to assess the suitability of the site for the study. Other colleagues involved with the study may be consulted in this process before making the decision to proceed or to reject the site. Although it can be embarrassing, the rejection of a site is not usually a major problem provided that the study specifications have been carefully explained at the outset. If there are any doubts over the suitability of a site, a decision to reject may be more appropriate than to proceed with a site that is not fully committed to the study. The monitor should not be forced into a decision because of time pressures or having to select a certain number of sites, otherwise sites that are not completely suitable will be included simply to make up the numbers.

Once the decision to continue has been made, the monitor should write to the investigator, informing him/her of the decision, detailing any agreed actions, and outlining the important issues and (if appropriate) the date of the next meeting.

INVESTIGATOR MEETINGS

It has become accepted practice to bring all investigators and support staff together for a joint meeting prior to study initiation. These meetings are an opportunity to explain GCP, the practicalities of the investigators' responsibilities, procedures for serious adverse event (SAE) reporting, CRF correction and query resolution, SDV and auditing. Investigator meetings provide an ideal platform for training the investigator in specific study procedures (e.g.

completion of rating scales), or for demonstrating study-specific techniques or systems (e.g. electronic data capture). Discussions amongst the assembled group of investigators can often identify problems with the protocol or other issues that have previously gone unnoticed. The meetings should address practical issues within the study, reinforce timelines, and be a good team-building exercise. If they are well conducted and held in a good location with excellent social arrangements, such meetings can be a key motivator for the investigators and a valuable public relations opportunity for the sponsor.

RETROSPECTIVE REVIEW OF THE SITE

Once the study has been completed, it is useful to review how the site has performed. Performance metrics are informative and provide a good indicator for selection of the site for future studies. It is useful to consider the requirements of the study at the selection stage and then to compare them with what the site actually achieved during the study. Typical parameters for review would include subject recruitment numbers, timelines, number of data queries, number of drop-outs, quality of laboratory samples, and adequacy of staffing and facilities.

If the investigator met the timelines, if there were few drop-outs, and if a good rapport existed between the site staff and monitor(s), the site was well selected. If there were major problems in finding suitable subjects, despite reassurances to the contrary from the investigator, and if insufficient staff were available to conduct the study, the site was definitely not suitable and should be considered carefully before being selected again. In reality, most sites perform somewhere between these two extremes and sound judgement needs to be exercised to assess whether performance was sufficiently good for the site to be recommended for future studies.

CONCLUSION

The selection of successful investigators is a difficult and time-consuming task that requires sound judgement. However, it is a critical exercise affecting the entire clinical research project and should not be undertaken without adequate training and support. When careful consideration and time are invested in the process, it can be a major factor contributing to the successful outcome of the clinical trial.

REFERENCES

Getz, K (1999a). SMOs invade Europe. *CenterWatch* **6**, 1–13.
Getz, K (1999b). The changing face of hybrid providers. *CenterWatch* **6**, 1–8.

12

Monitoring

John Illingworth

INTRODUCTION

This chapter will review the responsibilities, duties and procedures to be performed throughout the conduct of a clinical study by the monitor. Use of this role title is in accordance with the terminology of the ICH good clinical practice (GCP) guideline (ICH Guideline, 1996), although monitors are often referred to in the industry as clinical research associates, assistants, executives or scientists, with further sub-classification by seniority grade. Indeed, some aspects of the monitoring function may also be handled by people with more diverse job titles, e.g. clinical research co-ordinators, medical monitors, project managers and study managers.

This review will cover study preparation and pre-initiation activities, study conduct and monitoring during the active phase of the study, and study close-out or closure. The important topic of investigator selection is dealt with separately in *Chapter 11*. The intention here is to illustrate how the protocol, the paper document, is translated into a practical study involving human subjects.

In the sections that follow, the assumption is made that the relevant government approvals have been obtained from the appropriate regulatory agencies. This includes, for example, the clinical trial exemption (CTX) certificate in the UK or the Notice of Claimed Investigational Exemption for an investigational new drug (IND) in the USA.

Widespread agreement has now been reached concerning the responsibilities of the monitor's role and these are well documented both in the EC Note for Guidance on GCP (Committee for Proprietary Medicinal Products, 1991) and more recently in ICH Topic E6: Good Clinical Practice – Consolidated Guideline (ICH Guideline, 1996). However, monitors involved in international studies should be aware that specific local regulations or guidelines may also be applicable (*see Chapter 2*). In addition, monitors must comply with all internal sponsor standard operating procedures (SOPs). Potentially, there exists a large body of documentation of which the monitor must not only be aware but also have a sound working knowledge.

The monitor's role is one in which 'multi-tasking' is the norm. There is a responsibility not only to ensure that all study aspects are performed correctly according to all regulations and guidelines, together with any applicable local requirements, but also to cultivate good relationships, both with internal departments and with the study site staff. A positive relationship with the study site is vital for maximising co-operation and for ensuring the smooth running of the study. Starting with the very first visit, it is essential to develop a solid working relationship with the research team, and particularly with the research nurse and the clinical trials pharmacist, since these are the individuals at the study site who are also likely to be involved with the day-to-day running of the study. This can make the difference between a successful study and one that is hampered by poor execution and documentation. Effective communication between all involved is essential and the monitor has a pivotal role, often having to display consummate political skills to ensure optimal study performance.

STUDY PREPARATION

The steps followed during the preparation of a clinical study site prior to the initiation visits should be laid down in a sponsor SOP. This will direct the monitor not only during the visits themselves but also in the weeks (and sometimes months) leading up to them.

Once the decision has been made to use a certain site and investigator, the preparations can begin. At this stage the protocol may still be in an early draft form, in which case input from the investigator, research nurse and study site staff is invaluable. The first opportunity for such input will usually be at an investigator meeting organised specifically so that all the study site team can meet with sponsor staff to discuss and agree about the scientific and practical aspects of running the study. Feedback at this stage is often vital so that potential pitfalls can be avoided. Similarly, feedback should be sought on the draft case record forms (CRFs). However, for the purposes of this chapter, it will be assumed that a final agreed/approved protocol is available (*see Chapter 8*).

At one of the first pre-study visits, following site assessment but prior to initiation, the investigator should be given a copy of the investigator's brochure (IB) and its contents should be discussed and understood by all parties. It is essential to ensure that investigators who have previously used the investigational product possess the current version of the IB and that any recent changes are brought to their attention. This is particularly important for safety updates and information on the adverse event profile of the investigational product: in the early stages of product development, these sections of the IB are likely to be updated with each new version. The IB should be discussed not only with the principal investigator but also with the study site team, and particularly with those who will have day-to-day medical responsibility for the subjects in the trial. It is important that the instructions for handling the investigational product and any other trial-related materials (e.g. a drug delivery device) are clearly communicated to the study site team, either in the IB or in a separate document.

The final protocol should be discussed in detail with the entire study site team and should be signed by the investigator before it is submitted to the ethics committee (*see Chapter 3*). The patient information sheet and informed consent documents should also be ready at this stage because they need to be included in the submission to the ethics committee.

Depending on the particular study and the expected timelines for study initiation, the ordering and preparation of clinical trial supplies should be timed so that the study can start promptly once the formalities of correct documentation have been handled. This may mean that clinical trial supplies have to be ordered even before the submission for ethics committee approval. This is especially the case in large multinational companies whose clinical trial pharmacies may be dealing with several hundred studies at any one time. This aspect must be planned well in advance, and a six-month lead time for ordering clinical trial supplies is not uncommon. Randomisation codes should also be requested in a timely manner, since these will be required by the pharmacy preparing the supplies. Drug packaging may be performed either at the sponsor's own facility, at the study site, or possibly at another location by an independent contractor. However, a copy of the randomisation code may also need to be held by the investigator, study site pharmacist, and possibly others, depending on the study design. If the study is single-blind, unsealed codes may be provided; for double-blind studies, however, sealed and tamper-proof code breaks will be required. Specific instructions must also be provided to the study site concerning decoding procedures in an emergency; should this become necessary for any subject, the procedures must not allow the randomisation code for other subjects to be broken.

It is the monitor's responsibility to ensure that drug accountability forms required for the study are designed, ready in good time and understood by those who are responsible for completing them. Sponsor companies often have standard forms for this purpose but many studies require variations to the standard forms due to study-specific design features.

If external or central laboratories are to be used, whether for specialist tests or for standard safety tests such as routine clinical chemistry and haematology, the laboratories should be informed of the details of each study site and where and to whom laboratory supplies should be sent. This information must be provided well in advance so that dispatch of the necessary supplies is not rate-limiting. Ideally, the analytical laboratory will receive written instructions on what to provide, including number and type of collection vessel, number of request forms, type of packaging materials, etc. Prior to an initial assessment visit, the laboratory should provide confirmation of its certification or accreditation status, and a copy of reference ranges for the population to be studied in the protocol, together with details on methodology.

The laboratory documentation should be included in the investigator file, as should the documents detailed in section 8 of the ICH GCP guideline (ICH Guideline, 1996), and this file should be prepared by the time of the final initiation visit.

The following section summarises the duties to be performed and the appropriate supporting documentation to be collected by the monitor before the study is initiated.

Pre-initiation documentation

All relevant curricula vitae (CVs) should have been collected from the study site prior to the initiation visit. Many monitors wrongly treat this activity as a box-ticking exercise: its purpose is vital, namely to document the qualifications and experience of the staff who will be involved in the study. This being the case, each investigator CV (personally signed and dated) must be reviewed for adequacy and completeness. All CVs should be up-to-date and include details of the individual's current position. Sponsor SOPs may define up-to-date as between 6 months and a maximum of 2 years old. In addition, a CV should be collected for all other staff involved in the study, including those responsible for clinical aspects, informed consent, pharmacy matters, and laboratory procedures. Where applicable, CVs should also be obtained from staff in specialist units, e.g. those involved in reading pathology slides, performing computed tomography (CT), magnetic resonance imaging (MRI) scans or radiological assessments, or responsible for any other procedures relevant for the study.

Ethics committee approval must be obtained prior to initiation. There must be documented evidence to confirm that the final protocol has been approved, together with the informed consent and patient information documents. All documents reviewed by the ethics committee should be listed, together with version numbers and document dates, so that there can be no ambiguity in document or version control. This review will include not only the protocol, informed consent and patient information documents, but also the IB, subject recruitment procedures, documents relating particularly to payments and compensation to subjects, and any other documents specifically requested (e.g. a copy of the CRF and/or subject diary cards). Ethics committee approval is commonly subject to certain conditions. It is essential that the ethics committee review letter is seen prior to study initiation because additional work may be required to satisfy the ethics committee before the study can commence. The final approval letter from the ethics committee must be on headed paper showing the name and address of the committee and clearly identify the study and the investigator(s) approved.

Each ethics committee is required to maintain a list of its members and their qualifications. It is typically the monitor's role to obtain a copy of this documentation, of the committee's operating procedures and minutes of relevant meetings. The ethics committee must also provide a document listing the members who voted on the research proposal in question. This demonstrates that the committee is properly constituted, as defined in section 3.2.1 of the ICH GCP guideline, and will confirm that any member of the study site team who is also a member of the ethics committee did not take part in the deliberations or voting procedure on the research proposal.

Given the diverse range of documents that need to be submitted to the ethics committee, it is clear that considerable organisational work must be undertaken long before an initiation visit can be planned. The financial agreement or formal contract may require approval, not only from the investigator but also possibly from others within the hospital as well as personnel within the sponsor company. Similarly, an insurance or indemnity statement will be required to document appropriate compensation in the event of clinical trial-related injury.

Signed agreements may be required, not only between the investigator and the sponsor but also with other related hospital departments. It is advisable to draw up a single agreement to cover all aspects of the study at any one study site. However, if facilities from different departments are used, it may be necessary to have separate agreements. It is advisable to include payment schedules in any financial agreements to pre-empt any unforeseen requests during the study.

The delivery of the clinical trial supplies to the study site must be arranged to coincide with the initiation or 'kick-off' visit (and not before). This is done to prevent subjects being enrolled in the trial without all the necessary documentation. This practice is also useful to ensure that the clinical trial supplies provided are the most suitable in terms of shelf-life: in the early phases of clinical development, it is not unusual for only limited stability data to be available. The shipping records for the investigational product should document the site to which the supplies have been delivered, together with details of the delivery date, batch numbers and expiry dates. These documents should also allow for shipping and storage conditions to be tracked. If an investigational product needs to be stored within a certain temperature range, it should be possible to document adherence to this requirement throughout the study (*see Chapter 10*).

STUDY INITIATION

Once all the above steps have been accomplished, the study site can be initiated, although in practice this usually takes more than one visit. It is vital that all study site staff are made fully aware of their duties and this may frequently involve individuals from several departments. Consequently, although the ideal is for the study site to be initiated in a single visit, this is not absolutely necessary because it is usually not logistically possible.

At the final initiation visit the monitor should ensure that all study materials are either taken for the visit or have been delivered in advance. All present should be reminded of the background to the study and the protocol should be reviewed in full, including the expected recruitment rate and study duration. The CRF should also be reviewed comprehensively, together with any global monitoring conventions that may be specific either to the sponsor company or to the protocol. This is particularly relevant for international studies.

The monitor has the responsibility to ensure that the informed consent procedure is understood by all involved; details of those performing this procedure should be documented. A study site staff responsibilities form should be completed at the initiation visits, and specimen signatures and initials for study staff should be obtained.

Key GCP issues should always be covered with the study site team, even if they have previously conducted numerous studies. However, if the same investigator and site team have recently conducted studies for the same sponsor, it may suffice to highlight certain selected aspects of GCP pertinent to the study in question.

Good source documentation is the key to good data and the method, location and forms for recording study data should be discussed in detail with the site staff. It could be that more information than usual is to be recorded in the patient notes and it may be appropriate to provide source document sheets to assist with this process.

The timely and accurate reporting of adverse events is of vital importance in any study. The definitions of adverse events and serious adverse events (SAEs) should be reviewed with site staff prior to initiation and the reporting procedure must be explained in detail. It is helpful to provide a chart to document the adverse event reporting process and the time frame to be followed in the case of SAEs. Reporting of SAEs may necessitate breaking the randomisation code, with implications for the treatment to be administered. It may also be appropriate to reinforce this message with reminders during the study.

The initiation visit agenda will include discussion of the storage and preparation of study medication, and the subject of drug accountability must be carefully and clearly explained. If the procedures involved are at all unusual, it may be helpful to take a 'dummy' example for demonstration purposes. It is also important to emphasise any concurrent medications that should be avoided during the study. The pharmacy will play a key role in ensuring that the protocol is adhered to in this respect and good communication between the monitor and the study pharmacist is paramount.

Issues relating to the storage and shipment of specimens/samples obtained during the study must be explored in detail, and responsibilities must be agreed for arranging the mechanics of transport of analytical samples, dry ice or any other materials.

PRE-STUDY VISIT REPORT NUMBER/INITIATION VISIT REPORT (delete as applicable) Page 1/1				
Investigator:		Study site:		
Protocol no.:	Centre no.:	Study drug:		Indication:
Visit date:		Date of last visit:		Monitor:

Personnel present:

		Yes	No	ND/NA	*	#
A	**Were the following discussed and understood by the investigator?**					
1	Background information					_/_/_
2	Protocol, recruitment rate, study duration					_/_/_
3	Case record form (CRF)					_/_/_
4	Informed consent procedure and data protection issues					_/_/_
5	Good clinical practice (GCP)					_/_/_
6	Source documentation					_/_/_
7	Adverse event reporting procedure (to sponsor and ethics committee)					_/_/_
8	Randomisation procedure (if applicable)					_/_/_
9	Financial agreement					_/_/_
10	Preparation, storage and accountability of study drug					_/_/_
11	Storage and shipment of specimens (e.g. serum samples)					_/_/_
12	Records retention					_/_/_
13	Local regulatory requirements, e.g. potential for regulatory authority audit					_/_/_
14	Annual ethics committee review/approval (if applicable)					_/_/_
B	**Have the following been provided to the investigator?**					
1	Investigator's brochure (IB)					_/_/_
2	Final protocol and amendments					_/_/_
3	Copy of regulatory approval/notification					_/_/_
4	CRFs					_/_/_
5	Informed consent forms – written?					_/_/_
6	Study drug					_/_/_
7	Drug accountability forms					_/_/_
8	Serious adverse event (SAE) forms					_/_/_
9	Randomisation envelopes (if applicable)					_/_/_
10	Sample tubes and/or other specific material					_/_/_
11	Investigator file					_/_/_
C	**Have the following been provided by the investigator?**					
1	All relevant CVs					_/_/_
2	Laboratory certification/accreditation, normal values					_/_/_
3	Written notification of ethics committee approval with list of voting members					_/_/_
4	Ethics committee approval of informed consent form					_/_/_
5	Signed protocol and amendments					_/_/_
6	Signed letter of agreement					_/_/_
7	Signed letter of indemnity (if applicable)					_/_/_
D	**Was the proposed frequency of monitoring discussed?**					_/_/_
	Specify weeks					

ND/NA Not done/not applicable (specify which)
*Further information overleaf
#Addressed on a previous occasion – give date of visit/correspondence

Send original signed report to for trial master file and retain one copy	
Copies (specify initials or name) – these may be sent electronically to the following:	
Sponsor company:	Others:

Figure 1. Sample initiation visit checklist.

Records management is key to a successful study and the requirements for appropriate records retention should be pointed out at the initiation visit, with reminders given both during and at the end of the study. Records retention is important to confirm the reproducibility of data and the transparency of study conduct. It is especially relevant in terms of audit and inspection.

The investigator must also be reminded that the ethics committee will review the study annually at least. More frequent review may be necessary, especially for earlier phase studies or those in which levels of risk are perceived to be higher. The responsibility for providing updates to the ethics committee must therefore be clearly documented.

The monitor should also reach agreement with the study site team concerning the proposed frequency of monitoring visits. The schedule will depend on the intensity and type of the study, the expected recruitment rate and many other factors. The monitor should provide the study site with a copy of the initiation visit report or checklist for inclusion in the investigator file. This report confirms that initiation activities have been completed at this important visit. An example checklist that may be used for an initiation visit is shown in Figure 1.

STUDY CONDUCT AND MONITORING

It is recommended that the first monitoring visit should take place immediately after the first subject has entered the study. Any problems identified and rectified at this stage will save considerable time, resource and cost. However, if the first subject is not entered within a reasonable time from study initiation, a visit should be planned anyway to ascertain the reasons. In those instances where sites are clearly under-performing, either in terms of recruitment or data quality, the contractual agreement should allow for early closure of the site, where appropriate.

The purpose of monitoring is to verify that reported trial data are accurate, complete and verifiable from source documents. Monitoring further ensures that the rights and well-being of subjects are protected and that the conduct of the trial is in compliance with the approved protocol (and amendments), GCP and applicable regulatory requirements.

The protection of subjects' rights is an issue that many pharmaceutical companies are currently having to reconsider in the light of the EU Data Protection Directive (Directive 95/46/EC, 1995) that was incorporated into UK law, for example, in the Data Protection Act 1998 which came into force in March 2000 (The Stationery Office, 1998). The Act states that personal data should be transferred outside the EU only if there is a similar level of data protection in the country to which the data are transferred. It is likely that such data may be transmitted to the Food and Drug Administration (FDA) in the USA or to other authorities outside the EU. This has led to consent being requested from subjects in order for their data to be transferred. It is the monitor's responsibility to ensure that the study is conducted correctly and that all activities relating to data protection and transfer are properly documented.

The full responsibilities of the monitor are detailed in section 5.18.4 of the ICH GCP guideline. However, during the peak activity phase of a study there may be insufficient time to perform all these activities in a single visit. Sometimes, therefore, it may be necessary to make separate visits to focus on specific study conduct issues, e.g. drug accountability.

The monitor must always scrutinise recruitment rates; if these are too slow, the reasons should be ascertained. It may be possible to rectify practical restraints on recruitment, either by changing the way in which the site operates or, if necessary, by protocol amendment. If the recruitment rate is faster than anticipated, the monitor should consider looking more closely at the eligibility criteria and ensure that ineligible patients are not being recruited.

Consent forms for all subjects should be checked to ensure that they have been completed in full and that the form has been personally signed and dated by the subject and by any others involved in the informed consent process. The date of consent should be checked to ensure that the subject has not undergone any trial-related procedures prior to consenting.

The eligibility criteria should be reviewed to ensure that the subject is truly eligible for the study and that all the source documents adequately support his/her inclusion. Any ineligible subjects must be brought to the attention of the investigator and a plan of action must be agreed for handling this eventuality. The investigator agreement should stipulate clearly that no payment will be made for ineligible subjects who are included in the trial.

Source documents should be meticulously checked for evidence of adverse events, and SAEs in particular. If such events have occurred, the monitor should ensure that they are reported using the correct procedure as defined in the protocol and any local country procedures, as applicable. Concomitant medications should also be reviewed carefully, both for routine use and for the treatment of any adverse events.

A number of monitoring activities have been greatly facilitated by advances in technology and by the widespread availability of laptop computers and new software. For example, subject's visit dates can be predicted to ensure that visits are undertaken within the correct time windows, as specified in the protocol. As another example, SAEs can be tabulated electronically to provide the monitor with a full record of such events at any given time that will serve as a prompt with regard to any follow-up required.

Subjects who are withdrawn from the study should be detailed in the monitoring visit report and the reasons for withdrawal should be documented. The monitor must distinguish between withdrawals due to safety issues and withdrawals for other reasons, such as lack of efficacy.

For randomised studies the monitor should ensure that the correct randomisation procedures have been followed and that subjects have been randomised at the correct time with respect to the timing of other trial-related activities.

The thorough checking of CRFs is a time-consuming process that accounts for the bulk of the monitor's time during site monitoring visits and places great demands on the monitor's skills in terms of attention to detail. Each individual CRF should be checked for completeness, accuracy and legibility. All signatures should be checked to ensure that the CRFs and any associated laboratory reports have been signed by a person authorised to do so. The CRFs should also be checked against the source documents. While some companies continue to perform 100% source data checks, with large-scale studies this activity can be extremely time-consuming and cause focus to be lost. Therefore a study-specific SOP may be written to reduce the volume of source data to be checked. Nevertheless, source data must still be checked for all subjects to ascertain eligibility and to corroborate primary efficacy data and adverse events. For more routine and less critical data, a set procedure may be agreed to reduce the workload without sacrificing scientific validity. Irrespective of any study-specific procedure, each subject's source data should also be checked to ensure that all adverse events have been appropriately recorded and reported.

Clinical trial supplies accounting is another important task for the monitor. A complete check should be maintained on the associated documentation to verify that a detailed paper trail exists to account for all movement of study drug from the sponsor company to the study site, with documentation of usage and eventual destruction, whether performed at the study site, at the sponsor company, or by a third party.

The monitor should check that any biological samples taken for analysis during the study have been obtained correctly, and that they are correctly labelled, stored and delivered for analysis. Cross-checks should be performed to ensure that what is written on sample labels is also reflected in any associated data items on the CRF. If samples are collected or delivered to the analytical laboratory, this should be fully documented either in the monitoring report or elsewhere.

Protocol amendments may become necessary, either while a study is in progress or even before the study begins. If the monitor identifies the possible need for a protocol amendment, this should be recorded in the monitoring visit report and the monitor should follow the matter up with the appropriate personnel in the sponsor company.

The monitor should be aware of and report any changes in study site personnel who are to be involved in the trial. CVs for new study site staff should be reviewed to ensure that they have the qualifications and appropriate experience to perform their designated role in the study, and copies should be placed in sponsor and investigator files. It is also vital that new study site staff are correctly trained in all study procedures. The monitor should therefore review all study procedures with new staff, just as was done originally at the initiation visit. Such training needs to be recorded in the monitoring visit report.

The monitor should be aware of servicing requirements for any equipment or analytical processes used in the trial. This is particularly important in cases where a biochemical value is a primary end-point and analytical reagents have expiry dates. Similarly, to change a biochemical method may alter the normal range for an end-point variable, and this may have significant consequences. Changes in equipment or methodology used may have a profound effect on the trial: in a multiple sclerosis study, for example, a change in MRI scanner may alter the ability to correlate changes in demyelination patterns with physical signs assessed during the course of the study. If liver lesions are being monitored by CT scans in an oncology study, changing the scanner may negatively impact the study. If such changes are unavoidable, a measurement with the new and the old equipment at the same time point would identify potential problems or confirm equivalence. While such changes should be avoided if at all possible, these matters are usually outside the monitor's control. All changes in equipment and methodology must be documented and the information forwarded to those who will be involved in the interpretation of the data from such assessments.

The monitor must check the investigator file at regular intervals through the study to ensure that it is being maintained correctly. In particular, it should be established that the correspondence section is up-to-date and that any electronic mail between the parties has been correctly filed. This is an area that is frequently ignored through a lack of sponsor procedures for dealing with e-mail correspondence. The monitor must also verify that the subject identification log is being updated as subjects enter the trial. The monitoring visit log must also be updated.

During the course of the trial the monitor must continually ensure that the site has sufficient materials to allow the smooth running of the trial. The term 'materials' includes everything from CRFs and copies of the protocol to blood sample request forms and boxes for dispatching these to the laboratory. Such issues can be addressed not only during routine monitoring visits but also when the monitor contacts the study site by telephone. For example, it would be unfortunate if a subject was not recruited to a trial simply because insufficient blood sampling kits were available.

Following the monitoring visit, a detailed report must be prepared covering all the issues addressed. An example of a monitoring report checklist is provided in Figure 2. In addition, if specific issues are identified that require follow-up by the investigator (or a member of the study site team), a letter defining the issues to be clarified or resolved should be sent by the monitor to the investigator, detailing actions required and decisions agreed.

STUDY TERMINATION

If the monitoring process has been executed meticulously and correctly over the preceding months or years, many of the activities to be performed at the termination visit (also known as study close-out or closure) will already have been completed. Nevertheless, it is always essential to check that this is indeed the case. Since post-study activities can be quite drawn out from the time of

MONITORING VISIT REPORT NUMBER — Page 1/1

Investigator:		Study site:	
Protocol no.:	Centre no.:	Study drug:	Indication:
Visit date:		Date of last visit:	Monitor:

Personnel present:			
Patient recruitment information			
Recruited since last visit:	Total no.:		Target no.:
Ongoing:	Completed:	Withdrawn for safety:	Withdrawn for other:

		Yes	No	ND/NA	*
1	Is recruitment on schedule?				
2	Are patient consent forms in order?				
3	Are eligibility criteria adhered to and supported by adequate source documents?				
4a	Were the correct adverse events procedures followed for serious adverse events (SAEs)?				
4b	Were the correct adverse events procedures followed for non-serious events?				
4c	Did any subject withdraw for safety reasons? If so, specify details.				
5	Were the correct randomisation procedures followed?				
6a	Were clinical observations correctly completed?				
6b	Were laboratory tests correctly completed?				
6c	Were CRFs checked for completeness, accuracy, legibility, signatures etc.?				
6d	Were CRFs compared against source documents? Specify details.				
7a	Are study drug supplies correctly stored, dispensed and accounted for?				
7b	Are there sufficient unexpired study drug supplies on site?				
7c	Were any study drug supplies collected or was destruction authorised?				
8a	Were samples (e.g. serum, biopsies) taken, labelled and stored correctly?				
8b	Were samples (e.g. serum, biopsies) collected / was delivery arranged?				
9	Are protocol amendments necessary?				
10a	Are there any changes to study site staff? If so, specify details.				
10b	Were there any changes to facilities (e.g. change in normal laboratory values)?				
11	Was the investigator file checked for completeness?				
12	Are there sufficient study-specific supplies (e.g. sample tubes) on site?				

ND/NA Not done/not applicable (specify which)
*Further information overleaf

Send original signed report to	for trial master file and retain one copy
Copies (specify initials or name) – these may be sent electronically to the following:	
Sponsor company:	Others:

Figure 2. Sample monitoring report checklist.

the last subject visit to the last data query, and again from the last data query to availability of the clinical study report, it may be appropriate in many cases to perform more than one termination visit. An example checklist for a termination visit is provided in Figure 3.

The ethics committee must be informed of the completion of the study and must receive a final report to this effect. Some ethics committees also ask for a copy of any publication resulting from the study.

If the study was randomised, both the unopened and any opened randomisation envelopes should be collected (if this randomisation method was used) and returned to the sponsor. If randomisation envelopes have been opened, this fact and the reasons for doing so should be documented (although this will probably have been done previously at a routine monitoring visit).

Once it has been confirmed that all documentation is in place, the monitor will initiate the process for the final investigator payment to be made. The monitor should also ensure that any other departments at the study site with separate agreements have also received or will receive their final payments.

TERMINATION VISIT REPORT NUMBER — Page 1/1				
Investigator:		Study site:		
Protocol no.:	Centre no.:	Study drug:		Indication:
Visit date:		Date of last visit:		Monitor:

Personnel present:
Address of investigator at termination visit:
Telephone number of investigator at termination visit:
Fax number of investigator at termination visit:

1	Have the following been performed and adequately documented during the study?	Yes	No*	NA
a	All informed consent forms checked			
b	All CRFs checked and completed			
c	All data clarification forms checked and completed			
d	All drug accountability forms checked and completed			
e	All drug destruction forms checked and completed			
f	All SAE forms completed and followed up (if applicable)			
g	Adequate follow-up of all withdrawals/adverse events			
h	Adequate documentation of communication/correspondence with the ethics committee			
i	All randomisation envelopes collected (if applicable)			
j	If any double-blind envelopes were opened, are the reasons documented?			
k	All specimens (e.g. serum samples) collected/delivery arranged			
l	All changes in normal values and methods documented			
m	All payments made to the investigator in accordance with financial agreement			
n	All other applicable payments made (e.g. pharmacist, laboratory, hospital administration)			
o	All relevant documents filed in the investigator file			
p	Has a final check of the investigator file been made for completeness and, as far as possible, for consistency with the trial master file?			
2	Have the following been discussed with the investigator?			
a	Records retention (including investigator file and patient log)			
b	Potential for regulatory authority audit			
c	Obligations of the investigator to the ethics committee, e.g. report (if applicable)			
d	Preparation of technical report			
e	Publication policy			
3	Are the following adequately filed at the study site?			
a	Copies of all completed CRFs			
b	Copies of all completed data clarification forms			
c	Results of relevant central laboratory analyses			
d	Randomisation reconciliation list			
4	Have the following been collected from the investigator?			
a	Signed protocol amendments			
b	All unused documents, e.g. CRFs, diary cards, informed consent forms, SAE forms			
c	All remaining drug supplies (if destroyed, please document)			
d	All materials/equipment loaned to the investigator, e.g. fax machine, refrigerator, centrifuge			
5	Have all other administrative tasks been performed?			
a	All rental agreements terminated (if applicable)			
6	Is any post-study follow-up required?			
7	Are further termination visits anticipated?			

*If No, a follow-up report must be prepared once the issue has been resolved
NA Not applicable

Send original signed report to	for trial master file and retain one copy
Copies (specify initials or name) – these may be sent electronically to the following:	
Sponsor company:	Others:

Figure 3. Sample termination visit checklist.

As at a routine monitoring visit the investigator file should be reviewed for completeness, in particular to establish that any recent e-mail correspondence or notifications to the ethics committee have been correctly filed. If at all possible, consistency should be verified between the sponsor trial master file (TMF) and the investigator file. The list of all essential documents from section 8 of the ICH GCP guideline should be referred to and cross-checked against the TMF and investigator file to ensure that the correct original documents and/or copies are appropriately filed.

The monitor should check that all necessary documents are correctly filed at the study site. In all cases this will include CRFs (and e-CRFs, where used) as well as central laboratory results, randomisation reconciliation lists and any other appropriate documents. The precise list of documents to check will be study-dependent but can be compiled prior to the termination visit. Similarly, a list should be made of any documents or other items that need to be collected from the site. Often the sponsor may loan equipment (e.g. centrifuge, fax machine) to study sites for specific studies; such equipment will need to be collected and appropriate receipt/return documentation completed.

A variety of issues, including records retention, should be discussed with the investigator at the termination visit. To support this, sponsor companies may provide labels for patient notes to state that a subject has taken part in a clinical study. Since the local regulatory position varies concerning the length of time that patient notes should be kept, the study site should be instructed to contact the sponsor company before destroying such documents. Some hospitals may have a policy of destroying patient notes after a fixed period that may be shorter than the retention period required for clinical trial purposes. After study termination, the possibility of regulatory audit remains, especially for pivotal trials and high-recruiting centres. Even if an audit has already taken place, the investigator should be advised of the possibility of audit from a second authority. The monitor should make appropriate file notes to confirm local requirements regarding record retention and take time to remind investigators of their responsibilities.

The timetable for the preparation of the clinical study report and any publications must be outlined to the investigator. Details of the publication policy already discussed at the initiation visit will be reiterated.

At the end of a study, once all the results have been obtained, the laboratory must not be overlooked. The monitor should ensure that any contracts and equipment rental agreements are terminated.

After the closure visit, a full report should be prepared, documenting the visit in detail and confirming any outstanding follow-up actions required either by the monitor or another party. If further visits are anticipated by any party, the report should document this fact and the reasons for it. Finally, the investigator and study site team should be thanked for their efforts in the study. This is best done formally in writing and may be taken as a useful opportunity to document again the responsibilities of the investigator following the completion of the study.

CONCLUSION

The monitor's role is central in ensuring that the study runs smoothly and that all trial-related activities are performed as laid down in the protocol and in relevant guidelines, regulations, SOPs and monitoring conventions. Through close attention to administrative detail and the application of positive inter-personal, motivational and negotiating skills, the monitor is able to influence directly the successful running of the clinical trial and to make a key contri-bution to the drug development process. The details presented in this chapter are not exhaustive and will often need to be supplemented by individual company procedures. As a general guide, however, it should help monitors to perform their essential role in encouraging high-quality clinical research.

REFERENCES AND FURTHER READING

Applied Clinical Trials (various issues).

Clinical Research Focus (various issues).

Committee for Proprietary Medicinal Products (CPMP) Working Party on Efficacy of Medicinal Products (1991). *Good Clinical Practice for Trials on Medicinal Products in the European Community* (111/3976/88-EN Final), European Commission, Brussels.

Directive 95/46/EC (1995). On the protection of individuals with regard to the process-ing of personal data and on the free movement of such data.

ICH Guideline (1996). *Topic E6: Good Clinical Practice – Consolidated Guideline*, International Federation of Pharmaceutical Manufacturers Associations, Geneva (Issued as CPMP/ICH/135/95).

The Monitor (various issues)

The Stationery Office (1998). *The Data Protection Act 1998*, The Stationery Office, London.

13

Drug safety in clinical studies and pharmacovigilance

John C.C. Talbot

INTRODUCTION

Determining the safety profile of a new medicine is an integral and continuous part of the drug development process. Animal pharmacology and toxicology studies provide some information about the safety of a new drug and are a prerequisite for administering the drug to man. However, animal data are only partially predictive of what will happen in humans; hence the first dosing of volunteers or clinical trial subjects is a critical step in the process.

Adverse drug reactions (ADRs) can be classified simply into type A, those that are normal but augmented actions of the drug, and type B, those that are bizarre (Rawlins and Thompson, 1991).

Type A reactions are:

- the results of an exaggerated pharmacological action of a drug;
- largely predictable on the basis of the drug's pharmacology;
- usually dose-dependent;
- common;
- generally not serious or fatal.

Examples are numerous and include bradycardia with beta-blockers, bleeding with anticoagulants, and drowsiness with benzodiazepines.

Type B reactions are:

- totally aberrant effects that are not expected from the known pharmacological actions of the drug;
- unpredictable in a particular patient or subject;
- independent of dose;
- rare;
- usually serious and may have a high mortality.

Examples include anaphylaxis or hypersensitivity that can occur with many drugs (e.g. penicillins), some types of hepatotoxicity, and blood dyscrasias, such as aplastic anaemia and agranulocytosis.

Some type A reactions will be predictable from animal work and knowledge of the drug's pharmacology and will be confirmed by Phase I studies in healthy volunteers and by early studies in clinical trial subjects. On the other hand, type B reactions will not be identified until relatively large numbers of subjects have been exposed to the drug; some may be identified in Phase III but many type B reactions do not come to light until after the drug is marketed.

CLINICAL STUDIES

All clinical studies should have a safety component as a primary or secondary objective. In early Phase I and Phase II studies, safety and tolerability are often a primary objective and the main reason for conducting the study. In later Phase II and Phase III studies the primary objective is usually efficacy but safety and tolerability must also be included as an objective.

Safety data from clinical studies can be broadly divided into the following three types, although these can overlap:

- adverse events
- laboratory safety data
- vital signs and physical findings.

Safety monitoring in clinical studies can be considered as non-specific, i.e. general safety monitoring, or specific, i.e. looking for particular safety issues based on animal data or experience with other similar drugs.

Clinical studies have some general safety goals:

- to detect and characterise common ADRs, usually type A,
- to determine tolerability in volunteers or subjects, i.e. how the ADR is tolerated, does it resolve or improve on repeated dosing, is it so unpleasant that the subject has to stop treatment or can the subject put up with it?
- to identify any pre-disposing or risk factors for particular ADRs.

In studies where a range of doses is used and in studies with a pharmacokinetic component, the safety goal will be to determine the relationship between ADRs and dose or plasma concentrations of the drug.

The nature and frequency of the safety monitoring used in a study will depend on experience with the drug and the type of study being conducted. In early Phase I safety and tolerability studies in volunteers there will be extensive and frequent monitoring (ECG, blood pressure, etc.), blood sampling and questioning of the subjects. In large Phase III studies, standard questions and routine laboratory screens at appropriate time intervals are typically used. In some Phase IV studies only certain clinical outcomes, e.g. death, hospitalisation or stroke, may be collected.

ADVERSE EVENTS

The term adverse event was defined by Finney (1965) as 'a particular untoward happening experienced by a patient, undesirable either generally or in the context of his disease' (see also ICH Guideline, 1994). Adverse events are not necessarily recognised drug reactions and a causal relationship to treatment is not implied as it is in the term ADR. Thus, all ADRs are adverse events but only some adverse events are ADRs.

The concept of collecting adverse events rather than ADRs was adopted after the failure of clinical trials to detect skin and eye problems with practolol. Skegg and Doll (1977) proposed that the value of clinical trials in detecting unwanted effects of new medicines would be enhanced if doctors recorded all adverse events experienced by subjects, not just those regarded as adverse reactions to drugs. All events should be reported to the centre co-ordinating the trial and analysed in treated subjects and controls. This is the basis for how adverse event monitoring in clinical studies is conducted today. Events should be treatment-emergent. This can be defined as an event that was not present before the start of treatment and became apparent after treatment began, or an event that was present before the start of treatment but worsened after treatment began. In controlled studies, the profile of adverse events in the different treatment groups can be compared, see Figure 1 and the section on *Presentation of safety data*, below.

How adverse events are to be elicited by the investigator must be carefully considered when designing a study. The following options are available:

- Wait for the subject to volunteer information.
- Ask the subject a standard open question, e.g. have you had any medical problems since your last visit?
- Go through a symptom checklist with the subject.
- Use a self-administered questionnaire.
- Review the subject's diary card for adverse events.

Checklists and questionnaires collect adverse events in a structured fashion so that statistical comparisons can be made between treatment groups. They can elicit certain adverse events that may otherwise not have been mentioned by the subject, e.g. sexual events such as loss of libido or impotence, and can be designed to identify and quantify ADRs known to occur with similar drugs (see below). However, these methods will collect more symptoms than an open question and should be used only in controlled studies.

To evaluate different methods of collecting adverse events, Wallander *et al.*

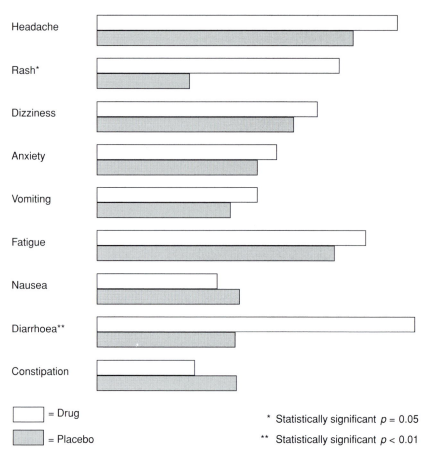

Figure 1. An example of an adverse event profile – drug v. placebo.

(1991) used a standard open question, a compliant score and a subjective symptom assessment profile in a hypertension study. Fifteen different adverse events were reported by all three methods, 16 by two methods and 35 by one method only. The two questionnaire methods collected far more adverse events.

Angiotensin converting enzyme (ACE) inhibitors, such as captopril and enalapril, are used to treat hypertension and are found to cause a persistent, dry cough in many patients. To determine whether this was also a problem with candesartan, a selective angiotensin type I (AT_1) receptor blocker, Tanser *et al.* (2000) compared the incidence and severity of dry cough in a double-blind study of candesartan, enalapril and placebo. Cough and other symptoms were evaluated using a symptom assessment questionnaire (5–point Likert scale: not at all, a little, moderately, quite a bit and extremely), a visual analogue scale and a quality of life instrument. The proportion of patients found to have cough was 26.9% on placebo, 35.5% on candesartan and 68.2% on enalapril (p < 0.001 v. candesartan). The incidence, frequency and severity of dry cough were shown to be significantly lower with candesartan than with enalapril and no different from those found with placebo.

When designing protocols and case record forms (CRFs) it is vital to consider how adverse events are to be elicited from trial subjects and what question or questions should be used. There must be clear definitions and instructions and a standard reporting form should be employed. Investigators and study monitors must be trained in these procedures if they are to succeed.

Serious adverse events

Serious adverse events (SAEs) are important and need to be reported quickly to appropriate personnel in the company responsible for the study. SAEs may have implications for the safety of subjects and the conduct of the study and they need to be reported to regulatory authorities within strict time frames on an expedited basis (e.g. seven calendar days for fatal or life-threatening cases and 15 days for other serious cases if other criteria are met). According to ICH (ICH Guideline, 1994), and based on older definitions, serious has been defined as any untoward medical occurrence that at any dose:

- results in death;
- is life-threatening (the subject was at risk of death at the time of the event);
- requires inpatient hospitalisation or prolongation of existing hospitalisation;
- results in persistent or significant disability/incapacity; or
- is a congenital anomaly/birth defect.

Medical and scientific judgement should be exercised in other situations, such as important medical events that may not be immediately life-threatening or result in death or hospitalisation but may jeopardise the subject or may require intervention to prevent one of the other outcomes listed above. Such events should also be considered serious.

Serious adverse events are described in a narrative format in the clinical study report and may require further discussion (see *Presentation of safety data*, below).

Other significant adverse events

Another significant subset of adverse events concerns those that result in discontinuation of investigational drug administration. These events may or may not be serious but are an indication of the drug's tolerability. They should be collected in all clinical studies conducted before marketing and should be described in a narrative format and discussed in the study report. Adverse events that result in a reduction of drug dosage and events specific to a particular drug or study may also be considered as other significant adverse events in the study report.

LABORATORY SAFETY DATA

As part of the non-specific safety monitoring in pre-marketing clinical studies, a range of haematology, clinical chemistry and liver function tests is usually performed before treatment, at intervals during treatment and after treatment is complete. The purpose of these tests is to assure continuation of baseline status in volunteers or trial subjects with regard to variables that are precursory of possible adverse effects on vital organ systems (e.g. blood, kidneys, liver) and of other systemic toxicity. Table 1 shows a suggested limited range

Table 1. Suggested laboratory tests for non-specific safety monitoring.

Group of tests	Laboratory parameter	ADRs that may be identified
Haematology	Haemoglobin	Anaemia
	Haematocrit	
	Red blood count (RBC)	
	Mean corpuscular volume (MCV)	
	Platelet count	Thrombocytopenia
	Total white count	Neutropenia
	Differential white count	
	Neutrophils	
	Lymphocytes	
	Monocytes	
	Eosinophils	
	Basophils	
Clinical chemistry	Sodium	Electrolyte and fluid imbalance
	Potassium	
	Calcium	
	Phosphate	
	Total protein	
	Albumin	
	Uric acid	
Renal function	Urea	Nephrotoxicity
	Creatinine	
Liver function	AST (SGOT)	Hepatotoxicity
	ALT (SGPT)	
	Alkaline phosphatase	
	Total bilirubin	
Urinalysis	Protein	Nephrotoxicity
	White blood cells	
	Red blood cells	
	Glucose	Abnormal glucose metabolism

of tests that could be performed routinely and the possible ADRs that may be identified.

The timing of these tests should be carefully considered. It is essential to establish baseline values and further tests must be timed so that treatment-related effects can be detected. For instance, changes in serum potassium and glucose are maximal 2–6 hours after dosing with a beta-agonist; sampling must therefore be timed to quantify these changes. Hepatocellular damage can manifest itself by increases in aspartate aminotransferase (AST) and alanine aminotransferase (ALT) 1–3 days after a single dose. ALT in particular has a fairly long half-life; sampling only one day after dosing could miss such an increase.

For some drugs, specific safety monitoring should be done in addition to these routine screens. For instance, if a new drug showed mild renal toxicity or toxicity only at high doses in animal studies but it was considered ethical to give the drug to humans, additional sensitive tests of kidney function and damage should be included in volunteer and patient studies, e.g. urinary microscopy/cytology, quantitative albumin excretion, beta-2-microglobulin and N-acetylglucosaminidase (NAG). Expert advice should be sought on which tests are appropriate. Stephens (1998) provides excellent background on the collection and reporting of laboratory data.

The clinical study protocol must state how abnormal laboratory results should be collected and reported. Consideration must be given as to whether they should be reported also as adverse events if they are outside normal limits, outside extended limits (e.g. three times the upper limit of normal for AST and ALT), result in discontinuation of the drug, or meet one of the criteria for a serious event.

A post-treatment sample, taken perhaps 7–14 days after treatment has been stopped, is also important for evaluating whether a change that occurred during the study might be due to the drug and for determining the outcome of any abnormal values.

VITAL SIGNS AND PHYSICAL FINDINGS

Collection of vital signs and physical findings data is another non-specific method of safety monitoring used in many pre-marketing and some post-marketing studies. This data category includes:

- pulse,
- blood pressure,
- ECG intervals,
- body weight, and
- body temperature.

As with laboratory data, baseline measurements and the appropriate timing of data collection are essential. Since food, rest, posture and other factors can affect these data, it is essential that the protocol describes a uniform method for data collection.

INVESTIGATOR'S BROCHURE

A current investigator's brochure (IB) should be available for all drugs in clinical development. The IB must be regularly reviewed and updated and, for reasons of patient safety, it is particularly important that the section describing the emerging safety profile is up to date. The IB also helps to identify those events from clinical studies that require reporting to the regulatory authorities. Generally, expedited reporting is required for serious, unexpected, possibly related events. An unexpected ADR is one whose nature, severity, specificity and outcome are not consistent with the information in the IB. Thus, if a reported event is unexpected in the IB, it may require expedited reporting.

CAUSALITY ASSESSMENT

The determination of whether an adverse event is causally related to a particular drug is a matter of judgement and opinion based on knowledge of what happened in the case in question and on experience with the drug. Almost all ADRs mimic normal symptoms, signs and diseases that patients suffer; only rarely are ADRs specific and clearly recognisable as being drug-induced. Causality assessment of individual reports is thus a practice of differential diagnosis.

Because of their individual knowledge and experience, different physicians may come to different judgements about the same case. To overcome this problem, a number of algorithms and scoring systems for assessing adverse events have been devised for use by clinical pharmacologists, regulatory authorities and pharmaceutical companies. Generally, these tools give greater consistency of assessments (unlikely, possible, probable, etc.) but are they more accurate? While this is difficult to determine, less emphasis is now placed on the individual evaluation of single cases in terms of possible or probable causality, and more on evaluating a collection of similar cases and looking for common factors.

There are a number of important factors to consider when making a judgement about adverse event causality, namely:

- *Temporal relationship:* was the time from the first dose of the drug to the onset of the adverse event consistent with a drug effect, considering the kinetics of the drug and the possible mechanism etc.?
- *Dechallenge:* was the drug stopped or the dose reduced and did the adverse event resolve or improve?

- *Rechallenge:* was the suspect drug re-administered and what happened? See *Drug rechallenge* below.
- *Alternative causes:* are alternative causes such as underlying disease, new disease or environmental factors likely, and to what extent have these been excluded?
- *Specifics:* are there any specific investigations (e.g. to detect drug antibodies) or characteristics such as a reaction at the site of application that would strongly suggest a causal relationship?
- *Consistency with drug profile:* was the adverse event a recognised ADR (expected) or could it be anticipated from the drug's pharmacology?

Causality assessment of individual cases in clinical studies still has an important role for SAEs. Investigators should be asked to evaluate each SAE. Some companies will request a 'Yes' or 'No' response to the question 'Do you consider that there is a reasonable possibility that the event may have been caused by the drug?'. Other companies use ordinal scales, e.g. unrelated, unlikely, possible, probable, almost certain. Causality assessment is recognised to be imprecise but the investigator is in the best position to make this judgement. SAEs for which there is a reasonable possibility of a causal relationship (or possibly, probably related, etc.) represent a safety signal and, if unexpected, will require expedited reporting to regulatory authorities. The causality assessment is thus used to alert the company to safety signals and to determine which SAEs need expedited reporting.

BREAKING THE TREATMENT BLIND

In a blinded clinical study, the investigator should break the treatment code only for appropriate medical reasons, i.e. to manage the subject in an emergency. The treatment code can also be broken by the company responsible for the study, but only for specific and specified reasons.

Although it is advantageous to retain the blind for all subjects prior to final study analysis, when a serious ADR is reportable to the regulatory authorities on an expedited basis, the ICH standards for expedited reporting recommend that the blind should be broken for that specific subject (ICH Guideline, 1994). The procedure used should maintain the blind for those persons (e.g. biometricians) responsible for analysis and interpretation of results at the study's conclusion. The code break and expedited reporting to the authorities is hence usually done within the drug safety department and the information is restricted to drug safety personnel. However, some believe that unblinding for this purpose is not appropriate and suggest that expedited reports should be submitted blind (Gait and Goldsmith, 2000). When a fatal or other serious outcome is the primary efficacy end-point in a study, the integrity of the study may be compromised if the blind is broken. Under these and similar circumstances, it is appropriate to reach agreement with regulatory authorities in advance concerning SAEs that will be treated as disease-related and not subject to routine expedited reporting. Data Safety Monitoring Boards also have a role in this respect.

DATA SAFETY MONITORING BOARDS

In some situations, such as large outcome studies in high morbidity or mortality disease states, it may be appropriate and helpful to use a safety committee or Data Safety Monitoring Board (DSMB). The main role of a DSMB is to protect subjects and to ensure the integrity of the study. Typically, these are responsibilities of the company conducting the study but they can be delegated to the DSMB. This can help to avoid difficult situations in the event of safety issues emerging during the study (Hampton, 2000).

DSMBs are initiated by the company responsible for the study but should be largely independent of the company and the study investigators. The decision to employ a DSMB is strategic and should be made at a senior level within the company and involve drug safety personnel. DSMBs must have a clear written charter outlining their responsibilities and mandate and their role should be described in the study protocol. In some studies, the DSMB will use pre-determined rules on the limits of benefit and harm at which the study should be stopped.

The format and frequency of the safety data required by the DSMB should be defined before the study starts and drug safety personnel should be involved in this process.

DRUG RECHALLENGE

Rechallenge is the re-administration of a drug that has been suspected as the possible cause of an adverse event. The result of the rechallenge can be positive, i.e. a recurrence of the adverse event, or negative, i.e. no recurrence of the adverse event. Amongst groups interested in ADR causality assessment, drug rechallenge with a positive result is generally regarded as the most important single factor in attributing causality. However, unless there is reliable, objective, temporally-related evidence of drug effect, the results of drug rechallenge can be misleading. For example, if the event is entirely subjective (e.g. nausea or headache), subjects can anticipate experiencing such symptoms. This can be overcome by using a blinded placebo control. Variability in underlying diseases can also give false negative or false positive results.

Drug rechallenge may occur inadvertently, without the subject or investigator realising, either because the drug is administered intermittently or because the subject stops treatment following an adverse event but resumes it later to relieve the symptoms the drug was prescribed for. Drug rechallenge can also be conducted deliberately to help to determine whether an adverse event was drug-related or not. Deliberate drug rechallenge is ethical provided that:

- the patient or subject consents to the rechallenge;
- it is performed in such a way that the results are valid;
- the original adverse event was not life-threatening;
- the adverse event is unlikely to be more serious if it recurs after rechallenge and there should be no sequelae;
- the patient or subject will benefit from knowledge of the result, i.e. if rechallenge is negative, the individual can receive a useful drug, in particular when alternative treatments are not available.

The decision to conduct drug rechallenge lies with the patient and the patient's doctor or, in a study, with the clinical investigator. Companies may be asked to supply drug and possibly a placebo control and they should do this provided that they are satisfied that the rechallenge is ethical and has a rational medical purpose.

PRESENTATION OF SAFETY DATA

Safety data collected in clinical studies (adverse events, laboratory data, vital signs and physical findings) will need to be presented in the clinical study report and possibly in a marketing authorisation application (MAA) and new drug application (NDA). How the data are to be presented should be considered when designing protocols and CRFs. What is collected and how it is collected will determine what can be presented.

ICH Topic E3 provides guidance on the structure and content of clinical study reports and has a substantial section on safety data (ICH Guideline, 1995). Analysis of safety data should be considered as follows:

- The extent of exposure (dose, duration, numbers) should be examined to determine the degree to which safety can be assessed.
- The more common adverse events, laboratory changes, etc., should be identified, classified, compared for treatment groups and analysed for factors that may affect their frequency, e.g. time, relation to demographic characteristics, dose or drug levels.
- Serious and other significant adverse events should be identified.

Three kinds of analyses are called for:

- *Summarised data*, often using tables and graphical presentations (cf. Figure 1).

- *Listings of individual subject data:* for adverse events these should include the subject identifier and details of age, race, sex, weight, severity, seriousness, action taken, outcome, causality assessment, time to onset, dose, concomitant treatment, etc.
- *Narrative descriptions* of events of particular interest: deaths, serious adverse events and other significant adverse events.

All tabulations and analyses should display events associated with the test drug and placebo or active control. In Figure 1, two of the adverse events, diarrhoea and rash, are significantly more frequent on the test drug compared with placebo. This might suggest a drug effect but, with multiple comparisons, some events are significantly different by chance. If the frequency of 100 different adverse events was compared, five would be significantly different by chance at $p = 0.05$. Events that are significantly different, particularly at low p values, should also be evaluated for possible mechanisms (they are likely to be type A reactions) and common characteristics before concluding that they are new ADRs.

The results of safety-related laboratory tests should be available in tabular listings, tests should be grouped logically, and abnormal values should be identified. For each parameter over the course of the study, the group mean or median values, the range of values and the number of subjects with abnormal values or values of a certain magnitude should be described. Shift tables are useful for analysing individual subject changes by treatment group. Table 2 is a simple shift table for a variable where only high values are relevant. In this study of one hundred subjects, nine who had normal values at baseline developed high values on treatment; these cases should be scrutinised more closely. Seven subjects who had high values at baseline remained high; these cases should be checked to see whether their values became further elevated. Figure 2 shows a graphical shift table for a variable where only high values are relevant. Individual changes can be seen and, if required, particular subjects can be identified; patient A has the most pronounced change on drug and, if clinically significant, this case should be discussed in detail.

The analyses of laboratory data should be designed to identify:

- small changes in many subjects – use means or medians;
- larger changes in some subjects – use shift tables and values beyond extended limits;
- changes across organ groups, e.g. liver function tests;
- changes associated with symptoms;
- serious or significant changes in occasional subjects.

Vital signs and other physical findings related to safety should be analysed and presented in a similar way to laboratory variables. If there is evidence of a drug effect, any relationship to dose, drug level or patient variables should be identified and the clinical relevance discussed. Attention should focus on changes not evaluated as efficacy variables and on those thought to be adverse events.

Table 2. Basic shift table showing numbers of patients with values going from/to.

Normal → High	High → High
9	7
Normal → Normal	High → Normal
80	4

n = 100 patients.

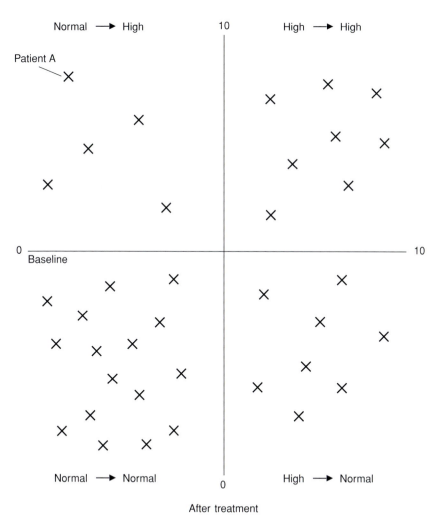

Figure 2. Shift diagram for a hypothetical variable (normal range: 0–5) showing change after drug treatment.

The overall safety evaluation of the drug should be reviewed with particular attention to deaths, SAEs, discontinuations and other significant adverse events. Any groups at increased risk should be identified and attention paid to potentially vulnerable subjects who may be present in small numbers, e.g. children, the elderly and patients with marked abnormalities of drug metabolism or excretion.

The integrated safety summary

An integrated safety summary (ISS) is an important component of the clinical summary for the MAA within Europe and for the NDA in the USA. The ISS integrates safety information from all sources, including animal data, clinical pharmacology studies, controlled and uncontrolled clinical studies in all indications, any marketed experience and epidemiological studies. It is an overall analysis, bringing together all studies to allow examination of differences among population subsets that is not possible with the relatively small numbers in single studies.

The ISS should describe the nature, frequency, seriousness and severity of adverse events, identify contra-indications and groups of individuals at risk. It should discuss drug interactions on the basis of clinical cases, drug–drug interaction studies, population kinetics and theoretical possibilities. It should determine what safety issues are included in the initial product information and summary of product characteristics (SPC, see below).

PHARMACOVIGILANCE

Pharmacovigilance has been defined as the process of identifying and responding to drug safety issues with marketed medicines. The principles apply equally to the pre-marketing period but the term pharmacovigilance originated in the post-marketing arena. The objectives of pharmacovigilance within the industry (Talbot and Nilsson, 1998) are essentially the same as those of regulatory agencies, namely:

- to protect patients from unnecessary harm by identifying previously unrecognised drug hazards;
- to elucidate predisposing factors to ADRs;
- to refute false safety signals; and
- to quantify risk in relation to benefit.

Pharmacovigilance is a shared responsibility. Companies are legally and morally responsible for monitoring the safety of their products, and regulatory authorities can be held responsible for the safety of the drugs they license for use. Individual doctors and pharmacists have a responsibility to patients at large to become involved in monitoring drug safety and to report suspected ADRs to the regulatory authorities and/or the manufacturer.

Pharmacovigilance is now seen as a specialist discipline within the industry and most large pharmaceutical companies have sizeable pharmacovigilance departments. In small companies, however, individuals may combine the role with clinical research or regulatory tasks. Some contract research organisations (CROs) have now established pharmacovigilance groups to offer this service to companies (Chukwujindu *et al.*, 1999).

Limitations of pre-marketing clinical studies to identify safety issues

In terms of their power to detect rare (particularly type B) ADRs, programmes of clinical studies conducted before the granting of an MAA are limited for several reasons:

- The relatively small number of patients/subjects studied before marketing (see Table 3) compared with the larger numbers exposed after marketing. Studies are usually powered to determine efficacy not safety; to have a high degree of certainty of detecting rare reactions requires large numbers of patients (see Table 4).
- The frequent exclusion of individuals who may be at greater risk of ADRs, e.g. the young, the elderly, pregnant women and patients with significant concurrent diseases and taking other medication.

Table 3. Median number (and ranges) of volunteers and patients exposed to new chemical entities during pre-marketing studies (applications submitted to the CSM during the period 1987–1989) (Rawlins and Jefferys, 1991).

	Healthy volunteers	Efficacy studies	Safety database
All applications	68 (0–819)	861 (41–4906)	1171 (43–15 962)
Successful applications	92 (0–819)	1126 (122–4906)	1480 (129–9400)

Table 4. Number of patients required in order to be 95% certain of detecting one, two and three cases of an adverse reaction when there is no background incidence of the reaction (Lewis, 1981).

Incidence of adverse reaction	Number of patients required to detect:		
	One ADR	Two ADRs	Three ADRs
1 in 100	300	480	650
1 in 200	600	960	1300
1 in 1000	3000	4800	6500
1 in 2000	6000	9600	13 000
1 in 10 000	30 000	48 000	65 000

- The structured nature of clinical studies where drugs are given at specific doses for limited periods with careful monitoring by experienced investigators. In clinical practice, a drug is unlikely to be used strictly in accordance with the SPC and there is less monitoring.
- The possibly long latent period between starting the drug and the development of the ADR.

Only with wider experience during routine clinical practice will it be possible to identify the rare ADRs and other groups of patients 'at risk' for ADRs. Post-marketing surveillance (PMS), which can be defined as the systematic detection and evaluation of adverse reactions occurring in association with pharmaceutical products under customary conditions of use in ordinary clinical practice, is therefore essential.

The first step in PMS is signal generation and this can be done by spontaneous reporting, publication of case reports, cohort studies and post-marketing clinical studies. While there may then be a period of signal strengthening, the next step is to subject such signals to hypothesis testing, e.g. by conducting case-control studies, to determine whether the signal does indeed indicate a new ADR.

According to Waller and Lee (1999), the following factors determine whether or not a signal should be investigated further:

- the strength of the signal;
- whether the issue or some aspect of it is new;
- its clinical importance, i.e. seriousness and severity;
- the potential for preventive measures.

SPONTANEOUS REPORTING

Spontaneous or voluntary reporting involves a doctor describing his or her own clinical observation of a suspected ADR with a marketed drug. Unlike reporting in clinical trials, spontaneous reports are unsolicited apart from the general invitation to use the national reporting system such as the UK 'yellow card scheme' (see below). Spontaneous reporting depends on the individual doctor recognising a possible ADR, suspecting a possible causal link to a drug or drugs, and reporting this observation.

Spontaneous reports can be made to the regulatory authority, to the pharmaceutical company that markets the product, or to medical or scientific journals. The pattern of reporting varies considerably between countries. In the UK most doctors report to the Committee on Safety of Medicines (CSM)/Medicines Control Agency (MCA) using yellow cards; conversely, in the USA and Germany, about 90% of reports to the regulatory authority are from companies. In practice, many reports to pharmaceutical companies come initially from non-medical health care professionals, such as hospital pharmacists and nurses, or directly from patients. Company sales representatives should also be instructed to pass verbal reports from doctors and others to the appropriate department. Company pharmacovigilance staff endeavour to obtain medical validation by the patient's doctor and seek detailed information on each case. This would include patient demographic details (age, sex, etc.), medical history, dose, route of administration and details of suspected ADR (symptoms, signs, timing, dechallenge and outcome). Additional information such as allergies, laboratory data and alternative causes excluded are also helpful in interpreting individual case reports.

Spontaneous reporting commences immediately a new drug is marketed, continues indefinitely, and theoretically involves all doctors and covers the entire patient population receiving the drug. It is very good for generating new ADR hypotheses and has identified many new ADRs, including those that are rare or occur in a particularly susceptible sub-population. It can also detect and characterise common reactions, perhaps confirming suspicions aroused during clinical studies.

Limitations of spontaneous reporting

The main disadvantage of any spontaneous reporting system is under-reporting of possible ADRs. Inman (1980) suggested that this was due to 'seven deadly sins':

1. complacency – the mistaken belief that only safe drugs are approved;
2. fear of litigation;
3. guilt because the patient may have been harmed by the treatment;
4. ambition to collect and publish a personal series of cases;
5. ignorance of how to report;
6. diffidence about reporting mere suspicions; and
7. lethargy.

Many factors influence reporting, such as volume of sales, how long the drug has been on the market, the type and severity of the ADR and publicity about the drug and the reaction. The reasons for doctors reporting or not reporting are undoubtedly complex.

Another limitation of spontaneous reporting is the difficulty doctors have in recognising previously unknown drug reactions. Some well-established ADRs were not initially recognised as such because they are common symptoms in the patient population; examples in this category are eye effects with beta-blockers or cough due to ACE inhibitors. It often takes one or two astute doctors to make and report these initial observations before others submit similar cases.

Occasionally, a single (or small number of) spontaneous report(s) can identify a new ADR. This usually happens when an acute, recognised iatrogenic event (e.g. anaphylaxis) occurs almost immediately after drug administration. Some type A reactions can also be recognised from spontaneous reports when viewed in the light of the drug's pharmacology; for example, sudden, profound hypotension on starting a new antihypertensive drug. In most instances, however, spontaneous reports generate suspicion of a new ADR but do not confirm the hypothesis. Typically, this is where the possible ADR mimics naturally occurring diseases, symptoms or signs – i.e. background noise in the population. In such situations, hypotheses generated by spontaneous reports may be confirmed by two principal methods: case-control studies and cohort studies.

Unlike the situation in clinical studies, the incidence of an ADR cannot be determined from spontaneous reports; only a reporting rate can be calculated. Neither the numerator (number of case reports) nor the denominator (number of patients exposed) can be accurately known. By the same token, there is no way of knowing what proportion of ADRs has been reported, and uncertainty usually exists as to how many cases are in fact drug-related. The denominator can be estimated from sales figures or numbers of prescriptions but, because most drugs are given in varying doses and for different durations, such estimates are crude.

The UK yellow card scheme

The thalidomide tragedy in the early 1960s resulted in the establishment of drug regulatory agencies by many Western governments and led to the recognition that centralised collection of ADR reports was crucial to monitoring drug safety. In the UK, the Committee on the Safety of Drugs was set up, under the chairmanship of Sir Derrick Dunlop, who wrote to all doctors requesting reports of 'any untoward condition in a patient which might be the result of drug treatment'. He announced the establishment of a Register of Adverse Reactions and a system of yellow business reply-paid cards for reporting suspected reactions. The Committee was reconstituted as the CSM following the Medicines Act 1968, which provided it with statutory powers.

Yellow reporting forms are now available in the British National Formulary, the ABPI Compendium of Data Sheets and SPCs and in prescription pads. Doctors are encouraged to report any reactions that could conceivably be associated with new drugs, i.e. those indicated by a black triangle (▼), and any serious suspected reactions with established products. The MCA receives about 20 000 reports per year; every case is reviewed by an assessor at the MCA and is entered on the Adverse Drug Reactions On-line Information Tracking (ADROIT) database. Information from the reports sent directly by doctors is made available to the product licence holder, i.e. the pharmaceutical company, as anonymised single patient prints (ASPPs) and product analysis prints (PAPs).

The yellow card system has generated many new ADR hypotheses and has had numerous successes in identifying and characterising new ADRs, some very quickly, others after many years. Its notable failure was the delay in identifying the practolol oculomucocutaneous syndrome in the mid-1970s, but once the first case reports had been published, hundreds of yellow cards followed (Inman, 1980).

CASE-CONTROL STUDIES

In a case-control study, a group of patients with a particular adverse event (cases) is matched with a control group without the adverse event (controls) and their exposure to a risk factor, such as a drug, is compared. To reduce bias, the controls should be matched as closely as possible for all factors (age, sex, etc.) other than the adverse event; however, many possible biases exist (Sackett, 1979). The number of control patients is usually larger than the number of cases.

While case-control studies do not identify new ADR hypotheses, they can be an invaluable way of investigating drug reaction hypotheses generated by other methods, such as spontaneous reporting. They are most suitable for investigating a single outcome (for example, an ADR, cancer or death), but can also be used to look at the association with multiple exposures, i.e. drugs, smoking, etc. Case-control studies cannot determine the incidence of an ADR, but they provide a measure of relative risk compared with the control group; this is known as the odds ratio.

By studying patients with the event and matched controls, a case-control study might involve tens or hundreds of patients rather than the thousands required for a cohort study. They can hence be conducted quickly and at low cost if a suitable method of identifying the cases and controls is available. Case-control studies generally obtain their information on exposures retro-spectively from a database or by abstracting medical records or administering questionnaires or interviews. Unless the relative risk is substantial, they are unlikely to be of great value for drugs that are not widely used.

Classic case-control studies proved the association between lung cancer and cigarette smoking. The case-control approach can be particularly useful where the event under investigation is rare. For instance, to test the hypothesis that vaginal adenocarcinoma in young women was due to their mothers having taken diethylstilboestrol during pregnancy, Herbst et al. (1971) conducted a case-control study involving eight cases and four matched controls who were born within 5 days for each case. All mothers were interviewed using a standard questionnaire. A highly significant association was found between maternal treatment with diethylstilboestrol and the subsequent development of vaginal adenocarcinoma in the daughters. No significant differences were found for maternal age, smoking, X-ray exposure and breast-feeding.

Careful study design is necessary to reduce sources of bias, and for this reason the results of case-control studies are often challenged by other groups. Such studies should therefore be conducted by independent, experienced investigators using reliable databases and methodology.

COHORT STUDIES

In a cohort study, a group of patients receiving a drug is identified and observed over time to determine the rate of occurrence of adverse events or outcomes. Another group of patients not receiving the drug, or possibly receiving another similar drug, is usually identified for comparison (control group). Cohort studies can be performed prospectively, i.e. simultaneously with the events under study, or retrospectively after the relevant events have already occurred, by using a database or reviewing medical records or using questionnaires and interviews. They can generate new ADR hypotheses and can be used to test existing hypotheses. They are sometimes described as observational cohort studies for obvious reasons, but the act of observing must not modify what is being observed.

In some ways cohort studies resemble controlled clinical trials, but the key difference is that participants in clinical trials are allocated to the study or control groups by randomisation, whereas in cohort studies the decision about treatment has already been made. This can result in bias known as 'channelling' (see below). Cohort studies are good for monitoring a wide range of ADRs and different outcomes that do not have to be defined in advance; hence they can be a useful means of searching for ADRs with a new drug. Many PMS studies conducted by the pharmaceutical industry and CROs are of this type.

Cohort studies require large sample sizes to study relatively uncommon ADRs and outcomes. This makes prospectively conducted studies very expensive and time-consuming, especially for drugs taken long term, when the study must continue for months or years. Another disadvantage of long-term studies is that many patients are lost to follow-up, thus reducing the power of the study to identify rarer ADRs and possibly affecting the validity of the results. For statistical reasons, cohort studies cannot detect very rare ADRs (see Table 4); such ADRs are best identified by spontaneous reporting and confirmed by case-control studies.

Retrospective cohort studies are usually conducted by selecting the patient population from a database. As with case-control studies, unless the relative risk is substantial, they are of limited value for drugs that are not widely used. Retrospective studies are dependent on the databases available and may include hospital cases, patients in general practice or the total population. Using trained nurse and pharmacist monitors, the Boston Collaborative Drug Surveillance Program, started in 1966, collected data from a large inpatient population at several hospitals. Although no longer active, the database has been used for a number of cohort and case-control studies. One example was the identification of a cohort of 1189 patients who had received intravenous cimetidine; this cohort provided reasonable estimates of toxicity (Porter et al., 1986). Forty patients (3.4%) had experienced adverse reactions, the most frequently reported being neuropsychiatric disorders (19 patients), which occurred with greater frequency in the older age groups, and leucopenia (eight patients).

Prospective cohort studies are usually conducted by identifying prescriptions for the study drug, and any drug used as a control, after they have been written. This can be done by pharmacists or prescription-pricing organisations. A cohort study of cimetidine conducted in the UK used both these methods. After the prescription had been dispensed, monitors visited the general practitioners (GPs) to record simple patient details and to identify a control patient who had not taken cimetidine, matching them for sex and age group but not disease (Colin-Jones et al., 1982). Nearly 10 000 patients who had taken cimetidine and almost as many controls were followed for 18 months. Cimetidine takers were found to be twice as likely to die during the study period as the controls, and there was an increased frequency of gastric cancer, other cancers and morbidity generally in the cimetidine group (Colin-Jones et al., 1987). The study co-ordinators attributed this not to cimetidine, but to underlying disease and other factors such as smoking and alcohol. Comparisons with national mortality data suggested that the control group was reasonably representative of the general population, but that the cimetidine group was not. The authors concluded that cohort studies should be capable of detecting all events occurring within a defined group of individuals, but that interpretation is difficult or impossible for the majority of events that mimic those occurring in the ordinary community. This well-executed, large study illustrated the problems of selecting an appropriate control group in a cohort study.

Channelling

Channelling is a way of describing the form of allocation bias, inherent in cohort studies, where apparently similar drugs are given to groups of patients with prognostic differences (Petri and Urquhart, 1991). Drugs with similar actions that are marketed at different times, and thus in different competitive situations, may be channelled to different groups of patients. Claims of fewer or less severe ADRs with the new drug may result in it being given to patients who had problems during treatment with an earlier drug. Similarly, claims for greater efficacy may channel it to patients in whom previous treatment has failed.

Channelling appeared to occur with Osmosin, a controlled-release form of indomethacin, for which fewer gastrointestinal side-effects were claimed. The product was withdrawn from the market because reports suggested an unexpectedly high occurrence of gastrointestinal ulcerations, bleeding or perforation. However, it is likely that it was prescribed for patients who were most likely to develop these problems. Within-patient control data can be used in order to avoid channelling bias (Petri and Urquhart, 1991).

PRESCRIPTION EVENT MONITORING

Prescription event monitoring (PEM) is a method of post-marketing surveillance conducted by the Drug Safety Research Unit (DSRU) in Southampton, UK. The DSRU is a charitable trust supported partly by donations from the pharmaceutical industry. Its mission is to monitor, study and communicate the safety of medicines (Shakir and Wilton, 2000). PEM studies are conducted on new medicines that are likely to be used widely in general practice. The main objective is to generate new ADR hypotheses, and to test existing hypotheses; examples include visual field defects with the anticonvulsant drug vigabatrin (Wilton et al., 1999) and serotonin syndrome with antidepressants (Mackay et al., 1999).

All prescriptions written by GPs in England are sent to the Prescription Pricing Authority which then forwards details of prescriptions for the drugs being studied to the DSRU, including the patient's name and that of the prescribing GP. After a period of time, usually 6 months, a questionnaire (green form) is sent to the prescribing GP who is asked to record the patient's age, indication for treatment, starting and stopping dates of treatment, whether the drug was effective, reasons for discontinuing treatment and 'events' during or after treatment. An event is defined as any new diagnosis, any reason for referral or admission to hospital, any unexpected deterioration or improvement in a concurrent illness, any suspected drug reaction, any alteration of clinical importance in laboratory values, or any other complaint considered sufficiently important to be entered in the patient's notes.

PEM studies provide incidence rates for events reported in 'everyday' practice; for patients on the drug these rates can be compared with those of patients who have discontinued it, or with those of patients on other drugs studied by PEM, allowing hypotheses about ADRs to be generated and ADRs to be identified.

PEM studies have the following strengths:

- they are non-interventional and retrospective, and therefore do not influence prescribing decisions – a major criticism of many PMS studies;
- they allow large populations to be studied in 'real world' conditions (average cohort size 10 721 patients in 74 completed PEM studies);
- they prompt all prescribers to provide event data (the response rate averages about 60%); and
- the expanding database is a valuable research tool, holding data on over one million patients.

Their disadvantages include:

- the time taken to complete the study – data are usually collected for 18 to 24 months (Mackay, 1998);
- their limitation to drugs prescribed in general practice;

- their lack of randomisation – this can lead to biases (most notably confounding by indication), making comparisons inappropriate;
- their inability to measure patient compliance (although data are based on dispensed prescriptions only); and
- the assumption that unreturned green forms would not differ from those returned.

THE GENERAL PRACTICE RESEARCH DATABASE

The General Practice Research Database (GPRD) is the world's largest computerised database of anonymised longitudinal clinical records from general practice. Originally established in 1987 as the VAMP Research Databank, it contains more than 30 million patient years of data. In the year 2000, data will be collected on more than 2.6 million patients from a broadly representative sample of practices in the UK. The data will comprise:

- demographic information (age, sex, registration date);
- medical records:
    - symptoms, diagnosis;
    - hospital referrals and summaries of outpatient letters;
    - treatment outcomes, including discharge diagnoses;
    - selected tests and results;
    - birth and death registration information;
- drug history:
    - all prescriptions (drug, dose, quantity);
    - indications;
- miscellaneous patient care information (immunisation, contraception, smoking status, height, weight).

The history of the database has been documented by Lawson *et al.* (1998). Academics, government departments, medicines regulatory authorities, the UK National Health Service and the pharmaceutical industry have used the GPRD. The extensive bibliography of publications in peer-reviewed journals, available on the GPRD website (www.gprd.com), testifies to the quality of data. Examples of studies conducted using the GPRD include the association between selective serotonin reuptake inhibitors and gastrointestinal bleeding (De Abajo *et al.*, 1999); the risk of venous thromboembolism in users of postcoital contraceptives (Vasilakis *et al.*, 1999); and the prevalence and management of heart failure in general practice (Majeed and Moser, 1999). Whilst usage has focused on epidemiological and pharmacoepidemiological studies, researchers are using the database increasingly for prescribing analysis, health outcome studies, health service planning and the development of pharmacoeconomic models.

Management responsibility for the GPRD was transferred in April 1999 to the UK MCA and a major investment in the database was announced to secure its future viability and evolution to support a wider range of public health activities. The redevelopment plans include enabling on-line access to the data and a range of services and enhanced feedback to contributing GPs in autumn 2000.

INDUSTRY-SPONSORED PMS IN THE UK AND SAMM

In 1985 the CSM Adverse Reactions Working Party, chaired by Professor Grahame-Smith, recommended that PMS studies should be undertaken under voluntary arrangements between the CSM and pharmaceutical companies on newly marketed drugs intended for widespread long-term use. It also stated that the CSM would expect PMS studies to be carried out on most new drugs, with decisions to be made on a case-by-case basis concerning which drugs would be involved and what form the studies should take. These recommendations led to the 'quadripartite guidelines' formulated jointly by the APBI, the British Medical Association, the CSM, and the Royal College of General Practitioners (Joint Committee, 1988).

Four years later, MCA staff reviewed their files of all such PMS studies that had taken place and evaluated their contribution to monitoring drug safety (Waller *et al.*, 1992). Thirty-one studies were included in the review, 27 prospective and four retrospective, of which only nine had a comparator group. Planned sample sizes ranged from 200 to 30 000 patients (median 5600), but only five studies achieved at least 75% of their target. The median ratio of study sample size to patient exposure before marketing was only 1.6. The duration of follow-up ranged from 2 to 104 weeks and was generally appropriate to the type of treatment. The ADR profiles seen were generally similar to those available from the yellow card scheme. Only one study identified an important new safety hazard, and for one of the drugs a new safety hazard was identified by another method. The review authors expressed four main areas of concern:

- Most studies did not include any comparator groups.
- In most studies patients had been identified prospectively, i.e. before a decision to prescribe had been made.
- Patient recruitment was slow: hence hazards were more likely to be identified by other methods, thus reducing the value of the study.
- Companies were slow to provide the MCA with information about these studies.

The value of PMS studies would be improved by increasing sample size, by removing selection bias in recruitment and by using comparator groups. The authors also suggested that a variety of study designs is necessary and that there should be a greater emphasis on potential safety issues identified in clinical trials or from spontaneous reports. This review confirmed the findings of surveys conducted about 10 years previously that PMS studies were ineffective at identifying new ADRs. In the USA, FDA staff reviewed three large Phase IV studies and determined that none resulted in the detection of new ADRs (Rossi *et al.*, 1983). Stephens (1984) surveyed 60 company-sponsored PMS studies involving some 340 000 patients in 11 countries. None of the publications mentioned the discovery of new ADRs, but subsequently 106 spontaneous reports of new ADR hypotheses for the drugs were published.

As a result of the review by Waller *et al.* (1992), the 'quadripartite guidelines' were reviewed, with additional representation from the MCA, to form the 'quintapartite' working party. This resulted in the Safety Assessment of Marketed Medicines (SAMM) guidelines for the conduct of all company-sponsored studies that evaluate the safety of marketed products in the UK (Medicines Control Agency, 1993). Although the SAMM guidelines initially caused a decrease in the number of new PMS studies conducted, the design and quality of these safety assessments have probably improved as a result.

The American Society for Clinical Pharmacology and Therapeutics has also published guidelines, similar to those in the UK, for prospective pharmacoepidemiology studies (Strom, 1990). These guidelines state that anyone conducting a PMS study must be prepared to defend its objectives and scientific design to a legitimate scientific or regulatory body.

Seeding studies

Uncontrolled cohort studies that appear to be planned more for marketing advantage than for detecting new ADRs are known as 'seeding studies'. They aim to alter physician prescribing practice; since this objective is not mentioned in the protocol, they are inherently dishonest and bring discredit to the industry and to the doctors involved (Stephens, 1993).

PRODUCT INFORMATION

One of the ultimate aims of drug safety monitoring in clinical studies and PMS is to provide clear and helpful product information in the SPC and similar documents in order to promote safe use of the product (see Table 5).

CONCLUSION

Drug safety monitoring should be an integral part of all clinical studies involving drug treatment. There should be a clear strategy for the collection, analysis and presentation of the safety data in the clinical study report and, where applicable, in the MAA and NDA. Although much of the knowledge concerning the safety of a drug can be gained from the programme of studies

Table 5. Sections of product information relevant to safety (Waller and Lee, 1999).

Section	Examples
Indications/uses	Limiting indications to particular conditions with the greatest benefits. Removal of indications: (a) for which the benefits are insufficient to justify use, and (b) for which use is associated with a greater risk of ADRs
Dosing instructions	Reductions in dose (may be applied to specific groups, e.g. the elderly); limitations on duration or frequency of treatment (especially for ADRs related to cumulative dose); provision of information on safer administration
Contra-indications	Addition of concomitant diseases and/or medications for which the risks of use are expected to outweigh the benefits
Interactions	Addition of concomitant medications or foods which may interact; advice on co-prescription and monitoring
Pregnancy/lactation	Addition of new information relating to effects on foetus or neonate; revised advice about use in these circumstances based on accumulating experience
Warnings/precautions	Addition of concomitant diseases and/or medications for which the risks of use need to be weighed carefully against the benefits; additional or modified recommendations for monitoring patients
Undesirable effects	Addition of newly recognised adverse reactions; improving information about the nature, frequency and severity of effects already listed
Overdosage	Adverse effects of overdosage; methods of management, including the need for monitoring

conducted before marketing, this is limited in some respects. Active pharmacovigilance is therefore necessary throughout the life of the product. New safety signals must be properly investigated and evaluated and the safety information on the product must be continuously updated.

ACKNOWLEDGEMENTS

I thank Dr Sian Taylor of the DSRU for information on Prescription Event Monitoring and Dr Louise Wood at the MCA for information on the General Practice Research Database. I am most grateful to a number of my colleagues for their constructive comments on the drafts of this chapter.

REFERENCES

Chukwujindu, JI, Holman, C and Sanderson, P (1999). Pharmacovigilance: the role of a CRO. *Int J Pharm Med* **13**, 137–141.

Colin-Jones, DG, Langman, MJS, Lawson, DH and Vessey, MP (1982). Cimetidine and gastric cancer: preliminary report from post-marketing surveillance study. *Br Med J* **285**, 1311–1313.

Colin-Jones, DG, Langman, MJS, Lawson, DH and Vessey, MP (1987). Review: post-marketing surveillance of the safety of cimetidine – the problems of data interpretation. *Aliment Pharmacol Ther* **1**, 167–177.

De Abajo, FJ, Rodriguez, LAG and Montero, D (1999). Association between selective serotonin reuptake inhibitors and upper gastrointestinal bleeding: population-based case-control study. *Br Med J* **319**, 1106–1109.

Finney, DJ (1965). The design and logic of a monitor of drug use. *J Chron Dis* **18**, 77–98.

Gait, JE and Goldsmith, D (2000). Should serious adverse events requiring expedited regulatory reporting be unblinded? *Int J Pharm Med* **14**, 37–39.

Hampton, JR (2000). Clinical trial safety committees: the devil's spoon. *Br Med J* **320**, 244–245.

Herbst, AL, Ulfelder, H and Poskanzer, DC (1971). Adenocarcinoma of the vagina. Association of maternal stilbestrol therapy with tumor appearance in young women. *N Engl J Med* **284**, 878–881.

ICH Guideline (1994). *Topic E2A: Clinical Safety Data Management: Definitions and Standards for Expedited Reporting*, International Federation of Pharmaceutical Manufacturers Associations, Geneva (Issued as CPMP/ICH/377/95).

ICH Guideline (1995). *Topic E3: Structure and Content of Clinical Study Reports*, International Federation of Pharmaceutical Manufacturers Associations, Geneva (Issued as CPMP/ICH/137/95).

Inman, WHW (1980). The United Kingdom. In: Inman, WHW (Ed), *Monitoring for Drug Safety*, MTP Press, Lancaster, pp. 36–37.

Joint Committee of ABPI, BMA, CSM and RCGP (1988). Guidelines on post-marketing surveillance. *Br Med J* **296**, 399–400.

Lawson, DH, Sherman, V and Hollowell, J (1998). The General Practice Research Database. Scientific and Ethical Advisory Group. *Q J Med* **91**, 445–452.

Lewis, JA (1981). Post-marketing surveillance: how many patients? *Trends Pharm Sci* **2**, 93–94.

Mackay, FJ (1998). Post-marketing studies. The work of the Drug Safety Research Unit. *Drug Safety* **19**, 343–353.

Mackay, FJ, Dunn, NR and Mann, RD (1999). Antidepressants and the serotonin syndrome in general practice. *Br J Gen Pract* **49**, 871–874.

Majeed, A and Moser, K (1999). Prevalence and management of heart failure in general practice in England and Wales 1994–96. *Health Statist Q* **4**, 9–15.

Medicines Control Agency (1993). *SAMM Guidelines: Guidelines for Company-Sponsored Safety Assessment of Marketed Medicines*, Medicines Control Agency, London.

Petri, H and Urquhart, J (1991). Channeling bias in the interpretation of drug effects. *Statist Med* **10**, 577–581.

Porter, JB, Beard, K, Walker, AM, Lawson, DH, Jick, H and Kellaway, GS (1986). Intensive hospital monitoring study of intravenous cimetidine. *Arch Intern Med* **146**, 2237–2239.

Rawlins, MD and Jefferys, DB (1991). Study of United Kingdom product licence applications containing new active substances, 1987–9. *Br Med J* **302**, 223–225.

Rawlins, MD and Thompson, JW (1991). Mechanisms of adverse drug reactions. In: Davies, DM (Ed), *Textbook of Adverse Drug Reactions (4th edn)*, Oxford University Press, Oxford, pp. 18–45.

Rossi, AC, Knapp, DE, Anello, C, O'Neill, RT, Graham, CF, Mendelis, PS and Stanley, GR (1983). Discovery of adverse drug reactions. A comparison of selected Phase IV studies with spontaneous reporting methods. *JAMA* **249**, 2226–2228.

Sackett, DL (1979). Bias in analytic research. *J Chron Dis* **32**, 51–63.

Shakir, S and Wilton, L (2000). Drug Safety Research Unit and pharmacoepidemiology. *Int J Pharm Med* **14**,1–2.

Skegg, DCG and Doll, R (1977). The case for recording events in clinical trials. *Br Med J* **2**, 1523–1524.

Stephens, MDB (1984). Pharmaceutical company viewpoint. In: Walker, SR and Goldberg, A (Eds), *Monitoring for Adverse Drug Reactions*. MTP Press, Lancaster, pp. 119–125.

Stephens, MDB (1993). Marketing aspects of company-sponsored postmarketing surveillance studies. *Drug Safety* **8**, 1–8.

Stephens, MDB (1998). Laboratory investigations. In: Stephens, MDB, Talbot, JCC and Routledge, PA (Eds), *Detection of New Adverse Drug Reactions (4th edn)*, Macmillan, London, pp. 149–196.

Strom, BL (1990). Notes of the American Society for Clinical Pharmacology and Therapeutics. *Clin Pharmacol Ther* **48**, 598.

Talbot, JCC and Nilsson, BS (1998). Pharmacovigilance in the pharmaceutical industry. *Br J Clin Pharmacol* **45**, 427–431.

Tanser, PH, Campbell, LM, Carranza, J, Karrash, J, Toutouzas, P and Watts, R (2000). Candesartan cilexetil is not associated with cough in hypertensive patients with enalapril-induced cough. *Am J Hypertens* **13**, 214–218.

Vasilakis, C, Jick, SS and Jick, H (1999). The risk of venous thromboembolism in users of postcoital contraceptive pills. *Contraception* **59**, 79–83.

Wallander, MA, Dimenas, E, Svardsudd, K and Wiklund, I (1991). Evaluation of three methods of symptom reporting in a clinical trial of felodipine. *Eur J Clin Pharmacol* **41**, 187–196.

Waller, PC and Lee, EH (1999). Responding to drug safety issues. *Pharmacoepidemiol Drug Safety* **8**, 535–552.

Waller, PC, Wood SM, Langman, MJS, Breckenridge, AM and Rawlins, MD (1992). Review of company postmarketing surveillance studies. *Br Med J* **304**, 1470–1472.

Wilton, LV, Stephens, MDB and Mann, RD (1999). Visual field defect associated with vigabatrin: observational cohort study. *Br Med J* **319**, 1165–1166.

14

Outcomes research and health economics

Pippa Anderson and Adam Lloyd

INTRODUCTION

The importance of health technology assessment has grown enormously in recent years because it is one of the ways in which those who fund health care, for example governments, insurers and health care provider systems, try to keep health care spending under control.

The pressure for control of health care expenditure has arisen because demand for health care is increasing while budgets for health care are constrained. Technological advances and increased understanding of disease processes mean not only that more health care interventions are available but also that awareness of this increased availability is growing amongst patient populations. In addition, demographic changes mean that the potential consumers of health care are also increasing in number; for example, the proportion of older people (i.e. those likely to use more health care resources) is growing.

Governments have developed many strategies for handling the increase in demand for health care and its consequent impact on budgets. Many developed countries impose requirements ('hurdles') for safety, efficacy and quality data, before health technologies are granted reimbursement or access to the market. Many governments are now also seeking evidence of cost-effectiveness for health care interventions. This requirement is often referred to as the 'fourth hurdle'. Thus, health technology industries worldwide are now under pressure to produce evidence of economic value alongside clinical efficacy data. Failure to provide this evidence could result in restricted formulary listing, no reimbursement or no government-level approval for use of a particular health care intervention. Apart from evaluating value for money, governments use reference pricing and guidance on generic prescribing as additional strategies to achieve cost containment.

These initiatives are important for those involved in clinical research. If market access is to be optimised, studies must be designed to meet the information requirements of the agencies that will ultimately appraise health technologies. If those who design and conduct studies understand the techniques of outcomes research and economic evaluation, how to interpret the results and the uses to which study results are put, it is more likely that new health technologies will ultimately reach the market place where they may benefit patients.

This chapter provides an overview of outcomes research and health economics for the clinical researcher with little experience in these disciplines. These are complex, rapidly evolving subjects that cannot be covered fully here. The references and further reading at the end are intended to help those who would like to explore the subject in greater depth.

BASIC CONCEPTS

Value for money

Value for money is a concept that we can all appreciate and that we usually try to maximise within our household or business lives. Unfortunately, even if we are able to obtain value information on our desired purchase, we are not always in a position to enjoy those products that demonstrate the best value for money. For example, a Jaguar motor car may represent excellent value for money but not everyone can afford one!

It is usually easy to obtain information about the price or charges associated with a product, i.e. the acquisition costs. More thought and effort, however, are required to understand the true cost of a product. There may be delivery charges, maintenance costs and additional taxation and insurance associated with owning a car, and these raise the true cost of ownership to a level that may be very different from the purchase price. Neither is it always straightforward to identify and quantify in absolute terms the value of some aspects of a product. Getting to the heart of the matter may necessitate detailed discussion with the users and providers of that product (or health care intervention), as people often have different needs and different values. An everyday example will help to clarify some of the important concepts discussed in this review.

Costs and benefits

Some people might value the appearance of a product, in this example a toaster. Provided that the toaster performs its basic function, there might be other attributes that are valuable to a purchaser, who might be willing to pay more for a toaster with these attributes; perhaps it has to match other items in the kitchen or simply be a pleasing colour to look at. Other people might not care about colour, but be more interested in the technical aspects of the product.

When assessing the value of a product, it is also important to consider what measure of value is most appropriate and which costs are most relevant, both for the purchaser and for others who might benefit from the product. For example, the choice of toaster colour might positively impact the purchaser's quality of life (QoL), yielding a measurable increase on a QoL instrument. Alternatively, the technical aspects of one toaster compared with another may mean that it will produce many more perfectly coloured pieces of toast and, unlike a cheaper alternative, be width-adjustable for the thickness of the bread that the purchaser will want to toast. The cheaper model may be less reliable or more likely to jam when thicker slices are toasted, resulting in higher maintenance charges due to more frequent repairs. Thus, the true cost of the apparently cheaper model will be higher than the acquisition cost.

Effectiveness and efficacy

The rate of perfectly brown toast production per week might be the outcome measure of interest to someone with a big family that likes toast. This could be said to be a measure of the 'effectiveness' of the toaster to them. In our example, the manufacturers may not have thought through the full range of options that customers might want for their money and have only made 'efficacy' data available in their product information, i.e. the ability to produce a number of slices of toasted bread in a period of time. For the toasters under consideration, it appears that both toasters do this equally well. This may not be the primary or only feature of interest to prospective purchasers. In the absence of relevant information, the potential purchaser might ask friends and neighbours informally for information about the two different toasters before making a decision to purchase. Unfortunately, this information may be inaccurate, or based on limited or infrequent experience, and result in an inappropriate choice. Given the different acquisition costs, prospective purchasers might be unaware of the additional value of the more expensive toaster and might simply opt for the cheaper model.

Affordability

No matter how desirable the value aspects that enhance the more expensive toaster, this information will not influence a purchaser with limited financial resources. The cheaper model that performs less well against the above criteria will be purchased because that is all the purchaser can afford.

The issues described above in everyday terms should clarify some of the complex questions that frequently pertain to health care interventions, and are fundamental to the growing field of economic evaluation and appraisal of health care interventions. The value of an intervention may be wide-ranging: it may have an impact on disease progression, QoL, and life expectancy, or it may simply be easier or speedier to administer. It is not always easy to capture those value-for-money aspects of an intervention that are most important, what the real costs are, and how the intervention will affect the overall delivery of health care. This may be particularly so if changes are necessary to realise the full benefits of the intervention. However, it will continue to be important to address these issues because significant expansion of health care spending and reduced interest in value for money are unlikely scenarios.

This introduction to value measurement in a non-health care environment has raised the following important issues:

- Outcome measures must be chosen to ensure that the *effectiveness* of an intervention is captured as well as its *efficacy*.
- The choice of outcome measures depends on the perspective of those considering the intervention and the setting in which it is to be used.
- With budgetary limitations, the total cost of adopting the intervention is important and may well drive decision-making as much as or more than the effectiveness data.

OUTCOMES RESEARCH

Table 1 defines the terms and language of outcomes research that may be frequently encountered by the clinical researcher. However, the reader is warned that in the literature confusion sometimes ensues because these terms are not always used consistently.

As an umbrella term covering a research environment supported by many disciplines, outcomes research is the most inclusive of the concepts defined in

Table 1. Terms and definitions.

Term	Definition
Outcomes research	The process of identifying and measuring the health outcomes that are important to the target audience
Economics	The study of scarcity and choice
Economic evaluation	The *comparative* analysis of *alternative* courses of action in terms of both costs and consequences
Health economics	The application of economics to health care and medicine
Pharmacoeconomics (PE)	The application of health economics to pharmaceuticals
Health-related quality of life (HRQoL)	A multidimensional concept that encompasses the physical, emotional and social components associated with an illness or its treatments (Revicki *et al.*, 1992)

Table 1. A full-scale outcomes study would typically involve epidemiologists, clinical researchers, health economists, statisticians, psychometricians, health service researchers, and QoL experts.

Health outcomes

When setting up a health outcomes study, it is important to explore and then define the outcome(s) of a health care intervention of interest. An outcome is an end result but the application of this concept to health care is not straightforward. An outcome that the patient might consider to be important and relevant could well be different from an outcome of interest to the clinician or to the body funding the treatment.

The American Institute of Medicine defines a health outcome as 'achievement in relation to realistic expectations or targets' and the UK Department of Health defines a health outcome as 'an attributable effect of an intervention or its lack on a previous health state'. To a clinician, the main outcomes of care might be mortality and morbidity. The two main types of outcome relating to health economics are considered below.

Economic outcomes

Economic outcomes include medical resource use and the cost of care of a patient receiving a health care intervention, and also the economic impact on the patient's ability to work, to benefit employers, or to participate in normal family life. The subject of economic evaluations and measurement of economic outcomes will be handled more fully in a later section.

Health-related quality of life (HRQoL) outcomes

HRQoL outcomes associated with health care interventions focus on the patient's experience of the intervention and its effect, and how the patient might value the impact of the intervention. HRQoL measurement will be covered in more depth in a later section.

EFFICACY AND EFFECTIVENESS

Randomised controlled trials

The randomised controlled trial (RCT) is regarded as the gold standard for demonstrating the clinical efficacy of an intervention. The tightly controlled inclusion and exclusion criteria are intended to eliminate bias and give the trial its high internal validity. Nowadays, clinical studies do not generally report short- or long-term clinical outcomes because the expense of large-scale, long-term studies is prohibitive, and they may also be impractical or unethical. Thus, it is usual for RCTs in many interventions to utilise a surrogate marker (e.g.

viral load or CD4 cell count in human immunodeficiency virus studies) that has a well-established relationship with a clinical benefit (e.g. longer life and less morbidity). Another good example of a surrogate marker is blood pressure: this is known to be associated with risk of cardiovascular events. The link between surrogate marker and clinical outcome needs to be clearly defined and quantified if it is to be useful in generating efficacy and effectiveness data.

When the study comes to be analysed and reported, the clinical outcome is estimated from the change in the surrogate end-point. If the surrogate end-point has a value and clinical relevance, as well as a well-established link with the clinical outcome, this has to be accepted as a sensible way of optimising clinical research budgets. In our blood pressure example, there are data from the long-running observational cohort study in Framingham, Massachusetts, USA, to provide the evidential link that raised blood pressure is a risk factor for cardiovascular disease (Anderson *et al.*, 1991). Thus, if an intervention reduces blood pressure levels in clinical studies, it is reasonable to infer that this is a surrogate marker for a reduction in the risk of cardiovascular disease in the longer term.

However, for those who are interested in the effect of a drug in the real world, this practical use of surrogate markers can reduce the information available. Few surrogate markers are as well understood as blood pressure. Also, a small-scale study may not detect rare but important side-effects and therefore fail to capture the economic and QoL impact as well as the impact of the clinical benefit of the intervention.

In the context of clinical research, *efficacy* is how well an intervention works under ideal or controlled conditions. It is one of the important outputs of RCTs in Phase II and III drug development programmes.

In contrast to efficacy data, *effectiveness* data show how well an intervention works in a real-life setting. Effectiveness data can be generated from trials that have wide inclusion and exclusion criteria and reflect real-world conditions for the use of the intervention. These are often referred to as 'pragmatic', 'real-world' or 'naturalistic' trials.

Given the high internal validity of the RCT, efficacy does not always translate into effectiveness in practice. This does not necessarily mean that the intervention lacks an effect: instead the dosing of a drug may be sub-optimal in practice, due to patient non-compliance or a poor clinical understanding of drug regimens. The medical care surrounding the intervention may not reach the high standards practised in the clinical trial programme when the intervention was developed, and this can have a significant impact on effectiveness. While RCTs can provide an excellent opportunity for prospective collection of QoL or economic data, the relative ease of data collection has to be weighed against the lack of generalisability to 'real life' because of the controlled and possibly atypical setting from which the data were derived. In addition, the value of the data collected in the trial should be weighed against the burden of extra data collection on study investigators and subjects compared with alternative strategies for data collection.

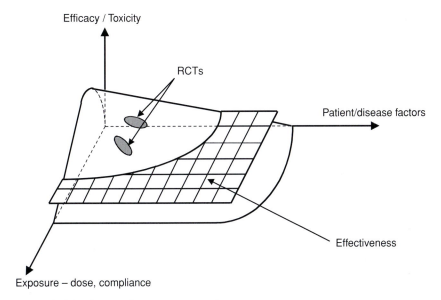

Figure 1. The dose–patient–response surface.

The relationship between RCT data, safety and efficacy and effectiveness is summarised in Figure 1.

Pragmatic trials

Pragmatic trials have less restricted entry criteria and allow recruitment of subjects with co-morbidities. Such trials are usually randomised, and blinding is not typically part of the design, thus reducing measurement bias, but at the expense of selection bias. The comparator in a pragmatic trial should be current care, and the setting and investigators should be representative of the setting in which the intervention will actually be used. The medical resources used should not be protocol-driven, meaning that laboratory tests and other procedures occur as they would normally. This design is far more useful to a researcher who is attempting to evaluate the cost of a disease and an intervention, or the patient's HRQoL.

Observational studies

These studies evaluate the outcome of a medical intervention, typically in a cohort of patients, and are usually run in the setting in which the intervention is intended to be used. The study population is heterogeneous and is not overly restricted by inclusion or exclusion criteria. There may or may not be a control or comparator group. Randomisation is not usually used. While these studies are very useful for evaluating real-life medical resource use and outcomes, they have a potential for confounding and bias, and data analysis should consequently be adjusted to reflect this.

Database studies

The use of electronic databases (also called automated or routine data) for outcomes research studies is increasing. Some Health Maintenance Organisations (HMOs) in the USA have large claims databases that can be used for research. In the UK, use of the General Practice Research Database (GPRD) is increasing, and in the rest of Europe there are a number of databases that support the growing outcomes research movement. These databases offer the opportunity to evaluate treatment outcomes and resource use on cohorts of patients selected from the database. The databases are not always set up as research databases; for example, the HMO databases exist for claims purposes and outcomes research is a secondary use. The extraction, analysis and interpretation of data on medical resource use and treatment outcomes is a specialist skill, and database research should be designed and executed in partnership with such specialists.

In summary, outcomes research is a broad area that involves collaboration between clinical researchers, health economists, statisticians, and epidemiologists. Study design and execution will always reflect a compromise between the desired goal of the evaluation, the research question, the extent of the budget available, availability of target population, and ease of measurement of the critical outcomes.

ECONOMICS AND HEALTH ECONOMICS

Economic evaluation

Unlike most goods and services, much health care is free at the point of delivery. Access in many countries is subsidised or insured so that the user does not have to pay the full cost of the service. A third party – insurer, sickness fund or government – pays the bill. This means that patients consume as much health care as they need, rather than as much as they can afford. It is up to the third party to allocate enough budget to pay the bills. It is unlikely that the allocated budget will meet all the health care needs of a population, and health care spending will inevitably be finite. The problem of prioritising interventions for funding is one result of this situation. The use of economic principles allows health care funders to evaluate the costs and benefits of the alternative uses of health care resources and, potentially, to organise spending to maximise the benefits. Efficiency – a state achieved when resources are allocated such that the maximum benefit is achieved with the resources available – is the desired goal when applying economic principles.

Health economics is the application of economics to health care and medicine. The information gained from applying economics to health care can be used to inform and support a wide range of decisions. For example, health economic information should help to answer the following questions:

- Should a new hospital be built, or should care continue to be given from existing older premises?
- How should health care funds be allocated between primary and secondary care?
- Which diseases should be treated as a priority?
- What are the most beneficial protocols for a disease management programme?
- What intervention is the best to use in a specific disease?

Economics is not only concerned with money or costs, or indeed solely the concern of economists; we all make economic decisions every day. Economic evaluation (or economic appraisal) is the *comparative* analysis of *alternative* courses of action in terms both of their costs and their consequences. It is a generic term that covers a number of techniques (described later in this section) and should encompass the costs and the benefits of an intervention.

Economic evaluation has a systematic and explicit framework in and of itself but it should also add to a wider evaluation process. For example, appraisals performed for the National Institute for Clinical Excellence (NICE) in England and Wales consider the clinical evidence and service delivery aspects of the intervention as well as its cost-effectiveness and patient benefits such as HRQoL gains.

Many health care decision makers can be involved in the introduction of a new intervention. In the UK, for example, this ranges from the Secretary of State for Health through health authorities and primary care groups to individual clinicians. To assist with decisions, a hierarchy of advisors is available, including NICE, specialty advisors, consultants in public health medicine, and prescribing advisors.

It is also important to consider the evaluation perspective from the outset. Should it be that of the individual patient, the health care provider, the health care purchaser, the regulators, the health care system, the government or society in general? The information users and other interested parties in each context may have quite different needs from an evaluation. The appropriate perspective will drive the choice of evaluation (as well as any decision) that is to be made.

In the context of wider health technology assessment, decision makers seek arguments that are sufficiently robust to pass more than a health economics test. Other relevant aspects of health technology assessment must be addressed. Given a clear context for assessment, a good health economics package should have a number of characteristics, including good evidence of effectiveness and a robust assessment of costs. Important though these are, the package also needs to offer solutions to any problems that might be caused by the new technology, e.g. reorganisation of service provision to ensure that the intervention is delivered to the right people at the right time.

Economic evaluation techniques

There are four main approaches to economic evaluation in the health care environment (see Table 2 and the following section).

Table 2. Summary of economic evaluation methods.

Type of analysis	Outcomes
Cost–minimisation analysis (CMA)	Outcomes identical
Cost–effectiveness analysis (CEA)	Outcomes measured in natural units, e.g. life years gained
Cost–utility analysis (CUA)	Outcomes weighted by utility, e.g. QALYs
Cost–benefit analysis (CBA)	Outcomes measured in monetary terms

Cost-minimisation analysis (CMA)

The purpose of CMA is to identify the intervention that costs the least. The outcomes of the interventions compared should be the same. An example might be an evaluation of day surgery versus inpatient surgery. Given evidence that the outcome (for example, 'successful operation') of each intervention compared is the same, the analysis should concentrate on identifying and quantifying the costs associated with each intervention. While this analysis sounds straightforward, it is vital to ensure that all the outcomes are indeed the same. For example, in the case of day surgery versus inpatient surgery, there may be an HRQoL difference associated with the differing management alternatives. Thus, the outcomes might be considered not to be the same. Determining the costs associated with the intervention in CMA can be difficult, and pragmatism is required in defining the level of detail of resource identification for the costing process.

Cost-effectiveness analysis (CEA)

CEA is used when the outcomes of interventions vary, but are measured in terms of a common natural unit, e.g. life years gained or days without symptoms. CEA is often useful for making choices and decisions about treatment alternatives within a single therapy area. For example, various interventions are available to lower blood pressure in people with hypertension. These interventions are associated with different levels of efficacy (lowering of blood pressure) and side-effects (possibly resulting in additional medical resource use). The impact on relative reduction in blood pressure translates into cardiovascular risk reductions and, consequently, life years gained. The common measure of outcome (life years gained) allows comparison of the effectiveness and cost per unit of effectiveness of the different interventions in different patient populations.

Effectiveness data for CEA can be obtained from clinical trial data, the existing research literature and epidemiological evidence. One way to obtain data is to conduct a prospective evaluation alongside a clinical trial so that relevant costs and effectiveness data can be collected in parallel with the trial. However, it should be borne in mind that the population here will be relatively narrow and may not always be the most appropriate (see below for further discussion of the pros and cons of data collection alongside clinical trials).

Assumptions about effectiveness evidence, whatever its source, mean that there may well be uncertainty about the true effectiveness of an intervention. Uncertainty may also surround the cost data collected for an evaluation. Sensitivity analysis can be used to test the robustness of the results of an evaluation, either by simply varying one or more key variables or by analysing extreme scenarios. Probabilistic sensitivity analysis uses more sophisticated, computer-based models to assign ranges and distributions to variables and to generate confidence intervals.

Cost–utility analysis (CUA)

CEA is limited in application because it is unable to inform decisions about allocation of resources to different interventions for different diseases. Cost-effectiveness methodology has therefore been extended to develop a 'utility'-based measure of outcome. Utility in this context is a term that encompasses a measure of satisfaction with, or preference for, health states resulting from an intervention (or lack of it). The advantage of having a utility value as an outcome measure is that it provides a single index that can be used to weight life years gained from an intervention and to yield an outcome expressed in quality-adjusted life years (QALYs) or cost per QALY gained. This means that, for any intervention in any disease area, there is a common outcome that can be used as a basis for comparisons.

Quality-adjusted life years. The QALY is a multi-dimensional measure of health. It is an attempt to combine quantity of life with quality of life in a single index score. This measure allows comparison of the QALYs gained for one intervention in one disease to be compared with those for another intervention in another disease (see CUA, above). More controversially, QALYs can be used to aid priority-setting across different health care programmes. In this case, resources are allocated to maximise the number of QALYs within a budget. This means in effect that we are 'buying' the cheapest QALYs first.

The idea of having intervention outcomes ranked in order of cost per QALY is appealing because it gives a consistent set of value-for-money information. In reality, however, health care decision-making is far more complex because issues of age, equity, access and affordability can influence decisions and are not captured in the QALY paradigm. These issues, as well as political priorities, mean that decisions cannot be based simply on QALY rankings.

A utility value associated with a state of health or an intervention can be derived using different approaches. This is because there are differences in the theoretical underpinnings of the methods developed to derive the utility values. When planning an evaluation, it is important to consider which of the approaches might be the most appropriate, and also to consider the practical aspects surrounding the methods of deriving utility values. Instruments, including multi-attribute utility instruments (MAUIs), have been developed that generate index measures in which a single score is derived by aggregating a number of single items or subscale scores. The choice of appropriate instruments for inclusion in a study is limited and is influenced by the disease area and country.

In deciding on which approach to employ, it is advisable to consult an expert when planning a study of this type. The EuroQol (EQ-5D) instrument is an example of a MAUI. There is a tendency for the EQ-5D to be used in Europe because much of the research to develop the instrument was performed there. Readers seeking further information on the EQ-5D should consult the list of websites at the end of this chapter.

Cost–benefit analysis (CBA)

CBA is a comprehensive form of economic evaluation that has been widely used in economics outside the health sector. Its application to the health care environment is logical because it takes the broad societal perspective and attempts to quantify and value both costs and benefits in monetary terms. The advantages of this method are clear because a decision on an intervention can be evaluated in terms of benefits exceeding costs. In some countries, patients pay for health care interventions and there is the opportunity to obtain a monetary value for an intervention. Most typically, however, health care systems do not charge for services, and so different methods for capturing the monetary valuation of an intervention have been adapted for use in the health care environment. One example of this approach to obtaining a currency valuation for an intervention is the 'willingness to pay' (WTP) methodology. Individuals' preferences for an intervention can be captured using a specially developed questionnaire that describes health scenarios and asks for a monetary valuation from the respondent. As with CUA, the measurement of WTP can vary and is fraught with methodological issues. CBAs are also complex and potentially expensive evaluations; it is best to consult a health economist if this form of analysis is deemed necessary. CBAs are still used infrequently in health care.

Readers seeking a more detailed description of the methods for economic evaluation should consult *Methods for the Economic Evaluation of Health Care Programmes* (Drummond *et al.*, 1997).

MEASURING COSTS

There are three categories of costs associated with the impact of a health care intervention: direct, indirect and intangible costs (see also Table 3).

Table 3. Jargon-busting: some terms used in costing.

Term	Definition
Direct costs	Medical, e.g. nurses' salaries. Non-medical, e.g. patient transport costs
Discounting	Technique for calculating the present value of costs and benefits of an intervention that falls in the future (the rate varies by country)
Incremental costs	The difference between the costs of alternative interventions
Indirect costs	Productivity gains and losses (e.g. loss of wages)
Intangible costs	Costs of pain, grief and suffering
Marginal costs	The cost of producing an extra unit of service
Opportunity cost	Value of the benefits forgone because the resource is not available for its best alternative use
Resources	Land, labour, capital, drugs, equipment

Direct costs are actual expenditures and are conventionally subdivided into:

● medical costs, e.g. the hotel costs of hospital care, drugs, clinical staff salaries and delivering the intervention; and
● non-medical costs, e.g. patient transport, social services expenditure.

Indirect costs are not actual payments but rather potential benefits forgone, such as changes in productivity that occur due to an intervention, e.g. losses to an employer due to sickness absence.

Intangible costs impact individuals because of the pain and suffering associated with their illness (and possibly its treatment). Compared with direct and indirect costs, intangible costs are more complex to value financially.

CMA should be used to inform a decision when the least costly option is being sought. Sometimes a decision concerns not whether a service should be provided, or a particular procedure undertaken, but rather how much of the service should be provided. In the day surgery v. inpatient surgery example above, an economic evaluation would help with the decision whether to expand day surgery and reduce inpatient surgery. In this case the decision would concentrate on *marginal costs* – the change in total costs resulting from a *change* in activity. The use of average costs compared with marginal costs might misinform the decision. The average cost of inpatient hospital stay does not reflect the fact that the initial days in hospital are generally more expensive than the later days. Hence, an intervention that reduces hospital days may reduce costs in terms of the charges associated with the cheaper days in hospital. In general the marginal cost is the appropriate cost to use in economic evaluation.

In CEA, the comparison is made between marginal cost and marginal outcome, i.e. the additional cost of using one intervention rather than the alternative, divided by the additional benefit. The differences between the interventions are expressed in *incremental* cost-effectiveness ratios.

Discounting and inflation

Many health care interventions cost money over a prolonged period and have an impact on health care costs well into the future. Interventions can also incur high costs now, but deliver their benefits well into the future. Discounting is a method of standardising differing cost and time profiles to bring them to present-day values. It works on the principle that costs and benefits now are more valuable than those in the future because people and society prefer to have things now (positive time preference). Economic evaluation weights costs by a discount rate, according to the year in which they accrue. Most countries are explicit about the discount rate that applies to costs in an economic evaluation. However, the discounting of outcomes is more complex and is still under debate among economists. Health and health care are not tradable resources and there is limited evidence to suggest that there is a positive time preference for health benefits. (However, there is a suggestion that people do not value highly future health benefits, as shown by activities such as smoking and drinking that have a negative impact on future health.) This is important because adoption of a zero or positive discount rate can affect the relative cost-effectiveness of different procedures. A zero rate will increase the cost-effectiveness of an intervention that costs a great deal initially but subsequently costs very little. For example, a vaccination programme has benefits over the lifetime of the recipient, while a health promotion campaign, e.g. to encourage people to stop smoking, may yield benefits at a remote future time.

ECONOMIC ANALYSIS ALONGSIDE CLINICAL TRIALS

Clinical trials present a convenient vehicle for evaluating a health care intervention and there is a temptation always to 'piggy back' an economic evaluation on to a trial. However, the potential advantages of this approach are offset by problems, and researchers planning or conducting such trials should be aware of them.

The trial being considered for the 'piggy back' study should meet the appropriate standards for trial design and have a sufficient sample size to detect at least the clinically important end-point. It is not easy to apply standard principles of statistical inference to economic variables; sample size calculations are problematic because the concept of an 'economically important difference' is not always easy to define. A pragmatic approach is usually adopted and the clinical end-point drives the sample size calculation. However, if little is known about the distribution of the key resource items and if the economic parameters show large variability, it is important to recognise that the trial may lack the statistical power to detect important differences in cost.

Clinical trials are usually conducted in tightly controlled settings with a homogeneous population. The trial protocol and tests employed may not reflect routine clinical practice and the comparator may not be relevant to usual practice. The data generated from these trials will have high internal validity, but often bear little relationship to the setting in which the intervention will be used in the real world. Late-stage drug development can include trials that are run in a more pragmatic manner and with broader inclusion and exclusion criteria in a setting that more closely reflects clinical practice.

As discussed above, the end-point of a clinical trial may not be ideal for an economic evaluation. Longer-term outcomes such as survival or interval between events may drive the economic analysis, but these outcomes are rarely collected in a study that is run for clinical evaluations, either because of cost, time and feasibility or simply because the objective of the study (perhaps a regulatory submission) does not require this information. Economic modelling can be used to overcome this, but is not always an ideal alternative for the health care decision maker who may prefer 'real life' data.

Clinical efficacy is very likely to be comparable nationally and internationally. The same is not always true of real-life medical resource use, costs, effectiveness and other economic data.

Conducting an economic evaluation alongside a clinical trial carries with it an additional burden for investigator and patients who have to complete the expanded case record forms (CRFs) and extra patient questionnaires. This then increases the burden for data handlers and analysts when the trial is complete. For this reason, it is important to consider how much of the data collection can be done outside the clinical trial and whether a reduced data collection load is appropriate within a subset of centres. This latter suggestion carries the important caveat that this data subset must be generalisable to all centres and to real life.

Assessment of a clinical trial programme to identify appropriate vehicles for an economic evaluation should take account of the above points.

Cost-of-illness studies

While cost-of-illness studies are not economic evaluations in the strict sense, they are an economic tool used to estimate the total cost or burden of a disease on the health service or society. They usually quantify the health care resource cost and the morbidity and mortality cost. While cost-of-illness studies are a very useful approach for estimating a baseline from which to plan economic evaluations, they do not provide information on the impact of a new intervention in terms of effectiveness or cost-effectiveness. Their usefulness also lies in identifying where an intervention might make most impact in terms of costs and likely benefits to the health care system. Such studies can make use of existing data or utilise clinical studies to collect more detailed data on costs and the burden of an illness on individuals and populations, for instance in terms of HRQoL.

HEALTH-RELATED QUALITY OF LIFE

Quality of life is a difficult concept to encapsulate. While many definitions exist, the common central theme is captured in the elements of the World Health Organization definition of health: 'Health – a state of complete physical, mental and social well-being and not merely the absence of disease or infirmity'. For the purposes of this chapter, QoL refers to HRQoL, as defined in Table 1 (Revicki *et al.*, 1992). This concept incorporates all the factors that impact upon an individual's health, and includes physical, sensory, cognitive, social and emotional functioning as well as experience of pain and the ability to care for oneself.

Disease impacts HRQoL in a number of ways and the effect on different dimensions of health depends on the nature of the disease. As when a stone is dropped into a pond, the effects ripple out into all areas of life (see Figure 2). How far the ripples reach and their size depend on the nature of the disease.

The evaluation of HRQoL in a clinical trial or in routine patient management recognises that there is more to disease than clinical signs and symptoms. For example, a patient asked about asthma will not mention inflammation of the lungs and bronchoconstriction, but will talk about being unable to run for a bus or being bothered by pollen. This translates into limitation of physical activity or curtailed social life through having to stay indoors in the hay fever season to avoid triggering an asthma attack.

HRQoL is an important and relevant indicator of benefit to a patient during or following a health care intervention. A clinical trial evaluating interventions using HRQoL outcome measures may pick up a meaningful difference in impact on QoL as a result of apparently small differences in clinical benefit, or may detect the presence or absence of HRQoL impact of an intervention in people who were previously untreated.

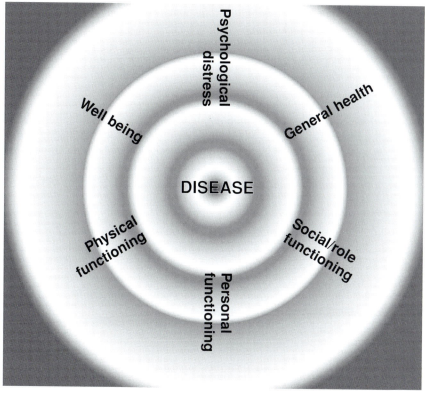

Figure 2. Disease and its potential impact.

In the context of health care delivery and the goal of improved health care for a patient population, clinicians, purchasers, providers and patients should also evaluate interventions by assessing the process of health care delivery as well as the outcome. Trade-offs between quality and quantity of life are important for assessing disease and treatment processes and outcomes, both for individual patients and for populations. Given the choice, one patient might feel that temporary loss of HRQoL (perhaps due to side-effects through a course of treatment) may not be 'worth it' despite potential improvement at the end of treatment; another patient may take the opposite view.

HRQoL is an important outcome measure for the person with a chronic disease such as multiple sclerosis or asthma, and has its place in clinical management. The team involved in disease management, the patient's caregivers and those who give treatment, support and rehabilitation all contribute to the HRQoL of the patient. In a disease where cure is not possible, the clinical team managing the individual's treatment and care seeks to improve or at least maintain the patient's HRQoL and to preserve independence and function as far as possible. Disease symptoms may be a barrier to a social life, continuing education or enjoying the social aspects of employment. Family life and the opportunity for leisure activities may decline. These problems, along with any loss in economic status, potentially affect the quality of the patient's life.

Measuring HRQoL

Most, but not all HRQoL instruments are designed to be self-administered, and such questionnaires should be completed by the patients wherever possible because they are the best judges of their own QoL. A study by Jachuck *et al.* (1982) illustrates the different results obtained (see Figure 3) when different people are asked about the HRQoL impact of a single intervention. A group of people with asymptomatic hypertension, their close relatives and their clinician completed an HRQoL questionnaire. The clinician thought that HRQoL must have been improved since the patients were being treated for their condition. While a few patients felt that there was a negative HRQoL impact, roughly half of the total patient population felt that HRQoL was about the same and half felt that it was better. The relatives' assessment of HRQoL was that HRQoL had diminished because the patient was an 'ill' person.

Some instruments are sufficiently simple to be included in a CRF or used in postal surveys as an adjunct to a prospective clinical trial. Other instruments designed to be administered by third parties, either face to face or on the telephone, are good for detailed data collection but this option has a significant impact on budget and time.

Broadly speaking, the existing approaches to HRQoL measurement can be placed into two categories: *generic* or *disease-specific*.

Many generic quality of life measures exist and some are available worldwide, translated and tailored for local use. The benefit of the generic approach

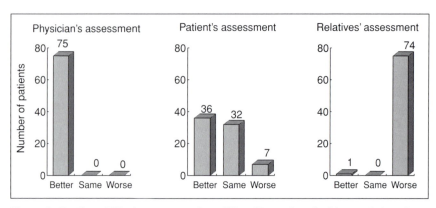

Figure 3. Quality of life: how perspectives differ. (Reproduced with permission, from Jachuck *et al.*, 1982.)

to measurement is that the impact on HRQoL of one disease can be compared with that of another. Care has to be taken when selecting a generic instrument for use in a particular disease. A generic instrument does not always pick up variability of symptoms amongst diseases and their impact on aspects of HRQoL. Disease-specific measures, however, can be more sensitive to particular problems and outcomes associated with specific conditions and their treatments.

The development of an HRQoL instrument is a rigorous scientific undertaking that includes a complete literature review, patient interviews, repeated testing of the instrument on the population of interest, and detailed statistical interpretation before the instrument can be accepted as a valid indicator of HRQoL. In the context of HRQoL instrument development, validity is defined as the extent to which the instrument measures what it is supposed to measure and does not measure what it is not supposed to measure. Instrument validation studies address the following criteria:

Reliability: analysis of the accuracy and precision of a measurement and the extent to which a measurement is reproducible on repeated administrations within the same subject and within the same temporal period it was designed to evaluate.

Content validity: an assessment of how well items in a measure sample the universe of possible measures within the intended domain.

Construct validity: the verification of expected theoretical relations between actual scale scores and external criteria known or believed to be associated with scale scores.

Criterion validity: the demonstration that actual scale scores correlate with an accurate or previously validated measure of the same concept.

Responsiveness: the ability to detect clinically significant within-patient changes over time.

The selection criteria for an appropriate instrument to be used in surveys and clinical studies are addressed in a review of HRQoL assessment by Cox *et al.* (1992). In the section that discusses HRQoL instrument selection, it is suggested that: 'Each context requires an assessment of the impact of ill health on aspects of the everyday life of the individual'.

The conclusions of Cox *et al.* (1992) highlight several points that are of particular relevance to the search for an HRQoL instrument:

- 'Simplicity should be the keynote wherever possible (whether with respect to design, analysis or presentation) ...'
- 'Despite the desirability of allowing (some) personalisation or special

choices for particular applications, the use of standard (evaluated) scales is advocated as a core with more detailed customised extensions.'

- 'A presentation of the results of QoL assessments should, as well as being as simple as possible, facilitate their use in treatment decisions for individual patients and interpretation of the clinical significance of events.'

- 'Despite practical and analytical difficulties, satisfactory assessment of QoL in clinical trials is worth pursuing, since the relevance of traditional approaches is limited and their objectivity to some extent illusory.'

The question of whether to use a disease-specific or a generic HRQoL instrument in a trial is hotly debated. Generic measures are applicable across different diseases and can be used to survey general populations with which diseased populations can be compared. These instruments generate descriptive profiles that create a rich picture of the impact of disease. A well-known example of a generic HRQoL instrument is the Short Form 36 (SF-36) Health Status Measure (Ware and Sherbourne, 1992; Ware, 1993; see also the list of useful websites at the end of the chapter). An example of a disease-specific HRQoL instrument is the Asthma Quality of Life Questionnaire (AQLQ) developed by Juniper *et al.* (1993).

One way of bridging the gap between the sensitivity of a disease-specific measure and the advantage of cross-disease comparison offered by a generic measure is to use both a disease-specific instrument and a generic instrument in the study, while recognising that the increased burden on respondents might diminish the completion rate. If available, another approach is to use an instrument that has a core containing a generic measure plus additional questions that address the specific impact of the disease. One example of this approach is the Multiple Sclerosis Quality of Life-54 (MSQoL-54) measure (Vickrey *et al.*, 1995, 1997).

HEALTH TECHNOLOGY ASSESSMENT AND MARKET ACCESS

This section describes the spread of health technology assessment (HTA) as a prerequisite for reimbursement and market access, and reviews the main information requirements of agencies that appraise health intervention.

Reimbursement and controls on market access

At the time of writing, the health care systems of many countries impose restrictions on the sale of health technologies. Health technologies include pharmaceuticals, medical devices and health care interventions such as surgical procedures. For the most part, however, the restrictions are focused on pharmaceuticals. As explained earlier, much of the motivation for these restrictions comes from the increasing cost of funding health care, and the desire of governments and others to control the growth in health care spending. In many countries this situation has led to the establishment of formal reimbursement procedures and other controls on market access.

Reimbursement applications typically take place after an intervention has been approved for marketing, for example, by the US Food and Drug Administration (FDA) or the European equivalent, the European Agency for the Evaluation of Medicinal Products (EMEA). Once this step, sometimes known as 'technical approval', has been completed, the efficacy, safety and manufacturing quality of a pharmaceutical or device can be regarded as proven. In many settings, however, this is not sufficient in itself to achieve market access. A further round of negotiation may be required to obtain the approval of the health service or health insurer that the intervention should be used in their system and that they are willing to pay for it.

Health care systems vary significantly, and each country has its own methods of controlling market access for new technologies. Some of the most common methods used and the settings in which they are found are described below.

Reimbursement negotiations are common in European countries. The developer of a pharmaceutical or medical device that has recently received technical approval must make a separate application to the health care system to request reimbursement status for the intervention. Negotiations between the manufacturer and the government or its agents may cover issues such as the patients in whom the intervention will be used; the effectiveness of the new intervention compared with existing therapies; and the price the government is willing to pay. If an intervention does not achieve reimbursement status then patients may only receive the intervention if they are willing to pay for it themselves.

Pricing may also be closely linked with market access. In certain countries (e.g. Spain) the price at which a new intervention can be sold must be negotiated with the government; and the sponsor company must provide evidence that the new intervention is desirable or else the health service will not grant a realistic price for the product.

Applications for formulary listing are the most common hurdle to market access in the USA. Companies there are free to set the price at which they will sell their technologies, but the insurance companies that pay for much of the health care provided are not obliged to pay for them. Many of the larger HMOs and similar bodies that insure against the costs of health care maintain formularies listing the pharmaceuticals that they will pay for. Many hospitals, primary care groups and primary care trusts in the UK also maintain formularies and expect physicians to prescribe only treatments that are included in these listings.

Other methods of controlling market access include treatment guidelines for particular disease areas and guidance from NICE and similar bodies.

The role of HTA in market access

Market access differs from technical approval in a number of important respects. While efficacy and safety are vital components of the decision and clearly relate to whether an intervention should be paid for, other telling considerations will form part of the negotiations:

- whether the intervention will provide real benefits to patients in practice (i.e. effectiveness as well as efficacy);
- its impact on overall expenditure;
- whether the intervention is an appropriate use of limited resources;
- political considerations; and
- the price that the sponsor company wishes to charge.

Because market access negotiations often determine who will pay for an intervention, value for money is a natural ingredient in these discussions. Payers are frequently not obliged to pay for new interventions, even if technical approval has been granted. In any event, they have a strong incentive to pay the lowest possible prices (even if this reduces the money available to pay for future research) because budgets are fixed, usually on an annual basis. Health systems also face pressures to show that they are spending their money wisely and to the benefit of patients. For all these reasons, recent years have witnessed an increase in the use of health economics in market access negotiations.

The spread of the 'fourth hurdle'

Australia was the first country formally to require companies to provide economic evaluations of new medical technologies. In the early 1990s the Australian Pharmaceutical Benefits Advisory Committee (PBAC) instructed pharmaceutical companies to prepare economic evaluations when requesting that drugs be included in their formulary, the listing that determines what will be reimbursed in the Australian public health care system. The Australian system of economic assessment of new medicines remains one of the most sophisticated and several other countries' systems reflect the Australian approach.

At present, health systems in the majority of developed countries either require economic evaluations or allow sponsor companies to present economic evaluations in support of reimbursement negotiations. Table 4 summarises the use of economic information in market access negotiations in a number of major markets. In most countries, the requirements for information to support applications for pharmaceuticals are more stringent than for other medical technologies.

Other markets that require or will consider economic information as part of their market access negotiations include: Sweden, Denmark, Norway, Finland, Portugal, New Zealand and several countries in Central and Eastern Europe.

Table 4. The requirements for economic information in market access negotiations.

Market	Economic information	Notes
USA	Required by some insurers	Each insurer has the right to set individual requirements. Many larger HMOs (e.g. Regence Blue Shield, Washington) have detailed requirements
Japan	Not required at present	The Ministry of Health and Welfare (MHW) has announced that it is considering introducing a requirement for economic evaluation
Germany	Not required	
France	Required for pharmaceuticals	A reimbursed price for new pharmaceuticals must be agreed with the transparency commission, which is willing to consider detailed economic arguments on the recommendation of the Economic Committee. Companies are required to re-submit their economic justification every 5 years to show that their intervention remains cost-effective in ordinary practice
Italy	Considered as part of reimbursement application for new pharmaceuticals	The Ministry of Health has requested economic justification for new pharmaceuticals although it is not yet clear how this information will be assessed
UK	Compulsory for technologies selected by NICE	NICE conducts assessments of the cost-effectiveness of both new and existing technologies, including pharmaceuticals, medical devices and other interventions
Spain	Not required at present	
Canada	Compulsory for some new pharmaceuticals	Companies must make submissions to health systems in several provinces. A central body, the Canadian Co-ordinating Office for Health Technology Assessment (CCOHTA), also conducts economic evaluations of established pharmaceuticals, devices and technologies
Australia	Compulsory	Very detailed guidance is available to companies for new chemical entities (NCEs), major new indications and major expansions of treated populations
Netherlands	Compulsory (pilot phase)	The sickness funds federation will require economic evaluation for selected new pharmaceuticals. Ther system is being introduced over the next 3 years.

Information required by agencies

The information required for market access varies from country to country, but a number of common patterns can be observed (see Table 4). The list of information required by NICE in England and Wales is fairly typical, and includes:

1. *Evidence of efficacy and safety.*
2. *Details of the population in which the intervention will be used.* Many agencies have the power to restrict reimbursement to a smaller group than the total population for which an intervention is indicated or might be used. For example, use of a new intervention can be restricted to a very severely ill group of patients or to a particular setting, or may be permitted only after other therapies have been tried and have failed.
3. *Evidence of the effectiveness of the intervention.* NICE prefers generic measures of health gain such as QALYs, symptom-free days or improvement in HRQoL.
4. *Evidence of cost-effectiveness using a recognised methodology.*
5. *Details of the impact on total expenditure if the new intervention is introduced.* Almost all markets require the sponsor company to estimate the likely total sales of the new intervention and the impact that its introduction will have on total expenditure. In general, interventions that are likely to have a large impact on budget receive more rigorous scrutiny than those indicated for small numbers of patients or likely to achieve limited total sales.
6. *Other important aspects.* For example, effect on health care service delivery.

The last five years have seen a rapid increase in the number of settings in which health economic information is used as part of the reimbursement negotiation process. Other countries are currently considering introducing similar controls, and the importance of economic information in this setting can only increase further. The possibility of introducing assessment of economic information at a European level is also being explored.

Implications

The increasing use of economic evaluation in the context of market access suggests that health economics is likely to become a more important part of clinical research over time. Clinical trials performed by the health technology industries must evolve to reflect the information needed to support market access negotiations, and one key change will be to include economic data collection. However, it is also important that these studies assess whether the selected patient population is relevant to that in which reimbursement will be sought, and whether the outcomes assessed will demonstrate the effectiveness as well as the efficacy of the intervention.

The situation is changing rapidly, but clinical development programmes extend over several years. Studies designed today must be sufficiently far-sighted to recognise that economic information will be increasingly important when the results of these studies come to be used in a few years' time. The team planning a development programme for a new intervention should there-fore include a health economist to ensure that the intervention is appropri-ately supported by economic and outcomes data when it reaches the market.

USEFUL WEBSITES

1. Information on the *EuroQol* and the algorithms available to generate utility scores from health states is available on the EuroQol website (http://www.euroqol.org).
2. Information about available versions of the *SF-36*, scoring rules and algorithms is to be found on the SF-36 website (http://www.sf-36.com) and in the *SF-36 Manual*: see Ware (1993). The UK English language version of the SF-36 has been widely used in the UK by a network of investigators who have pooled their experience to produce a rich database, including popula-tion norms and profiles for specific conditions: see Jenkinson *et al.* (1993).
3. The *National Institute for Clinical Excellence (NICE)* in the UK maintains a substantial website (http://www.nice.org.uk) that includes information on the purpose and content of the appraisal process for medical technolo-gies. New guidelines for manufacturers will be released in early 2001.
4. The *Pharmaceutical Benefits Advisory Committee (PBAC)*, the authority responsible for admitting new pharmaceuticals to the list of reimbursed products in Australia, has the best established and probably the most sophisticated system for assessing new medicines. The PBAC website (http://www.health.gov.au/haf/branch/pbb/pes.htm) offers detailed guidance about the information to be submitted.
5. The *General Practice Research Database (GPRD)* website is at http://www.gprd.com.

REFERENCES AND FURTHER READING

Anderson, KM, Wilson, PWF, Odell, PM and Kannel, WB (1991). An updated coronary risk profile: a statement for health professionals. *Circulation* **83**, 356–362.

Cox, DR, Fitzpatrick, R, Fletcher, AE *et al.* (1992). Quality-of-life assessment: can we keep it simple? *J Roy Stat Soc A* **155**, 353–393.

Drummond, MF, O'Brien, B, Stoddart GL and Torrance, GW (1997). *Methods for the Economic Evaluation of Health Care Programmes (2nd edn)*, Oxford Medical Publications, Oxford.

Jachuck, SJ, Brierley, H, Jachuck, S and Willcox, PM (1982). The effect of hypoten-sive drugs on quality of life. *J Roy Coll Gen Pract* **32**, 103–105.

Jenkinson, C, Coulter, A and Wright, L (1993). Short Form 36 (SF-36) Health Survey questionnaire: normative data for adults of working age. *Br Med J* **306**, 1437–1440.

Juniper, EF, Guyatt, GH, Ferrie, PJ and Griffith, LE (1993). Measuring quality of life in asthma. *Am Rev Respir Dis* **147**, 832–838.

Revicki, DA, Rothman, M and Luce, BR (1992). Health-related quality of life assessment and the pharmaceutical industry. *PharmacoEconomics* **1**, 394–408.

Spilker, B (1995). *Quality of Life and Pharmacoeconomics in Clinical Trials (2nd edn)*, Raven Press, New York.

Vickrey, BG, Hays, RD, Harooni, R, Myers, LW and Ellison, GW (1995). A health-related quality of life measure for multiple sclerosis. *Qual Life Res* **4**, 187–206.

Vickrey, BG, Hays, RD, Genovese, BJ, Myers, LW and Ellison, GW (1997). Comparison of a generic to disease-targeted health-related quality-of-life measures for multiple sclerosis. *J Clin Epidemiol* **50**, 557–569.

Ware, JE (1993). *SF-36 Health Survey. Manual and Interpretation Guide*, Nimrod Press, Boston.

Ware, JE and Sherbourne, CD (1992). The MOS 36–item short-form health survey (SF-36). I. Conceptual framework and item selection. *Med Care* **30**, 473–483.

15

Data management, now and in the future

Karen Grover and Roger Ashby

INTRODUCTION

'The truth, the whole truth, and nothing but the truth'. This phrase encapsulates the objectives of the clinical data manager, whose job it is to organise and ensure the collection of accurate data from the trial, to capture the data on a database, to validate and correct the data, and to provide the 'clean' data to the statistician in a form that will facilitate the statistical analysis. Because the data represent the results of the trial and provide the only basis for analysis and determination of its outcome, it is evident that the data manager performs a central and critical function in the trial and, ultimately, in the successful registration of the new drug.

Ideally, the data manager will be involved in all aspects of the trial's organisation that affect the data to be collected. In the case record form (CRF) design phase (*see Chapter 9*), the data manager can give guidance, for instance, on the format and internal consistency of the document and the suitability of text versus coded responses, and identify potential problem areas within the data. At the investigator meeting, the data manager can guide the investigators through the CRF, pointing out how entries should be made and highlighting aspects that could lead to query generation. At the monitors' meetings, the data manager can review the queries generated, identifying any systematic or site-specific problems. Involvement such as this is the best way to ensure the quality of the data recorded on the CRF and thus to minimise the time-consuming and expensive process of querying and correcting data.

DATA MANAGEMENT NOW

Planning for the trial

The practical aspects of work flow in data management (see Figure 1) indicate the high degree of interaction with other members of the clinical team. To ensure that the process works as effectively as possible, the data manager must be fully integrated into the clinical team and contribute to the logistical planning as much as to the specific aspects of data collection.

Planning the database

There are two principal formats in which data may be received for entry on to the database: paper-based and electronic. Paper-based data will include the

ACTIVITY	OTHER TEAM MEMBERS INVOLVED
CRFs received	Monitor
CRFs tracked, queries issued	Monitor/investigator
CRFs reviewed, queries issued	Monitor/investigator
Data entered	Data entry team
Electronic data entered	Laboratory/centre
Test datasets generated	Statistician
Validation checks, queries issued	Monitor/investigator, laboratory/centre
Medical and medication coding	Coding experts
Adverse event/serious adverse event reconciliation	Safety experts
Final edits	
Quality control checks	QC group
Database lock	
Quality assurance	QA group
Database release to statistician	Statistician

Figure 1. Data management work flow and clinical team members involved.

CRF and, possibly, patient diary cards, quality of life (QoL) questionnaires and laboratory data. Electronic data will include laboratory reports and, possibly, efficacy data such as ambulatory blood pressure measurements. The data manager must identify which parts of the data presented are to be captured by the database. In some cases, for instance, screening data will be collected in the CRF but not included on the database; some laboratory parameters, which are not required by the protocol, may appear on the laboratory reports because they form part of the routine of the laboratory.

The design of the database and the validation rules must take account of which data are to be manually entered and which are to be captured electronically. Having identified these aspects of the data, the data manager can start to design the database. The first step is to plan the way the data will be structured. This depends upon the relationship and interdependency of the data, and upon the way in which the statistician will wish to use the data for the analysis. Essentially, each piece of data (a variable) will form part of a subset of related data (the dataset). Thus, the adverse event dataset would contain all the variables collected on the adverse event pages of the CRF (e.g. description of event, when it occurred, when it ended, its severity, its relationship to the trial medication, what action was taken, what the outcome was, etc.) and any other pertinent data. The content and identity of the various datasets (on average 15–30 per study) may also be influenced by the design of databases for other studies with the same product, for example, to ensure that a 'global' safety database can be maintained, or to facilitate potential future combined analyses using data from several studies.

The variables and datasets are then identified using alphanumeric codes; typically, these codes are annotated on to a blank copy of the CRF to assist in the database construction, data entry, validation and analysis. The same process is followed with the electronic data. A quality control check at this stage will ensure that there are no duplications of variable names and that the variables are correctly assigned to the datasets.

Using the protocol and the CRF, the next step is to create the validation rules that will trap errors in the data as they are captured by the database. These validation rules are highly varied in their complexity. They may be as simple as not allowing a missing entry, and as complex as checking that the patient did not violate the protocol by taking prohibited medications, by falling outside the medication compliance rules or by breaking exclusion criteria during the trial. Although these rules will eventually be tested in the constructed database, it is advisable that a formal validation plan is written and that this is reviewed by the quality control group and the statistician, at least. The annotated CRF and the validation plan are the key tools for database design.

The data manager will also create a central data management file, in which the documentation can be retained in an orderly fashion. It is essential that there is supporting documentation to indicate how and by whom the database was designed and validated, any changes that have been made to the database structure, problems encountered and actions taken. This will allow the successful reconstruction of the data management process in the event of inspection by the regulatory authorities.

Planning the flow of data

In creating the time plan for the data management process, it is important for the data manager to establish how the data will be received and how queries will be handled. In general, the way in which the data are supplied will be determined by the size of the trial, the design of the CRF, and the monitoring plan. Thus, for a small Phase I trial with a small number of patients running simultaneously, the data manager would expect to receive completed CRFs for all subjects as one delivery. For larger trials, with staggered recruitment, longer durations and multiple visits, it will probably be convenient for the monitors to provide part CRFs, by visit. In such cases the data manager will need to obtain a monitoring plan, so that resources for data entry and query handling can be available when the data arrive.

The monitoring plan can also help the data manager to ensure that queries are generated at an appropriate time to fit with the monitor's visit. Query turn-round times should also be agreed so that the data manager can plan resource. This is especially relevant at the end of the trial, when the deadline of database lock looms.

The precise documents to be used must also be defined at this stage. The data manager must ascertain which copy of the CRF they will receive (typically, the second page of a no-carbon-required (NCR) CRF, or a photocopy of a non-NCR CRF) and whether annotation for secondary monitoring is permitted. The format and content of the query (data clarification form, DCF) should also be decided. Standard operating procedures (SOPs) and corporate standards may cover these aspects in the pharmaceutical company, but now that many contract research organisations (CROs) are involved in the data management process, it is important that the monitors and data managers are clear about and happy with the formats of the documentation.

Creating the database

There are several database systems used by data management groups, ranging from the large, commercially available, specialised data management software (such as Oracle Clinical® and Clintrial®) through to purpose-designed individual systems based on SAS®, Microsoft® Access or Microsoft® Excel, for example. The specific procedures for creating a database will depend, of course, upon the software. However, the underlying principles of clinical database design are common to all.

Security

Access control is an essential element of the database. Levels of access must be set so that people cannot interfere with aspects of the database for which they have no authority or responsibility. Thus, only data managers with editing responsibility should be able to enter the editing modules; when blind double data entry is used, the data entry technician making the first entry should not be able to gain access to the screens for the second entry; when the database is locked, there must be a formalised procedure for making any amendments that may be necessary.

Continuity and standards

As well as allowing the entry of trial-specific data, the database must also permit the trouble-free pooling of data from several trials for combined analysis or overall compilation of safety information. This means that standards must be applied for dataset content and variable naming.

Date formats should also be standardised. This should normally be achieved by the CRF design, but there may be multinational studies in which different date formats are used and the database must be able to cope with this. There should also be standard codes for 'missing', 'not required' and 'query'.

Audit trails

The data received for entry on to the database are commonly hand-written, and not always perfect. This means that the initial data entries may contain missing values, queries, or errors. The database must allow for the editing of its content, but must maintain an audit trail for all edits, retaining the original entry, the revised entry, and details of who made the change, why and when. It must be possible to amend the database structure, for instance, by adding new variables or extra visits, or changing validation rules. These changes must also be audit-trailed.

Null values

The database must allow null values to be entered (for example, if no adverse events are recorded). This can be achieved by the use of codes as described above.

Reporting

The database should have a reporting element that will enable progress to be checked and the interim publication of safety data, for example. This should also facilitate response to unexpected questions from regulatory authorities.

Data validation

The database should provide in-built validation to assure the accuracy of the data it contains. This involves cross-checking between two or more variables in one or more datasets. The validation can be run on a batch basis (i.e. performed by separate programs) or be on-line and respond to individual data entry.

System validation

The database itself should be validated. This includes assuring that the intrinsic validation rules work and are appropriate (usually achieved by entering data containing deliberate errors and data that are perfectly correct, in order to test the rules). The overall integrity of the database (access security, system stability) and the accuracy of its output (as tables and listings and as electronic files to be passed to other software, e.g. for analysis) must be tested and assured.

CRF receipt, checking and tracking

Although the CRF may not contain source data, it forms the data manager's raw data. This means that care must be taken to check what has been received, chase any part of the CRF that is missing or damaged, and store it in a secure, safe place. All these actions must be logged, either as a paper trail or electronically. It is an advantage if CRF tracking is part of the database software and if it is sufficiently flexible to record transactions at the full CRF, visit or CRF page levels.

If the study team has been successful in its planning, the data manager will know when to expect delivery of CRFs. Even then, it is essential for the data manager to be advised by the monitor that CRFs have been dispatched and by what route. This allows the data manager to warn the monitor if the CRFs do not arrive as expected, so that mis-delivery can be chased urgently. Along with the CRFs the monitor should provide a list stating which CRFs or pages have been sent; the data manager will check this as a first priority. The data manager will next review each CRF to ensure that all pages are present and that none is damaged, and an acknowledgement should be sent to the monitor, detailing what has been received.

Further checks (secondary monitoring) may be applied to the CRF, this time at the level of the data but before data entry. These checks will trap errors and omissions that may delay data entry, or will look at more complex inter-relationships between the data for errors that cannot readily be checked by the validation programs included in the database software. A further application of secondary monitoring occurs when text entries are difficult to decipher. An example of this may be seen in global trials where the CRF invites text entries of medical terms, bacterial species, etc. Because script and letter formation differ from country to country and the investigators are writing in a second language, secondary monitoring such as this can greatly facilitate data entry and reduce the number of queries generated. Any errors found in the data will be queried back to the monitor for resolution. With database systems that have substantial on-line validation, intense secondary monitoring may not be necessary unless specific problems are found in the data.

It is imperative that the CRFs are kept in such a way that pages are not lost or mixed up between patients or studies. Various methods are used; for example, lever arch files, colour coded by study, in which the CRFs are inserted and separated by transparent folders. The data entry area may be divided into units in which only one trial at a time may be worked on, and if this is backed up by secure storage and document control (i.e. CRFs are signed out and back), the opportunities for mix-up are minimised.

Data entry

Manual entry

There are two commonly used methods of manual data entry: single entry and double entry. There is an ongoing debate about the efficiency and effectiveness of these methods, although eventually, with the advent of direct data capture via the Internet or secure line, single data entry will surely become the norm.

Single data entry can be made by a specialist keyboard operator, for maximum speed of entry. If the validation step is performed when data entry is completed, then the database can be rapidly filled. However, considerable validation is required to ensure a clean and accurate database and this is potentially time-consuming and expensive. Often, an extensive (advisedly 100%) quality control check is necessary, and this is demanding of resource. Alternatively, single data entry may be performed by the data manager or the investigator, with on-line validation. This is slower, especially since the entry may be made by someone without a high level of keyboard skills, but there will be a greater level of insight into the data and interpretation of the CRF entry. Even with on-line validation there remains the potential for entry error, as an incorrect entry may fall within the validation criteria. Thus, extensive quality control checks are still required.

Double data entry is usually made by experienced keyboard operators, working blind of each other. Validation of the entry accuracy may be based on keystrokes (strokes that differ on second entry from the first are signalled to the second operator) or on file comparison (when the content of the fields for first and second entry is compared). This can be enhanced by providing on-line validation checks that prompt the operator when the rules are broken and permit 'internal' queries to be raised for resolution by the data manager.

When substantial text entry is required (e.g. for medical history, physical examination, adverse events), it is of great benefit if the keyboard operator has some understanding of the terminology that may be used for the particular indication or therapeutic class of test material, because significant delays can occur when interpreting the script. Also, access to drug dictionaries for entering concomitant medications can serve to enhance the entry process. Providing such dictionaries on-line, and even as pick lists, forms an even more substantial enhancement.

In general, a lower level of quality control checking is required for double data entry, especially if the 'blind' nature of the two entries can be maintained effectively.

The unique identity of the data for a given study, patient, visit and dataset must be maintained throughout the database. The requirement for these details to be entered against every CRF page or dataset is very inefficient and it is far better for the database software to 'fill in' these standard fields for the operator.

Further features that can facilitate accurate and rapid data entry include:

- making the data entry screens as similar as possible to the CRF;
- permitting table entries to be tabbed down the screen rather than across;
- minimising the use of the mouse and maximising keystroke use for travelling from one field to another;
- 'hiding' fields when an entry is not required.

Data entry may be performed off-line or on-line. In off-line data entry, the data are entered on to a system that is remote from the main database and the data thus entered can be up-loaded to it at convenient times. This is most appropriate when data entry is being performed at the investigator site because the system does not depend upon the slow response times and interruptions that may occur through an Internet or land line connection to the main database. Such a system may retain data entry validation checks and permit the raising of queries at source.

On-line data entry, direct to the database, is a more secure method and it means that the database is a real-time reflection of the data entry stage reached. All the validation routines available in the database can be made available at the entry level, if this is required. It is, however, vulnerable to system failure, which will mean that all data entry has to stop.

The most effective systems permit a combination of the two methods, with on-line entry when the main database is running, but providing an off-line fallback if the main database is down.

Electronic data capture

Increasingly, data produced by such devices as ambulatory blood pressure monitors and ECGs are generated in formats that permit electronic capture by the database. Previously, data from such devices were transcribed on to the CRF, resulting in delays and the potential for errors to be further compounded by the manual data entry process. It is important for the data manager to be aware at the outset of which data are to be transmitted electronically, so that the database can be set up to receive it and so that data format compatibility can be ensured between the equipment and the database. It is also imperative to run test transmissions of the electronic data to verify that the formatting is appropriate and that the database receives the data without corruption.

Typically, the data will be supplied to the data manager as files on disc or downloaded via a modem. Often, the equipment generating the data will produce more information than is required on the database and so close liaison is necessary between the data manager and the unit supplying the electronic information. The data manager must also determine the extent to which validation has been applied to the data before they are transmitted to the database. This is especially relevant when data of the same type are being transmitted from different centres or machines.

Laboratory data are now commonly entered on to the database electronically. If these data emanate from a single central laboratory, then the job of the data manager is made easier. The central laboratory will issue the data using common units for the analytes and single standards for flagging out-of-range and clinically abnormal results. The challenge to the data manager is in receiving laboratory data from several sites, each with different units and different normal and abnormal ranges. In such cases preparation is of the essence, and the data manager must ensure that each site has provided advance notification of the format of the data to be sent. The database can then be set up to receive and convert data to common units, and the data manager can generate global normal and abnormal ranges. Even then, laboratory data present hidden challenges. In Germany, for example, patients may go to the clinic of their choice for haematology and biochemistry tests, and it is therefore likely that the data formats will vary even within individual patients.

Trapping and correcting errors: validation and the query process

The data type and error type

The data contained in the CRF are essentially of seven types: checked boxes (i.e. 'Yes' or 'No'), numeric, dates, times, codes, alphanumeric, and graphics. These types each lend themselves to different kinds of error.

1. Checked boxes. The incorrect box may be checked, or more than one box is checked when only one choice is permitted, or no boxes at all are checked.

2. Numeric. There are many formats for numeric data. They may be whole or decimal values, dates or times. Errors in whole or decimal values include transposed values, values out of range (e.g. age), or values recorded in the wrong units (e.g. height in metres and centimetres instead of centimetres).

3. Dates. Many date errors are associated with use of the wrong year or format. The wrong year is typically entered around the turn of the year, or when the investigator inadvertently inserts the current year in the birth date or start date of a medical condition. Date formats vary, the commonest being dd/mm/yy (25/12/99); dd/mmm/yy (25/DEC/99); dd/mm/yyyy (25/12/1999) and mm/dd/yy (12/25/99). The first and last examples represent international differences in the way that dates are recorded and may be a source of errors when investigators are asked to provide the date in a 'foreign' format.

A further problem may arise with historical information (for instance, concomitant medication) when the full date is not known. In this case the incomplete data do not represent an error but provide as much information as is available. It is important, therefore, that the date field of the database can accept codes that allow partial dates.

4. Time. Time may be recorded as a 12–hour a.m./p.m. cycle or as a 24–hour clock. The 24–hour clock is a preferable standard, but errors may occur, for example, in patient diary cards when the patient is not familiar with its use. Time and date errors may also occur unless a strict convention is used for the time when the date changes (is it 24:00 on 24 December or 00:00 on 25 December?).

5. Codes. Codes provide a method for ensuring consistency when textual data are to be used for analysis; for example, the outcome of an adverse event may be coded as 1 = resolved, 2 = unresolved or 3 = death. Codes may be applied at CRF completion, CRF review, or data entry. The selection of a wrong code may be obvious (male code selected for patient with positive pregnancy test), but the greater the number of choices, the greater the potential for selecting the wrong code and the difficulty of detecting the error.

6. Alphanumeric. These data are textual and are thus prone to original spelling or transposition errors. Further, as data entry is often performed on the second sheet of NCR paper or on a photocopy, poor legibility can result in incorrect transcription.

7. Graphic. The graphic data most frequently confronting the data manager are visual analogue scales (VASs) in which a line is drawn between two extremes (e.g. 'no pain' and 'unbearable pain') and the patient or investigator is asked to indicate current status by marking the line at a point between these extremes. The distance of the marked point from one end of the scale is measured, and this measurement is entered into the database. Problems arise if the mark does not intersect the line, if a cross has been used that is not centred on the line, or if a tick mark has been used that intersects the line at two points. More subtly, if the CRF has been photocopied, the distance between the extremes on the VAS may not be faithfully reproduced, giving rise to variations from site to site. The data manager then has to apply an appropriate correction factor to each CRF.

There is a further type of error that is independent of the data type: inconsistency. Consistencies will be expected between different variables that may be in the same or different datasets. The relationships can be as simple as two actions occurring on the same day should have the same date recorded, or as complex as 'presumed infection = temperature above 38°C for three consecutive days or recurring at least twice, after three days of systemic antibiotic treatment, and with findings at X-ray or magnetic resonance imaging (MRI) indicative of infection'. Some relationships may be expressed in the protocol (as in the second case above). Others may not and the data manager is expected to anticipate them. It will be apparent that, in order to test these consistencies, the data manager must have a thorough grasp of the protocol and a good understanding of the science involved.

The source of error

The data manager's responsibility is to trap errors in the original data received from the centre, and to ensure that the data are faithfully transposed from the CRF to the database. This process has several inherent sources of error:

● the original recording of findings,
● their transcription from the source data to the CRF,
● the inputting of data into the database,
● the database itself.

1. The original recording of findings. This error source is beyond the data manager's control unless the recordings fall outside limits that the data manager can set; the most effective control here is good investigator and monitoring technique. An example of this type would be grades incorrectly assigned to a disease state for which degrees of severity are applied. In this case, the data manager would only be able to isolate major fluctuations from visit to visit as indicating potential recorder error. In laboratory data, haemolysis will affect some of the results, but the data manager can only detect this if the values fall outside the normal range. Thus, major errors in original recordings may be detected by the data manager's checks, but there can be no guarantee that all will be found.

2. Transcription from source data to the CRF. While the validation programs that the data manager designs for the database will highlight many such errors, some will escape detection. For instance, the data manager will certainly

detect fields that should contain an entry but do not. Checks are also possible between dates of birth, date of visit and age. The visit dates can be
checked against the protocol requirements and each other. However, no
validation check can detect a physical observation that is present in the source
data but not in the CRF. These errors can only be detected reliably when the
monitor checks the source data against the CRF.

3. Inputting of data into the database. Data entry errors can result from simple
miskeying, from missed fields or from misinterpretation of text comments.
Range checks performed by the database at the point of entry can pick up
miskeying that produces unreal values, but they will not detect plausible entries
that are incorrect. The database can also be designed to minimise missed fields
by preventing the operator from exiting the dataset unless all fields are filled,
or by automatically inserting a 'query' code in an empty field. The misinterpretation of text comments is a far greater problem but as with all the above
errors, double data entry with comparison of the two entries will often highlight
text comments that were difficult to interpret. To give the data manager the
best chance of identifying errors due to misinterpretation, double data entry
should be blind, and the operators should be prevented from discussing a difficult entry and arriving at a common, but erroneous, conclusion.

Although the database can be set to trap many entry errors, there is no
substitute for a cross-check between the CRF and the database content before
the database is locked.

4. The database itself. While it may not introduce new errors, the database can
perpetuate existing errors if its validation checks are inadequate. It is important therefore that the validation programs are checked thoroughly before the
database is 'validated' for use in the study. These checks will include challenging the database with false data that transgress the validation rules, entering
totally correct data, and performing trial entry of two or three real CRFs.

The output from the database, in the form of tables and listings, may be
produced directly from the database or via separate statistical software. If the
output is generated directly from the database, it is possible that the programs
written for this purpose may introduce error (for instance, the selection of an
inappropriate variable to filter the data). If separate statistical software is
used, the transfer of the data from the database must be checked, usually by
a sample check with the database. Again, the programs written in the statistical software can introduce error and it is important that adequate quality
control checks are run.

Validation checks

The available methods of data validation resolve into two types, visual and
programmed. Programmed validation will be more accurate and less resource-

consuming than visual validation provided that the program has been thoroughly checked and tested. However, 'sanity' checks should always be run on the computer output, especially when the program is designed to detect complex errors involving inter-related variables.

Visual checks will initially be made on the CRF at receipt, when the completeness of the data (all pages present, no missing values) and the correctness of CRF completion (data entered in the right place) will be examined. This initial check also allows a review of the CRF data against the protocol requirements and may thus permit early detection of errors in study conduct or violations of the protocol. In multicentre studies, the visual check provides an opportunity for comparing how the different investigators have completed the CRF and for highlighting inconsistencies.

If there is a significant amount of textual data, the visual check can be used to clarify illegible or ambiguous entries. In a multinational, multicentre study in which medical terms are handwritten on the CRF, it is more effective for the data manager to clarify the entries at this stage than to handle the many queries that will result from unaided data entry.

Visual checks are especially useful when dealing with patient diary cards and they are essential if the diary cards contain variables that will be used as measures of efficacy. It can be predicted with confidence that there will be more inconsistencies in the completion of these cards than there are patients in the study.

Programmed validation can be performed at two stages: on data entry or within the database, i.e. post-entry. In general, the more complex checks are performed post-entry because these tend to involve cross-checks between different variables and datasets that may not be on the database until a later stage of data entry.

Many data entry validation checks are based on the nature of the data and the structure of the database. Thus, if the database is set up for height to be expressed as x metres.yy centimetres, it will reject a height recorded as 180 centimetres. This ensures that the data for a given variable are consistent throughout the database. Further checks may relate to acceptable ranges for values (for instance, the database will reject the age of a patient if it falls outside the range stipulated in the protocol inclusion criteria, or a red cell count if it is above or below preset normal value ranges). In these cases the database is detecting probably spurious values. It is also possible to compare different variables for inconsistencies (e.g. the patient's age does not match the date of birth or the visit date, or the Visit 5 date is earlier than the Visit 4 date).

If double data entry is used, the first post-entry validation check is the merging of the two entries and the identification of fields where the two entries do not match. These mismatches will be a consequence of entry error or poor legibility. The merging will also identify missing fields and query codes. Further post-entry validation checks may be run as queries within the database or may necessitate the review of listings. Because the limits of the search may be defined, these programmed checks offer a considerable advantage over CRF review, for example.

Checks that can be run within the database are those that require no interpretation (e.g. overall medication compliance = tablets returned $\leq 20\%$ of tablets issued). Other checks may require interpretation (e.g. concomitant medication with a systemic antibiotic prohibited for five days before any visit). Interpretative checks can be performed by generating listings for review.

The query process

Having identified potential errors, the data manager is required to correct them. In general this means informing the centre or the monitor of the error and requesting a correction. However, this process is time-consuming, potentially costly if not managed properly, and can be frustrating for the monitor or investigator if the request is not clear or the answer is obvious.

One way to minimise the number of queries is to agree, at the outset of the study, changes to the data that may be made by the data manager without a query being generated. For example, these 'allowable changes' may involve correcting transposed date fields or spelling mistakes. It is important that these changes are audit-trailed in the same way as conventional edits.

The queries that are issued should be in a standard format and contain all the information that the monitor and investigator need to identify the problem and supply the appropriate answer. They should be individually identified and tracked, in the same way as CRFs. The queried field in the database can carry a query code, which permits a search before database lock to ensure that all queries have been resolved.

Paper-based queries are still the norm in data management because many companies and sites have not resolved the 'electronic signature' issue. However, fax and e-mail are being used increasingly to transmit the documents for printing and signing at the site, especially towards the end of the study as the database lock deadline looms. To facilitate the query process, it is advisable for the issue of queries to be linked to the visit schedule of the monitors, who can then deal with them as a batch and provide rapid turn-round.

On return of the query, the data manager acts upon it, amending the database content appropriately. Such amendments, and those made to the original data through the 'allowable changes' procedure, must be audit-trailed, preferably within the database. Because this editing is effectively 'single entry', special quality control procedures should be in place to ensure the accuracy of the amendment.

Communication

During the data collection phase of the trial the data manager is the only person who has all the trial data available in one place. It is therefore important that information about the conduct and the progress of the trial is relayed to the clinical team at appropriate intervals and it is essential that the data manager is a good communicator.

In addition to regular review meetings between the data manager and the monitors, the data manager should issue frequent reports on the progress of the trial. These may include information on:

- recruitment, by centre;
- data entry progress;
- queries raised, number resolved and time to resolution, all by centre;
- number of protocol violators, by centre;
- number of adverse events, by centre.

These parameters can be invaluable in the management of the trial. They will help monitors to identify problem centres or investigators and will provide excellent insight into the quality and responsiveness of the monitoring process.

Coding and coding dictionaries

The principle of coding is to ensure the consistency of the database in areas where different terms may be used to describe the same entity. Apart from the coding of data within the CRF, as described previously, the most frequent uses for coding are medications, medical conditions and adverse event descriptions.

In a multinational study, it can be immensely difficult to calculate the frequency of use of a particular medication when it is represented on the database under national brand and generic names for each country involved in the trial. Some companies have developed their own drug coding dictionaries, while others use 'off-the-shelf' dictionaries, for example, the *WHO Drug Reference List* or the *Read Codes*. Ideally, the medication dictionary should be hierarchical in nature and contain international drug names and synonyms, permitting coding by drug identity, therapeutic class and pharmaceutical class. It should also be regularly updated and, usefully, contain links to other dictionaries.

Medication coding lends itself to auto-encoding. In this process the medication dictionary is held on-line and linked to the database. Auto-encoding may be invoked at data entry or afterwards, when the drug entry is matched against the dictionary content. A perfect match enables the drug code to be extracted from the dictionary into the database. The dictionary may reject imperfect matches or offer alternatives. This process eliminates coding transcription error, a potential problem when coding is performed manually. It is substantially quicker than a manual process and it removes any possibility of bias or inconsistency in code attribution.

The use of dictionaries for coding medical conditions and adverse events is especially important in the overall safety review of the drug. It is essential that the same dictionary is used for every study on a given drug so that the data can be merged, if necessary, to provide an overall safety database. The description of an adverse event or medical condition is always made in text form on the CRF and is often open to misinterpretation. While some entries cannot be helped by a coding system (for example, does 'cold' mean hypothermia or viral respiratory infection?), others can. Identical events reported by two investigators ('swelling at injection site' and 'administration site swollen') would not be classified as the same by any computerised system sorting on a text string basis, but could be by a coding dictionary.

Several adverse event and/or medical condition coding systems are available (ICD 10, CO-START, WHOART, MedDRA). Of these, MedDRA (developed under the auspices of ICH) is gaining the ascendancy.

The principle of coding medical conditions and adverse events is to map the investigator's term to a 'preferred term' and then, through a hierarchical pathway, eventually to a broad category defining the body system involved. This then assures the consistency of terminology at the 'preferred term' level and permits sorting and frequency calculations at various levels from the specific to the more general. Unfortunately, because the original entry by the investigator is free text, medical coding does not readily lend itself to auto-encoding. Furthermore, there are several decision-making steps for the coder. The first step is to decide whether the investigator term describes one medical condition or more than one. For example, is 'sickness and nausea' a single event or (1) vomiting and (2) nausea? The second step is to find the appropriate preferred term for the investigator term; an exact match may exist but more frequently this is not the case. Finally, the coder may be offered routes to different body systems (e.g. 'headache' may be neurological or cardiovascular). It is important, therefore, that medical coding is performed or checked by someone with experience of the dictionary used and with a medical background so that accuracy and consistency are achieved.

Locking the database

The locking of the database is a significant event in the clinical trial; it marks the moment when the data may become unblinded and statistical analysis can begin. Several criteria must be satisfied before the data manager is able to lock the database.

- All queries must be resolved and all fields must contain an entry. The completion of all fields is achieved by having codes set for data that are missing (after querying has provided no value) or not required (e.g. a subordinate field that may or may not contain a value). The resolution of all queries is assured by a check of the query tracking system and a search for any query codes in the data.
- All medical and drug coding must be complete.

- Protocol violators must be identified, as must the different analysis populations (safety, intention-to-treat, per protocol). To prevent bias, this step must be performed before unblinding.
- Quality control checks must show that the error rate is within accepted limits. Quality control involves a review of the data contained in the database against the CRF and query forms. Usually, this review will be extended to 100% of the primary efficacy variable data, and to all withdrawals, adverse events and demography. There will then be a check on all the data from a proportion (usually 10%) of the patients. SOPs should specify the process and define acceptable error rates; these vary substantially between companies, and rates as high as 1% or as low as 0.05% are used. With double data entry, quality control of all text edits, and validation programs in the database, it is certainly possible to achieve very low error rates (typically below 0.05%). Sequential quality control checks are preferable to a batch procedure at the end of the process. These permit early identification of systematic errors or of differences between centres in CRF recording.

Once all these criteria are fulfilled, the database can be locked. This means that the database content or the database structure cannot be changed without a formal procedure that will include full documentation, and the database therefore becomes the data for the analysis of the outcome of the trial. At this stage quality assurance procedures become appropriate. Rather than simply checking the database content, the purpose of quality assurance is to assure that the processes used in the construction and completion of the database, query resolution, editing and quality control checks have been as claimed, as per SOPs, and have provided a product of acceptable quality. The quality assurance review will therefore include an examination of the data management documentation and of the quality control findings, and finally a sample check (usually 10%) of the database against the CRF.

Occasionally, there may be the requirement for an interim analysis, or the need for an urgent analysis of certain parameters before the full database is locked. In such situations there is an advantage if the database permits locking at the dataset level. The various checks listed above are still necessary and it is vital that the study is not unblinded by any of the staff involved in the data entry or data management processes.

After database lock

The data manager's responsibilities do not end at database lock. Documentation is needed to accompany the datasets that are sent to the statistician. Typically, this will include a data handling report that will address at least the following aspects:

- the name of each variable within each dataset, and the format of each variable,

- the validation rules applied,
- database structural changes that have been made,
- the number of patients present on the database,
- the number, identities and rules violated for all protocol violators, and
- anomalies or variations in the data identified by the data manager to assist the statistician in generating listings, tables and analysis.

Finally, the data manager is responsible for ensuring the archiving of all study data, including data management documentation and the CRFs.

DATA MANAGEMENT: THE FUTURE

This section will consider how data management as a process will change with the introduction of new technologies.

Within the next few years, the process of data collection will undoubtedly shift substantially from paper-based systems to on-line electronic data capture. The disciplines of data management will necessarily change, as the design of the data entry screens and in-built validation become significant elements of the data capture process. The data manager's role may well be combined with that of the monitor, providing training and ongoing guidance to the investigator and investigational site staff, the emphasis being that the *initial* recording of the data provides the final database.

However, there is a cost/benefit issue to be addressed. Remote electronic data capture is a relatively expensive procedure: it requires the provision of hardware and software to the contributing sites, the maintenance of a high degree of security, considerable training and support, and effective management to ensure that all sites are using the same electronic CRFs and software versions. It is likely that, for some time, the cost/benefit ratio will favour paper-based systems for smaller trials although, conversely, much of the testing of systems has been and will be done on such studies. An exception to this is Phase I centres, where several studies are performed to a similar format and where very rapid turn-round of safety data, for example, is required. These centres would clearly benefit from remote electronic data capture.

The corollary of the remote data entry process is the remote interrogation of the data as they are entered. Systems now exist that allow the sponsor to view the contents of the database in 'real time', down to the individual variable level, and to generate *ad hoc* reports.

The benefits of remote data capture therefore include:

- bypassing of transcription errors from source data to CRF and from CRF to database,
- on-line validation allows the investigator to generate complete validated data at entry,

- reduction in data processing resource required,
- fewer queries generated,
- real-time interrogation of the database by the sponsor (if appropriate),
- overall reduction in cycle time.

At the same time a number of problems surround the subject of remote data capture. The most obvious is that the study cannot start until the database is constructed and the entry screens and on-line validation have been programmed. In the conventional process flow for clinical trials, the database will be ready for entry sometime after the first patient has been recruited and often after the first CRFs have been completed. This is because the database cannot be constructed until the protocol has been finalised, and the CRF designed. Companies frequently compress this period (protocol finalised, ethical approval gained, study start) so that the CRF designer is working against a 'first patient, first visit' deadline. Since the construction of a remote entry database and entry screens is considerably more resource-intensive than the design and printing of the CRF, it is implicit that the data manager will have to be involved in the study planning stage considerably earlier than is commonly the case at present.

A further issue in remote data entry is to gain the acceptance of the investigators for the style of the entry screens and the process of on-line validation. The data manager will have to work closely with the investigators to learn what is, and what is not, acceptable. The entry screen must be simple to navigate, easy to enter data and have as many aids to entry as possible. Thus, a facsimile of a well-designed paper CRF might prove appropriate. Data entry should be designed so that the number of keystrokes is minimised. This can be done by using check boxes with underlying coding and providing drop-down picklists containing the allowed range of entries. Picklists could also be supplied for drug names and adverse event terminology. Coding dictionaries linked to the database could then be used to auto-encode the data, as the picklist would ensure that consistent terms were selected. On-screen validation must not be so extensive that the data entry process is constantly interrupted. Indeed, the data manager will probably need to work with the investigators in setting some of the validation rules so that the reasons for them are obvious.

Remote data entry becomes impossible if the computer fails or the system goes down. As this will inevitably happen when the investigator is dealing with a full clinic and cannot afford to wait for system repair, there must be some mechanism that will allow data recording on paper with eventual transcription to the database. The data manager will have to provide the investigator with paper CRFs to use in emergency. The main issue here is that the paper entries may be more prone to error than usual because of pressure of time and unfamiliarity with the paper system. Also, the investigator may have to enter information that is not necessary for the on-line system (patient identifiers, for example). In such circumstances, the CRF facsimile is a useful fall-back. If the paper CRF and electronic CRF are identical, the investigator will at least be able to navigate around the document. When the system is operating again, the investigator may then enter the data collected on paper. However, this is inefficient use of valuable time and it would be more productive for these data to be entered at base.

The data manager will also need to accommodate the investigator's work practices and to adapt the system accordingly. It is possible that the investigator will wish to enter clinical data at the time of the visit, but because of pressure of time at the clinic, may prefer to enter concomitant medications and adverse event data, for example, in batch mode at another time.

Substantial training will be required in the use of the system for individual studies, together with ongoing user support. The data manager will have to be involved in designing the training, if not in providing it, and certainly in the construction of help screens and prompts. However, a very high level of user support will be required, especially in the early days of the study, and it is difficult to envisage how the data manager could supply this service without assistance. Thus, the relationship between the data manager and the investigator will be key to the success of remote data entry, as will the quality of support services.

Now that electronic signatures are accepted, the way is open for electronic communication and resolution of queries. With the need to optimise the degree of on-line validation to which the investigator is exposed, the data manager will still have to design validity checks within the database and generate queries from base. However, these queries could be generated electronically and sent to the investigator by e-mail, or to the data collection software itself. In the first case, the investigator could either supply the answer to the data manager by e-mail, or answer the query directly into the database. In the second case, the data collection software could be designed to prompt the investigator with the query and to take the investigator directly to the entry field in question. In either case, if the investigator is making the entry to answer the query, the data manager must be able to view the response and check that it does indeed resolve the issue. The security levels of the system could be set so that only nominated individuals can amend the database in this way, and inbuilt audit trails would hold the requisite information about the change.

Another trend that will affect the work of the data manager is the use of central or virtual laboratories to generate the haematology, biochemistry and urinalysis data. The bonus here is consistency of data, units and limits. The potential exists for the laboratory equipment to access the database directly and download data without the intervention of the data manager. This demands, however, that other standards are maintained. For example, the identifiers used for patient, sample and time will have to be consistent between the laboratory and the database. It will also be essential for the data

manager and the laboratory to communicate before the database is designed
– currently a most unusual concept!

The advances in technology will also affect document management. It is
possible to make the protocol and other essential documentation available to
the investigator on-line, as read-only files. This is especially useful if the
system has a search facility to enable the investigator to go directly to the item
in question. The documentation could also be linked to the data entry screens
so that, as part of the in-built help process, the investigator could call up the
section of the protocol relevant to the field or dataset that is being entered.
Other documents, e.g. a data entry guide, could also usefully be linked to the
data entry screens. These linkages to the database would be managed by the
data manager, who would also be responsible for version control.

One of the continuing challenges for the data manager is patient diary data
and a number of computerised solutions are now available. The most effective are those that guide the patients by allowing them to enter only and
exactly what is required. However, these solutions are relatively expensive at
the moment, and it is probable that paper-based patient diaries will remain in
common use for some time to come.

It is clear that the data manager of the future will be working against quite
different deadlines from those of today. There will be far greater emphasis on
setting up the database to allow the study to start, and the increase in data
quality and the reduction in data query volume will facilitate much quicker
database locks after 'last patient, last visit'. An overall reduction in the time
from 'first patient, first visit' to database lock can be anticipated, with a saving
of up to one month compared with current practice. However, the duration
of involvement of the data manager in the trial will be much longer than at
present, with essential planning and design starting several months before the
trial begins.

CONCLUSION

Data management today is a complex process that involves anticipating,
trapping and correcting a variety of errors in a range of data types to generate an accurate database. The database is designed to allow the rapid entry
of data from paper and to detect errors using validation procedures that are
mainly performed after data entry. The error correction process creates a
substantial administrative burden for the data manager, monitor and investigator.

Increasingly in the future, the initial entry of data on to the database will
be made at the investigational centre, and through on-line validation this
single remote entry will be the final entry. The data manager, who currently
becomes involved in the trial as or just before it begins, will instead control
when the trial can start; database construction, validation and training of the

investigators in the use of the software will all have to be completed before the first patient makes the first visit. The administrative duties of the data manager as the trial proceeds will become less onerous, but interaction with the investigator will increase. The data manager currently plays a significant role within the clinical study team. The degree of involvement and interaction that will accrue through the advances in data capture techniques will result in the data manager having a higher profile within the team and a much greater involvement in the planning stage than at present.

FURTHER READING

Rondel, RK, Varley, SA and Webb, CF (Eds) (1999). *Clinical Data Management*, John Wiley, Chichester.

16

Statistical thinking for clinical trials

Richard Kay

INTRODUCTION

The purpose of this chapter is to introduce some of the basic ideas in the statistical design and analysis of clinical trials. In the space available it is not possible to provide more than an introduction, but hopefully the topics covered will provide a starting point for further study (see Further Reading). It is vital that everyone involved in clinical research should gain an overview of statistical methodology, and it is very difficult to make any progress without at least a basic understanding of this subject. Statistics is the science of the clinical trial. The clinical trial is not about the practice of medicine *per se*; it is an experimental environment, invented by statisticians, that allows a structured methodology for the evaluation of new treatments.

We will focus exclusively on comparative trials where the objective is to detect treatment differences. There is an expanding area of methodology associated with demonstrating the 'clinical equivalence' of treatments. This will not be addressed. Further, particularly in the early sections, we will focus on the analysis of continuous, normally distributed data. There are many issues associated with assessing the assumptions of normality and the use of non-parametric methods but these will not be discussed in this introductory coverage.

BASIC ISSUES IN CLINICAL TRIAL DESIGN

Between- and within-patient designs

The most commonly occurring study design is the *parallel-group design* where, in its simplest form, trial participants are randomised to one of two treatment groups, say A and B. Typically, we would then obtain a response measure from each subject and compare the average response in one group with the average response in the second group. Using mean $\bar{x}$ as a measure of average, this will then involve the numerical comparison of $\bar{x}_1$ and $\bar{x}_2$. Irrespective of any real treatment differences, it is almost certain that $\bar{x}_1$ and $\bar{x}_2$ will be numerically different as a result of natural patient-to-patient variation in response. Any differences seen between these two means will therefore be caused by natural patient-to-patient variation and by any real differences in treatments, assuming they exist. The purpose of statistical analysis is to decide which of those two factors has caused the observed difference. Is the difference indicative of a real treatment effect or has it been caused merely by patient-to-patient variation? This evaluation is very difficult and one way of making this distinction easier would be somehow to eliminate, or at least reduce, the impact of patient-to-patient variation. This could be achieved by making the subject mix in the first group identical to that in the second group. An alternative design, which moves us in this direction, is the *paired design*. For example, in a dermatology trial, the left hand receives cream of type A, while the right hand receives cream of type B; or in an ophthalmology trial, the right eye receives drops of type A and the left eye receives drops of type B. In these designs the mean response seen in group A is calculated on the same group of subjects as the mean response obtained in group B; the groups are identical in terms of mix. This greatly facilitates the evaluation of treatment differences but there is only a restricted set of situations in which this design is going to be possible. Nevertheless, when it is possible, it is a very efficient way of comparing treatments. In principle, the *cross-over design* attempts to achieve the same thing. In a 2 x 2 cross-over where 20 subjects receive A followed by B while 20 subjects receive B followed by A, the 40 response measures on A and the 40 response measures on B will have come from the same group of 40 subjects.

The parallel-group design is an example of a *'between-patient'* design while the paired design and cross-over are examples of *'within-patient'* designs. The within-patient designs have the advantage of better accounting for patient-to-patient variation so that any differences observed numerically in the mean responses in the two groups can be more confidently ascribed to real treatment differences.

Signal-to-noise ratio

The difference between the means may be referred to as the 'signal'. The bigger the difference, the stronger the signal in terms of suggesting real treatment differences. The patient-to-patient variation is termed the 'noise'. Noise is an obstacle to identifying real treatment differences; large amounts of noise make it more difficult to identify differences while small amounts of noise make the task much easier. The main purpose of any statistical analysis is to identify the signal in the presence of the noise, and indeed statistical analysis techniques are employed that highlight the signal while accounting for the noise. Clinical trial design is also chosen in such a way as to minimise or, at least, control the noise, as discussed earlier.

THE ROLE OF THE STATISTICIAN

Protocol development

Statisticians need to become involved in a number of different aspects of the design and analysis of a clinical trial and indeed prior to that, it is useful to involve statisticians in the formulation of the complete clinical drug development plan. In the context of a particular trial the statistician will be included in discussing general aspects of the design, the objectives of the trial, the choice and implementation of the randomisation scheme, the choice of endpoints and their measurement, the specification of the methods of statistical analysis, and the way the results are to be presented and reported. The statistical methods section of the protocol should contain details of the sample size calculation, the methods to be used for the analysis of the primary endpoint(s) and, in broad terms, the strategy to be adopted for the secondary endpoints and any additional specific analyses. It will further address any aspects of multiplicity which may arise, outline methods to be used for interim analysis, if any, and finally discuss in general terms how the safety data are to be evaluated and presented.

Statistical analysis plan

Once the protocol is completed and the trial is underway, the statistician will write a detailed statistical analysis plan. This plan will contain a more detailed specification of the analyses to be performed and will be finalised prior to any unblinding of the data for statistical analysis.

Blind review

Following the completion of the trial and locking of the database, the statistician should undertake a blind review of the data. During this blind review, decisions will be taken regarding the handling of protocol violations and deviations and missing data and the subsequent choice of analysis sets. The overall integrity of the data should also be reviewed at this stage. The blind review allows specific aspects of the statistical analysis plan to be revisited in the light of features that have been seen in the data. For example, if it is noted that one of the covariates that was to be included in the analysis has many missing values, a decision may be taken to redefine that covariate or to remove it from the analysis.

Statistical analysis and reporting

The statistician will undertake the detailed statistical analysis of the data and its presentation and this will result in a separate statistical report or, a more likely scenario, the statistician will work closely with medical writing to produce an integrated clinical study report. In the broader context, the statistician will also need to be involved in compiling the regulatory submission and responding to questions raised by the regulatory authorities.

SAMPLES AND POPULATIONS

The purpose of statistics is to draw conclusions about populations based upon samples taken from those populations. For example, let us suppose that we are developing a new drug for mild to moderate hypertension. The 'target population' is defined by the inclusion and exclusion criteria for the particular trial. We then take a sample of subjects from that target population and on the basis of the data collected on the sample, we draw conclusions, or in statistical terms make inferences, about the population from which the sample has been drawn.

There are usually two elements of the sample and population data that are of direct interest. First, it is important to know what is happening on average and this will usually be measured by either the median or the mean. The mean is the arithmetic average and the median is the middle value when the data points are ordered from smallest to largest. These averages form the basis of the signal. In a two-treatment, parallel-group design the signal will be the mean in Group 1 minus the mean in Group 2. Secondly, we need to have some measure of the patient-to-patient variation because this forms the basis for the calculation of noise. The most usual measure of variation is the standard deviation. Large standard deviations are indicative of a large amount of patient-to-patient variation while small standard deviations indicate that patients are giving consistent values for the variable under consideration.

Within the sample the symbols $\bar{x}$ and s are used to denote mean and standard deviation, respectively. In theory, these same values can be obtained for the population as a whole, in which case the symbols μ and σ are used to denote these quantities, respectively.

THE NORMAL DISTRIBUTION

The normal distribution has a special place in statistical methodology. It was discovered almost 200 years ago by a German mathematician, Karl Friedrich Gauss, and relates to the behaviour of randomness. In a purely random process where data values are the result of 'averaging', the histogram of the values for the complete population (the population distribution) will be normally distributed. In reality, clinical data never arise from such a random process; nevertheless, the normal distribution can often provide an adequate approximation to the distribution of the data values in the population. In fact, when data are analysed, it is frequently assumed that they are 'normally distributed'.

The normal distribution is a bell-shaped symmetric histogram centred at μ. The standard deviation for the population values has certain particular properties when the data are normally distributed:

- 90% of the data values lie within the range $\mu -1.645\sigma$, $\mu+1.645\sigma$;
- 95% of the data values lie within the range $\mu -1.960\sigma$, $\mu+1.960\sigma$;
- 99% of the data values lie within the range $\mu -2.576\sigma$, $\mu+2.576\sigma$.

SAMPLING AND STANDARD ERRORS

As has been mentioned previously, statistics is primarily concerned with sampling from populations and making inferences about those populations on the basis of the sample data. In order to make progress, it is therefore important to understand the sampling process: what happens when we sample from a population?

Let us suppose a population of patients whose systolic blood pressure is normally distributed with mean 118 mmHg and standard deviation 8 mmHg. Suppose too that a sample of 80 patients was taken from this population by computer simulation, and that the sample mean was calculated, giving a value of $\bar{x} = 117.2$ mmHg. The principal point to notice is that the sample mean $\bar{x}$ is not equal to the overall population mean μ. A second simulation might give an $\bar{x}$ value of 118.9 mmHg, again different from the population mean $\mu = 118$ mmHg. In any practical setting, μ is never known and any sampling process will always give a value that is different from the true value; the sampling process can never be 'exact'.

Provided that the trial is designed and conducted appropriately, the sampling process will give a value that is equal to the correct (population) value on the average (termed *unbiasedness*) but on any particular occasion the sample value will be away from the true value. The accuracy, or reliability, of the sampling process, however, can be calculated in terms of the standard deviation of the sample mean values which is given by the formula $\sigma/\sqrt{n}$ and the value of this expression can be calculated from data. In the first simulation above with a sample mean of 117.2 mmHg, the standard deviation (s) of the 80 sample values was 7.76 mmHg. In the expression for the standard deviation of the sample mean values, substituting s for σ (since that is also not known) gives $7.76/\sqrt{80} = 0.87$. Thus, in this particular setting, the estimated standard deviation of the $\bar{x}$ values, known as the standard error of $\bar{x}$, is 0.87.

This value measures the precision of the sampling process; a small standard error indicates that the $\bar{x}$ values are 'close' in an overall sense to the true mean μ whereas a large standard error is indicative of an unstable setting where some of the $\bar{x}$ values could be a long way from the true mean. In this case, the single $\bar{x}$ value obtained in practice could mislead as to the true value μ. With a small standard error, the single $\bar{x}$ value is likely to be close to μ.

There are formulae for calculating the standard error of any 'statistic' that is of interest. For example, in a placebo-controlled trial, the main interest will centre on the value of $\mu_1 - \mu_2$, the active treatment mean minus the placebo mean: the 'treatment effect'. In a particular clinical trial $\bar{x}_1 - \bar{x}_2$ is calculated as an estimated treatment effect. We know that this value will not be exactly equal to $\mu_1 - \mu_2$ but can we be confident that it is close? The standard error of $\bar{x}_1 - \bar{x}_2$ provides information on this and a standard error formula is available, involving n_1, n_2 (the sample sizes) and s_1, s_2 (the standard deviations) in the two groups. A small standard error again indicates that the estimate is reliable; a large standard error indicates that it is unreliable.

CONFIDENCE INTERVALS

The previous section has illustrated that $\bar{x}$, from the sampling process, never hits the true population mean. The confidence interval provides a compromise, a range of values within which we are fairly certain that the true value lies. For a single mean, the 95% confidence interval for large sample sizes is given by:

$$(\bar{x} - 1.96s/\sqrt{n}, \ \bar{x} + 1.96s/\sqrt{n})$$

In the first computer simulation above where $\bar{x} = 117.2$ mmHg, $n = 80$ and $s = 7.76$ mmHg, this interval is (115.5, 118.9). The interval is termed the 95% confidence interval because 95% of such intervals calculated from repeated samples through the sampling process will contain the 'truth', μ. Therefore, on any single occasion, there can be 95% confidence that the truth is within the calculated range. The 95% property results from the 95% coverage provided by the range $\pm 1.96\sigma$ around μ in the normal distribution. For a 90% confidence interval 1.645 should be used in place of 1.960 and for a 99% confidence interval 2.576 is used.

Strictly speaking, these multipliers are only valid for large sample sizes; for smaller samples the correct multiplying constant will depend on the sample size and is provided by the so-called t-tables. Finally, for the 95% confidence interval, using a multiplying constant of 2 will provide an adequate approximation for sample sizes of 30 or more.

The confidence interval concept can be easily adapted to yield confidence intervals for any quantity of interest. For example, for the difference between two means, $\mu_1 - \mu_2$, the confidence interval is $\bar{x}_1 - \bar{x}_2 \pm t \times se$, where the multiplying constant t is chosen from the t-tables and se is the standard error of the

$\bar{x}_1 - \bar{x}_2$ value. Again, for large samples, a multiplying constant of 2 often provides a good approximation.

HYPOTHESIS TESTING AND *p*-VALUES

Clinical trials usually pose some very simple questions: Are these two treatments different? Does this treatment work? In order to answer these questions in statistics, they are formulated in terms of statistical hypotheses. For example, in evaluating an active treatment to lower blood pressure, the intention would be to compare the mean reductions in diastolic blood pressure in the active treatment and placebo groups, and the null hypothesis (H_0) and alternative hypothesis (H_1) would be formulated as follows:

$$H_0: \mu_1 = \mu_2 \qquad H_1: \mu_1 \neq \mu_2,$$

where μ_1 is the active treatment mean and μ_2 is the placebo mean. In trials where the objective is to detect differences, H_0 is always equality while H_1 is inequality.

Data are now used to guide the choice between the two hypotheses and it is the *p*-value that formalises this decision-making process. The *p* in *p*-value stands for probability and, as such, lies between 0 and 1. Its calculation is organised in such a way that *p*-values close to 0 cause us to prefer H_1, i.e. that the treatment means are different, while *p*-values away from 0 cause us to prefer H_0, i.e. that there are no differences between the treatments.

Continuing with the blood pressure example, let us suppose that the mean diastolic blood pressure reduction in the active treatment group is 7.6 mmHg while that in the placebo group is 2.7 mmHg, giving a difference in the means equal to 4.9 mmHg. Suppose further that $p = 0.03$, or 3% in percentage terms. What precisely does this *p*-value signify? A common misunderstanding is that it is the probability that H_0 is true. However, the correct definition is as follows: there is a 3% probability of obtaining a difference between the treatment means at least as large as 4.9 mmHg when the null hypothesis is true (i.e. equal treatment means). In informal terms, since 3% is a small probability, it indicates that the observed data are unlikely to have occurred with equal treatments and it is on this basis that we conclude in favour of H_1, i.e. that the treatment means are different. Alternatively, let us suppose that the *p*-value is 0.72. This would indicate that, with equal treatments, there is a 72% probability of seeing a difference in the means as large as 4.9 mmHg. This is a large probability and consequently the data in the trial are consistent with equal means, and as such there is no reason to doubt their equality.

Thus, small *p*-values indicate that the data are not consistent with 'equal treatments' and lead us to conclude that the treatments are different (H_1) whereas *p*-values that are not small indicate that the data are consistent with equal means and lead us to accept equality (H_0). The operational definition of 'small' in this context is 0.05 (5%). If p falls below 0.05, the treatment means are significantly different at the 5% level, and if p does not fall below 0.05, then the treatment means are not significantly different at the 5% level.

In the definition of the p-value, the phrase 'by chance' is sometimes used in place of 'when the null hypothesis is true'; it should be noted also that the p-value calculation is in terms of seeing a difference at least as large as that observed *in either direction,* that is, Treatment A better than Treatment B or *vice versa.* This second point relates to the fact that differences are always sought in either direction using two-sided or two-tailed tests. Finally, the calculation of the p-value and all that surrounds it is known as a statistical test; we are 'testing' the hypotheses.

THE *t*-TESTS

The two-sample *t*-test

The two-sample *t*-test (or unpaired *t*-test) is the most commonly used test and is the basis of the example outlined in the previous section. This test compares two means in a parallel-group trial.

The null hypothesis (H_0) is $\mu_1 = \mu_2$ and the alternative hypothesis (H_1) is $\mu_1 \neq \mu_2$. The p-value calculation is based around the evidence, provided by the data, in favour of H_1 and as a general procedure this is expressed as the signal-to-noise ratio (see above). For the two-sample *t*-test, the signal is the observed difference between the treatment group means and the noise is the standard error attached to this difference between the means.

To continue with the earlier blood pressure-lowering example in which $\bar{x}_1 - \bar{x}_2$ = 4.9 mmHg: if the *se* of this difference is calculated as 1.95, the signal-to-noise ratio is then 4.9/1.95 = 2.51. In the context of undertaking a statistical test, the signal-to-noise ratio is termed the test statistic (the statistic on which the test is based).

In order to calculate the p-value, it is necessary to add up all the probabilities associated with seeing an observed difference of 4.9 mmHg or greater (either larger positive or larger negative) or, equivalently, with obtaining a value for the test statistic of 2.51 or greater (either larger positive or larger negative). The probabilities associated with all the possible values of the test statistic when H_0 is true are given by the *t*-distribution. There exists a whole family of these *t*-distributions and the particular shape chosen depends on the total number of subjects in the trial. For *n* subjects, the appropriate distribution to choose is the *t*-distribution with '$n-2$ degrees of freedom'. In general, the distribution of the test statistic when the null hypothesis is true is known as the null distribution.

In our example, if we suppose that the total number of subjects is 16, then the t-distribution on 14 degrees of freedom is used for the p-value calculation. The test statistic value was 2.51 and the probability associated with this value and larger values (larger observed differences) is 0.02. Computer programs perform these calculations because they cannot be done by hand.

This value is below the nominal 0.05 cut-off; there is therefore a significant difference at the 5% level. The data are not consistent with equal treatment means in that there is only a 2% chance of seeing a difference as large as that observed with equal treatments and so the conclusion is in favour of H_1, i.e. that μ_1 and μ_2 are not equal.

The paired t-test

The two-sample t-test is used for between-patient comparisons. In a within-patient design, the paired t-test is used. Instead of using the difference between the treatment means as the signal, the paired t-test uses the mean of the within-patient differences and the noise is given by the standard error of this mean. If μ denotes the mean of the within-patient differences in the complete population, then the null and alternative hypotheses for the paired t-test are: H_0: $\mu = 0$ and H_1: $\mu \neq 0$, respectively.

When the null hypothesis is true, the probabilities associated with the test statistic (signal-to-noise ratio) are given by the t-distribution on $n-1$ degrees of freedom, where n is the number of subjects in the trial. The p-value is then obtained as the sum of all those probabilities associated with the observed signal-to-noise ratio and larger values of the signal.

The paired t-test is used in one of three settings; the cross-over trial, the paired design and a comparison of baseline with final value in a single treatment group.

Type I and type II errors

Unfortunately, statistical tests do not always give the correct answer and from time to time we may be misled by the data.

Consider a two-sample t-test comparing two means. The true situation will be that either $\mu_1 = \mu_2$ or $\mu_1 \neq \mu_2$. Having obtained the data and calculated the p-value, the result will be either $p < 0.05$ or $p \geq 0.05$ (Table 1).

Table 1. Illustration of type I and type II errors.

Data	Truth	
	$\mu_1 = \mu_2$	$\mu_1 \neq \mu_2$
$p \geq 0.05$	✓	✗
$p < 0.05$	✗	✓

If $\mu_1 = \mu_2$, then we would hope that the data would yield a p-value ≥ 0.05, enabling us to conclude correctly that there are no differences between the treatment means. However, this does not always happen: it is possible to have $p < 0.05$, causing us to conclude mistakenly that there are differences. This mistake is called the type I error, sometimes referred to as the alpha error. It is the false positive, concluding that differences exist where there are none.

Conversely, let us suppose that the true situation is $\mu_1 \neq \mu_2$. We would hope that the data give a p-value < 0.05 which would justify the conclusion that differences do exist. Again, however, this does not always happen and there will be occasions when the resultant p-value is non-significant, leading to the erroneous conclusion of no differences when in fact $\mu_1 \neq \mu_2$. This mistake is called the type II error or the beta error and is the false negative; the treatment means are different but the difference has been missed.

It is well known in statistics that these mistakes cannot be eliminated completely; the best that can be hoped for is to minimise the chance that they will occur. The type I error is conventionally fixed at 0.05, the level at which differences are declared to be significant. This is because the null distributions indicate exactly what will happen when the treatments are equal and extreme values of the test statistic *will* be seen purely by chance on 5% of occasions. On such occasions, however, a result of $p < 0.05$ will lead to the (incorrect) conclusion that the treatments are different, the type I error.

The type II error is controlled by modifying a related quantity – power. Power is 100% minus the type II error: if the type II error is 10% then power is 90%, if the type II error is 20% then power is 80%. The type II error corresponds to missing a real difference; power is a measure of the ability to capture a real difference. In order to control type II error at an acceptable level, power must be made sufficiently high. Usually, confirmatory trials are designed in such a way that power is at least 80%. More will be said about power in a later section.

EXTENSIONS OF THE *t*-TESTS

Multicentre trials

Many large trials involve several centres. The method of statistical analysis in such cases, an extension of the two-sample *t*-test, is known as two-way analysis of variance. The comparison of the two treatment groups remains the main focus of interest in these trials but there is also a secondary question and this concerns the homogeneity of the treatment difference across the centres. If the treatment effect is not homogeneous, there is said to be a treatment by centre (or treatment $\times$ centre) interaction and it is far more difficult to generalise the results of the trial under these circumstances.

Two-way analysis of variance gives p-values for two sets of hypotheses. First, assuming a consistent treatment difference, it provides a test of the (composite) null hypothesis that the treatment means are equal in each of the centres. This is achieved by calculating the observed difference between the treatment group means in each centre and comparing the 'average' difference (a weighted average where more weight is given to larger centres) to zero. Secondly, two-way analysis of variance provides a comparison of the treatment differences over the centres to evaluate the possible presence of a treatment by centre interaction.

If a treatment by centre difference is identified, further work is needed to try to understand why it has occurred; otherwise it is very difficult to predict the precise nature of the treatment difference in the population as a whole.

Analysis of covariance

In many cases it is of value when comparing treatments to take account of factors measured at baseline that are predictive of outcome. These factors are referred to as covariates. First, this gives more power; it increases the chance of detecting differences if they exist. Secondly, the technique can compensate for minor imbalances in subject mix across the two groups at baseline that may occur even though the trial is randomised. Finally, analysis of covariance allows the investigation of 'treatment by covariate' interactions and indicates whether the treatment effect is consistent over the different values of the baseline covariate.

The technique of analysis of covariance is now widely used. Those factors to be included as covariates should be specified either in the protocol from the outset or in the statistical analysis plan. Baseline values of the outcome variable are frequently used as covariates, together with the 'change from baseline' in the outcome variable as the focus for the treatment comparison. The technique often leads to an analysis that is summarised in terms of 'adjusted means'. These are sample means that, through the analysis of covariance technique, have been adjusted to correct for baseline imbalances in the covariates between the two treatment groups.

THE CHI-SQUARED TESTS

Data types

The data discussed in this chapter have been almost exclusively continuous, i.e. data measured on a continuous scale, such as blood pressure, forced expiratory volume in 1 second (FEV_1), cholesterol level and so on. Not all data are collected in this way and this section will consider methods of analysis for binary, categorical and ordinal data. Binary data are simply yes/no data, success/failure, cured/not cured, etc. Categorical data are binary data extended to more than two categories: for example, primary cause of death could be classified as death from cancer causes, death from cardiovascular causes, death from respiratory causes or death from other causes. In clinical applications, however, categorical data have an implicit ordering. For example, in classifying pain a simple four-point scale may be used: none, mild, moderate and severe. In such cases the data are termed ordinal or ordered categorical data.

Binary data

The chi-squared (χ^2) test is used for a two-group comparison with binary data. Such data can be expressed in terms of a 2×2 contingency table, as shown in the example below (taken from Pocock, 1983). In this case, the binary outcome is survival beyond 90 days/death up to and including 90 days following acute myocardial infarction and the two treatment groups are metoprolol and placebo. The χ^2 test in this example is based on the comparison of the observed (O) frequencies (Table 2) and the expected (E) frequencies (Table 3). The expected frequencies are based on what would be expected to happen if there were no differences between the treatment groups in terms of the probability of 'early' death. They are calculated by dividing the total numbers of deaths and survivors according to the proportions of patients in the treatment groups as a whole.

Table 2. Deaths and survivors – observed data.

	Died	Survived	Total
Metoprolol	40	657	697
Placebo	62	636	698
Total	102	1293	1395

Table 3. Deaths and survivors – expected data.

	Died	Survived	Total
Metoprolol	51	646	697
Placebo	51	647	698
Total	102	1293	1395

The signal on which the χ^2 test is based is $(O-E)^2$ while the noise is the standard error formula for the O values. Note that the $O-E$ values are numerically the same, and equal to ± 11, whichever cell in the table is used. To obtain the p-value, the signal-to-noise ratio (test statistic) is then compared with the χ^2 distribution on one degree of freedom, the null distribution in this case. In the above example, the signal-to-noise ratio is 5.12, giving a p-value of 0.024, significant at the 5% level, and indicating differences between the probabilities of early death across the treatment groups.

The odds ratio

The odds ratio is often used as a summary statistic to indicate the magnitude of the treatment difference. It is the ratio of the odds in favour of the event of interest. In the above example, the odds in favour of survival in the metoprolol group are 657/40 = 16.4/1 while in the placebo group they are 636/62 = 10.3/1. The odds ratio is then 16.4/10.3 = 1.60. An odds ratio of 1 indicates that there are no differences between the treatment groups, while an odds ratio away from 1 is indicative of differences. It is also a straightforward exercise to obtain confidence intervals for odds ratios.

Categorical and ordinal data

The χ^2 test extends in a simple way to categorical data. Again this involves a comparison of observed and expected frequencies and the test statistic is a sum of the separate signal-to-noise ratios over the outcome categories and is compared with the χ^2 distribution, with degrees of freedom equal to the number of outcome categories minus one.

However, a completely different technique known as the Mantel–Haenszel χ^2 test is used when the categories are ordered. This test, sometimes termed the 'one degree of freedom test for trend', exploits the ordering of the categories to produce an appropriate comparison of the treatments in terms of a shift in the frequencies across those categories. The test statistic for this test, for two treatment groups, is always compared with the χ^2 distribution on one degree of freedom, irrespective of the number of outcome categories.

POWER AND SAMPLE SIZE CALCULATIONS

Power

The concept of power was introduced earlier as the opposite of type II error. Power measures the ability to detect differences between treatments when differences exist. Typically, in a statistical test, differences are detected by observing $p < 0.05$; to be precise, therefore, power is the probability of observing $p < 0.05$.

In advance of running a clinical trial, it is possible to calculate the power of the trial to detect certain levels of effect. Let us take as our example a hypertension trial comparing the mean reduction in diastolic blood pressure between two active treatments, using a two-sample t-test. Let us further assume that the standard deviation for reduction in blood pressure in each group is 5 mmHg, that the group sizes are 50 and that differences will be declared if $p < 0.05$. The power calculated on the basis of various levels of true difference is shown in Table 4.

Table 4. Power for group sizes of 50 subjects.

True difference between means (mmHg)	Power
1	0.166
2	0.508
3	0.844
4	0.977
5	0.999

Thus, if the true difference between the two active treatment means is 2 mmHg, there is a 50.8% probability of emerging from this trial with a significant p-value, i.e. having 'detected' an effect. If the difference were 3 mmHg, this probability would be 84.4%, and so on. In these two cases the type II errors are 49.2% and 15.6%, respectively.

In a head-to-head comparison between one company's treatment and that of its direct competitor, let us assume that a difference between the means of 2 mmHg would be an important difference to detect. Under these circumstances, this design would be very unsatisfactory because the chance of detecting a difference of 2 mmHg is only approximately 50%. The only option for redesigning the trial is to increase the sample size. The power for group sizes of 100 patients is shown in Table 5.

Table 5. Power for group sizes of 100 subjects.

True difference between means (mmHg)	Power
1	0.290
2	0.804
3	0.988
4	1.000
5	1.000

This appears far more acceptable because there is an 80.4% probability of emerging from the trial with a significant p-value if a difference of 2 mmHg actually exists.

Sample size calculation

These considerations of power provide the basis for the sample size calculation. The power required to detect a defined difference is specified and the sample size that confers that power can be calculated. From the example above, if the requirement is to have 80% power to detect a difference of 2 mmHg, then a sample size of 200 (i.e. two groups of 100 subjects each) would be adequate.

When calculating sample size, four quantities invariably need to be specified: the significance level, the power required (the regulators advise that this should be at least 80%), the level of difference looked for (denoted the 'clinically relevant difference'), and some quantity that permits calculation of the 'noise'. For the two-sample t-test, this would be the anticipated standard deviation of the end-point, while for binary data and the χ^2 test, this would be the expected 'event' rate in the control group. Once each of these aspects is specified, the sample size calculation is straightforward.

The specification of the clinically relevant difference is a clinical or commercial decision, not a statistical one, while the specification of the standard deviation for the t-test or the 'event' rate for the χ^2 test will usually be made on the basis of past data. These latter quantities, although sometimes difficult to pin down, are unfortunately critical to the sample size calculation. In the two-sample t-test, a doubling of the standard deviation leads to a four-fold increase in the required sample size; the relationship is an exponential one. It is therefore important to pay careful attention to the standard deviation value. If the standard deviation is understated, the sample size will be too small and this could have a major impact on the ability to detect important differences.

CONCLUSION

The purpose of this chapter has been to outline some of the basic concepts in clinical trial design and the statistical analysis of data from clinical trials. There is a perception that statistical methods are difficult. This is not the case. There are admittedly some tricky issues that need to be studied carefully in order to gain understanding, but the methodological development is entirely logical. In providing a basis for an understanding of the methodology, I hope that this brief chapter will motivate readers to explore the subject in greater depth (see Further Reading).

FURTHER READING

Altman, DG (1991). *Practical Statistics for Medical Research*, Chapman and Hall, London.

Armitage, P and Berry, G (1994). *Statistical Methods in Medical Research (3rd edn)*, Blackwell, Oxford.

Chow, S-C and Liu, J (1998). *Design and Analysis of Clinical Trials: Concepts and Methodologies*, John Wiley, New York.

ICH Guideline (1998). *Topic E9: Statistical Principles for Clinical Trials*, International

Federation of Pharmaceutical Manufacturers Associations, Geneva (Issued as CPMP/ICH/363/96).

ICH Guideline (1999). *Topic E10: Choice of Control Group in Clinical Trials*, International Federation of Pharmaceutical Manufacturers Associations, Geneva (Reached Step 4 in July 2000).

Piantadosi, S (1997). *Clinical Trials: A Methodological Perspective*, John Wiley, New York.

Pocock, SJ (1983). *Clinical Trials: A Practical Approach*, John Wiley, Chichester.

Senn, SJ (1997). *Statistical Issues in Drug Development*, John Wiley, Chichester.

Spilker, B (1991). Statistical issues. In: Spilker, B (Ed), *Guide to Clinical Trials*, Raven Press, New York, pp. 497–501.

17

Project management of drug development

Bryan C. Hurst and Gill Pearce

INTRODUCTION

The development of a new drug is a lengthy, costly and complex process. This chapter focuses on the project management of the clinical components of a drug development programme, the life cycle of which is well-defined (Figure 1).

The size, complexity and cost of drug development have been increasing consistently since the 1970s. The need to be first to market, combined with the need to meet detailed regulatory requirements, has resulted not only in increased time pressures but also in more extensive drug development programmes. Additionally, the pharmaceutical industry has come to operate more on a global scale, and this has brought new logistical challenges. These

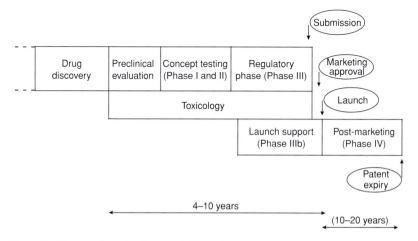

Figure 1. Typical drug development life cycle.

needs have precipitated the implementation of effective project management using formal project management methods that have previously proved successful in other industries.

HISTORY OF PROJECT MANAGEMENT IN THE PHARMACEUTICAL INDUSTRY

Project management theory was born in the 1950s and was further developed throughout the 1960s and 1970s by the manufacturing and construction industries. In essence, however, any project will have three basic targets – deliverables, time and cost. A project may also be broken down into sub-projects and each sub-project, in turn, into a list of tasks. While these fundamental project management concepts can be used effectively across a number of industries, it is important to remember that successful implementation will require some adaptation. To fully understand why such adaptation is necessary, it will be helpful to understand how the pharmaceutical industry differs from the construction or manufacturing industries. Some key differences are shown in Table 1.

Table 1. Differences between a production line and clinical research.

Production line	Clinical research
Identical, repetitive tasks	Similar, non-repetitive tasks
Well-defined outcome	Ultimate outcome may require learning
Duration easy to define	Duration difficult to define, e.g. unforeseen problems with ethical or regulatory approval of a protocol
Many relatively straightforward steps	Fewer more complicated steps
Resource mostly under the direct control of the project manager	Key resources, e.g. investigators, not under the direct control of the project manager

In a production line environment, similar tasks tend to be repeated over and over again. However, this is not the case with clinical research where planning has to be done for each 'novel' task: this may present its own set of problems and issues, some of which may not have been encountered before. Likewise, production line tasks tend to be straightforward and the complexity arises from the large number of tasks that need to be executed in a precise sequence. In clinical research, the tasks are often less well-defined, may be interlinked and are modified as a result of learning (heuristic process). Often, progress and cost information will predict new or unforeseen problems and ideally these need to be resolved as they arise. Additionally, clinical projects often encompass input from many different departments across the organisation. This necessitates that work and resources are coordinated in a matrix across normal line management structures.

Clinical task durations are more difficult to define, e.g. regulatory and protocol approval times depend on external, independent committees which usually respond badly to time pressures imposed from outside. As a result of these uncertainties, project management of clinical research is as much an art as a science. A skilled project manager knows how to apply the theory appropriately and how to adapt project management tools, largely developed for other industries, for use in clinical research. More detailed information on basic project management theory is available in Kerzner (1998) and Meredith and Mantel (1999).

SCOPE OF THE PROJECT

What is a project? A project is a defined piece of work which has agreed timelines and requires a team of people with diverse skills to work together to achieve a common set of objectives.

The scope of any project needs to be carefully defined from the outset (Posner and Applegarth, 1998) and this is especially important if any part is to be outsourced (Lewis, 2000; *see also Chapter 22*). Definition of the project scope should clearly lay out the anticipated deliverables, timelines and cost estimates. A critical success factor in any project is having an appropriate 'sponsor' who is of sufficient seniority to be able to exert influence at the cross-functional level. The sponsor needs to ensure that:

- the project aligns with the business need;
- key stakeholders are committed;
- sufficient resource is available.

Stakeholders are those who will be affected by the project: they may benefit as a customer or be required to contribute as a resource provider. Stakeholders will be involved in key decision-making, e.g. stopping the project or approving major changes in its scope. Sponsors and stakeholders need to 'own' the scope of the project, i.e. the definition of its boundaries. With the scope defined and stakeholder support in place, planning and scheduling can begin.

Planning the project

Project planning entails planning, scheduling and controlling project activities to achieve performance, cost and time objectives for a given scope of work, while using resources efficiently and effectively within quality and budgetary targets.

A project first needs to be broken down into manageable pieces or tasks. A task has a start date, an end date, attached resources and links to other tasks. For very large projects, the first division may be into sub-projects; these

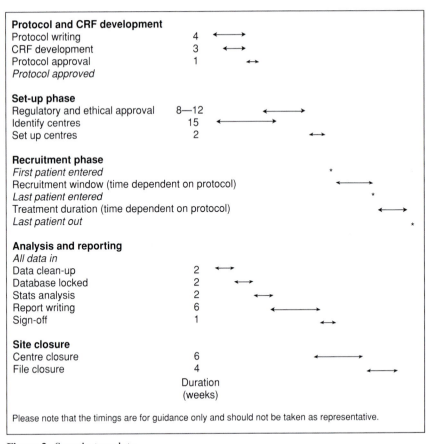

Protocol and CRF development
Protocol writing   4
CRF development   3
Protocol approval   1
Protocol approved

Set-up phase
Regulatory and ethical approval   8—12
Identify centres   15
Set up centres   2

Recruitment phase
First patient entered
Recruitment window (time dependent on protocol)
Last patient entered
Treatment duration (time dependent on protocol)
Last patient out

Analysis and reporting
All data in
Data clean-up   2
Database locked   2
Stats analysis   2
Report writing   6
Sign-off   1

Site closure
Centre closure   6
File closure   4
                                   Duration
                                   (weeks)

Please note that the timings are for guidance only and should not be taken as representative.

Figure 2. Sample template.

are further divided into lists of tasks. Each task can be viewed as an individual building block of the project as a whole. By establishing those that are related and interdependent, the tasks need to be organised into a work breakdown structure (Lewis, 2000). Within clinical research, for example, the project could equate to the development/registration of the new therapeutic drug; one of the sub-projects could be a large Phase III clinical trial, and this would then be divided into the following phases:

- protocol and case record form (CRF) development;
- set-up;
- recruitment;
- analysis and reporting; and
- site closure.

Within each phase there will be a number of tasks, milestones, links and dependencies that are specific for each project.

A sample template that could be used with any commercially available software is provided as a guide (Figure 2), but most major companies have their own software template, which usually includes resource forecasting by skill group (Gwede *et al.*, 2000).

PROJECT MANAGEMENT TOOLS

It is worthwhile to reflect on what is required of a project management tool in general terms, as a basis for choosing an approach. In the early phase of a clinical project the main tool is planning software to describe the process and help predict resource demand and timelines (Michael and Burton, 1992). Although many kinds of tools are available, some variant of project management software is used almost universally, and the next most useful tool is probably a spreadsheet (see the section below on 'Effective use of project management tools'). These tools can be incredibly effective in managing/tracking information. However, it should not be forgotten that the information is only as good as the people who provide it. These management systems cannot evaluate problems, make decisions or indeed define the overall strategy. Our attention will therefore turn to the teams of people that are required to be involved in project management. Effective teams rely on quality people management. However, since many entire books are already devoted to the subject of teams and team structures (e.g. Andersen *et al.*, 1998), this aspect will only be touched upon here

Team structures

Within the last decade there has been an increasing trend to merge pharmaceutical development companies into global organisations. As a result, clinical development programmes have become worldwide projects that are run across international boundaries by multidisciplinary international clinical development teams (ICDTs). An ICDT may involve a number of highly qualified and technically skilled individuals who reside in different locations. Typically, the ICDT is led by a full-time project leader and together the team is responsible for the successful delivery of the project. It is the responsibility of the ICDT to create and implement the international clinical development plan (ICDP): this will outline the major features of the project and the estimated time to completion. The ICDT's activities will involve planning, monitoring, reporting, evaluating, re-directing or in some cases even terminating the project. To terminate a project at the right time can be one of the most important recommendations the ICDT can make. Within the competitive environment of a large organisation it is imperative that the project team communicates effectively to senior management on an ongoing basis to ensure that correct prioritisation/resource is allocated.

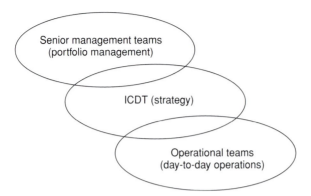

Figure 3. Reporting structure.

The ICDT reports upwards to senior management and will generally be supported by smaller 'operational teams', as shown in Figure 3.

ICDT membership will tend to evolve as the project moves through the different clinical development phases; however, the core development team will usually encompass the major development disciplines.

The ICDT may be supported by a number of operational teams (e.g. the clinical development team, product launch team, business development team, external communications/publications team, etc.) with responsibility for ensuring that the ongoing day-to-day activities are carried out within the time frames laid out in the clinical development plan. Typical team compositions are summarised in Table 2.

It may be that additional 'task force teams' are assembled and dissolved *ad hoc* to ensure that any new issues arising (e.g. particularly slow recruitment in a pivotal Phase III trial) are addressed swiftly.

Team meetings

The ICDT will meet on a regular basis (every 4–8 weeks depending on the issues at hand), either face to face or more frequently, given the cost constraints of international travel, by videoconferencing, PC conferencing or teleconferencing. Team meetings should be well disciplined with a planned, primarily issue-driven, agenda. Minutes from team meetings should be short and reflect the agreed action points. Routine updates should not be given at the ICDT meeting as these can be circulated beforehand for information. One of the keys to a successful ICDT is the ability to make decisions: in order to get this right, it is imperative to have the right information and the right people making the decision. The ICDT also needs to have clear direction on those decisions for which it can take responsibility and those which require the authorisation of senior management.

Table 2. Typical team composition.

International clinical development team	Clinical operations team	Launch operations team
Project leader	Clinical pharmacology (Phase I)	Sales/marketing
Research	Clinical research (Phases II–IV)	Commercial strategy
Chemical development	Clinical statistics	Regional territories
Formulation development	Clinical monitoring	Communications
Toxicology	Clinical data management	Media relations
Drug metabolism/ pharmacokinetics	Clinical report writing	Visual communications
Clinical development	Clinical trial supplies	
Regulatory	Clinical safety	
Marketing	Clinical auditing	
Health economics		
Genetics		

Matrix management

What is meant by matrix management? In pharmaceutical development, a matrix organisation brings the project and the functional organisations together. Within today's pharmaceutical industry, international project management co-ordinates the assembled team of individuals selected from different parts of the organisation.

In a line management structure, each function or department would hold part of the project budget; in a matrix organisation, skill groups are still managed within functional groups but the budget is owned by the project.

The ICDT is a matrix team, with team members each being experts in their project-related discipline. For instance, the regulatory team member of the ICDT will probably work within the international regulatory department and may be the ICDT member for more than one clinical development project. Within the regulatory department he/she may manage a small team of regulatory personnel while still reporting to the departmental head who in turn will report to a more senior line manager. Within the matrix organisation, however, their role has responsibilities to the project team. The line management and matrix structures are illustrated in Figures 4 and 5.

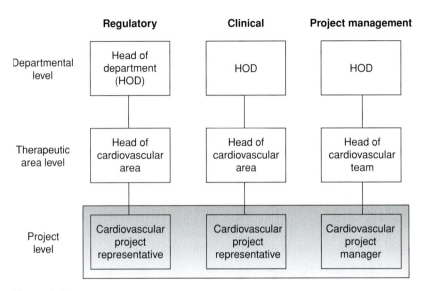

Figure 4. Line management structure.

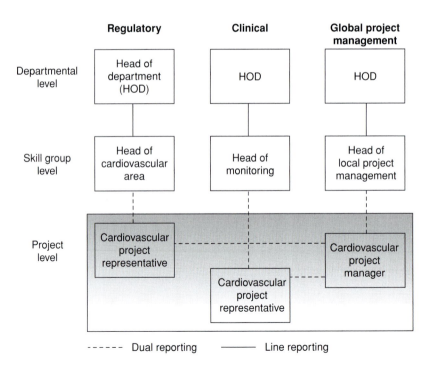

Figure 5. Matrix management structure.

This means that the ICDT regulatory representative will report to at least two managers (and possibly more): the regulatory department manager through the line management reporting structure and the individual project leaders through the matrix management system. This can sometimes lead to conflict if the project leader and the departmental manager disagree on the direction the project is taking or on the priorities of one project versus another. Such conflict can often be avoided if the departmental manager is identified from the outset as one of the key stakeholders of the project. As a key stakeholder his/her 'buy-in' should be sought at the beginning of the project and he/she should be kept updated on the progress of the project on a routine basis. Additionally, a good team leader will clarify when a team member has authority to make a decision and when he/she has to go to line management for a decision. The advantages and disadvantages of the line management structure and the matrix organisation are enumerated in Tables 3 and 4.

Table 3. Line management structure.

Advantages	Disadvantages
● Good information flow within the function	● Limited cross-functional interaction
● Supporting skill groups to achieve excellence	● Slower development for multi-functional projects
● Maintaining quality and standards within the function	● Increased bureaucracy
	● Conflict between function and project

Table 4. Matrix structure.

Advantages	Disadvantages
● Flexibility around day-to-day problem-solving	● Greater ambiguity and uncertainty
● More rapid decision-making by taking functions out of the loop	● More complex to operate
● Maximises available resource by having greater flexibility to move people around	● More than one boss for many team members
● Avoids overloading top management by having a single channel of communication	
● Promotes cross-functional interaction by removing barriers	
● Decisions are made by those closest to the data rather than those at the top of functional hierarchies	

The pros and cons of each of these approaches need to be weighed for each project. One novel alternative to the two management systems described above is to form a separate 'venture group' to encompass the project team. This would have the effect of making the team independent of line management authority: the project team would then operate as a completely separate entity and be empowered to make its own decisions. This type of management system would only be put in place for a top-priority project that needed to be progressed very quickly. The project team would need to be highly experienced and probably to have demonstrated a successful track record. To operate in this way the ICDT of the venture group would need to be fully resourced and funded prior to project initiation.

Managing resources

Throughout the life span of a project it is important to plan and track the resources required to support its successful completion. Resources can be divided into budget and manpower. The overall budget can generally be agreed up front and the expenditure forecast can be easily automated by inserting a timing factor.

Manpower can be tracked in different ways:

- amount of resource for each time unit (e.g. a varying number of people in each day); or
- a total effort, assumed to be spread evenly over the activity (e.g. 20 man days spread over a six-week task).

Most project management software can handle these inputs. Network analysis can identify flexibility in activity timing and therefore be used to reschedule tasks to give a more even workload. When tasks are on the critical path, or multiple tasks need to be conducted at the same time, this flexibility is lost. In this case, activities must be rescheduled within the resource available according to priority, to give the best possible compromise between completion time desired and what is possible with the available resources. However, most computer systems will perform this task, usually termed 'resource levelling'. This information can then be used to procure additional resources ahead of time from senior or line management.

Strategic planning

Optimal global product development requires thorough long-term strategic planning. Strategic planning will generally encompass a five- to 10-year planning horizon and will take into account the entire portfolio of drugs within an individual therapeutic area. As such, it allows a cross-product strategy to be developed to ensure that the maximum potential of each product is achieved. Current information on the disease area and market segments is used to predict the likely future environment. Strategic plans outline any competitive advantage, help to differentiate the organisation from its competitors, and are often used to achieve review and agreement at a senior level; as such, these plans need to be kept concise and direct. Once the overall strategy has been agreed, this is converted to individual operational plans.

Operational planning

Following the decision to move forward into a full-scale clinical development programme, the ICDT is charged with creating an international clinical development plan (ICDP). This is an operational plan that will list out the schedule of activities required over the following 3–5 years to enable successful registration of the product. This operational plan should be developed, focusing on the intended commercial product, outlining the key characteristics of the product (i.e. the product profile) and then mapping this to the pivotal data that will be required to support registration and the therapeutic claims. Once all the key activities have been laid out in the clinical development plan and agreed, the individual sub-projects can be assigned time and resources, taking care to clearly identify individual tasks that are interlinked and time-dependent on each other. As a simple example, we can review the individual tasks involved in setting up a single clinical study, estimate how long each task may take and identify the order in which they must be completed to achieve the final goal of recruiting patients. The following five tasks would be required:

1. Study protocol finalised (time estimate = 6 weeks);
2. CRF produced (time estimate = 4 weeks);
3. Ethical review and approval (time estimate = 4 weeks);
4. Drug shipped to study site (time estimate = 6 weeks); and
5. First subject recruited.

Tasks 1 to 4 above (Figure 6) must be completed prior to subject recruitment. If each task were completed before the next is begun, the entire process would take 20 weeks. However, effective identification of those tasks that are independent of each other (Figure 7) will reveal the steps that are rate-limiting or on the critical path: protocol finalised (6 weeks) – ethics review (4 weeks) – drug shipped to site (6 weeks) – recruitment.

By overlapping those tasks that are not time-dependent on each other and allowing CRF production to take place at the same time as ethics review, it is possible to save 4 weeks by removing this task from the critical path. Similarly, if it were also possible to ship drug to site (or to a location nearby for immediate release once ethics approval had been given), another task could effectively be removed from the critical path, thus saving an additional 6 weeks. This simple example shows how effective planning can help to highlight improved processing of individual tasks. It also becomes clear that planning the hundreds (or even thousands) of individual tasks required in

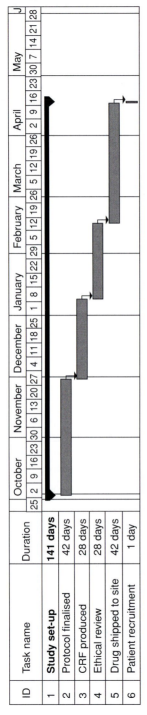

ID	Task name	Duration	October	November	December	January	February	March	April	May
1	**Study set-up**	**141 days**								
2	Protocol finalised	42 days								
3	CRF produced	28 days								
4	Ethical review	28 days								
5	Drug shipped to site	42 days								
6	Patient recruitment	1 day								

Figure 6. Sequential task completion.

ID	Task name	October	November	December	January	February	March	April	May
1	**Study set-up**								
2	Protocol finalised								
3	CRF produced								
4	Ethical review								
5	Drug shipped to site								
6	Patient recruitment								

Figure 7. Removing CRF production from the critical path.

multiple sub-projects, which then form part of an overall project such as the development of a new therapeutic agent, often requires all the skills of a full-time project planner. The project planner is often responsible for providing programme evaluation and review technique (PERT) and Gantt charts which can map down to the very detailed level of individual tasks.

The project team will not often become involved in individual task management because this will be left to the operations team or, in the case of an individual study, perhaps to the study team leader in charge of that particular protocol. The project team will, however, focus its attention on the development and timely implementation of the ICDP.

The ICDP is effectively an operational plan that can be used on an ongoing basis to identify major milestones or decision points and to highlight at an early stage where bottlenecks may occur and where additional resources will be required. The ICDP generally covers the following topics:

Brief rationale for development

Scientific. This section should give a brief overview of the compound to be developed. It should review any *in-vitro* data with regard to activity or toxicity. If animal data are available for evaluating the drug's bioavailability and toxicity, these should also be included.

Medical. This section should give a brief update on the therapeutic area for which the drug is intended and should include any clinical trial data obtained with the therapeutic compound under development.

Commercial. This section requires an overview of the current market situation, together with a predicted view at the time of launch. Likewise, a review of any other competitor drugs currently licensed within the same therapeutic class (or those currently under development by other companies) should be included.

Chemical development/manufacturing

In the early stages of development, this section of the ICDP can be of paramount importance to the success of the project. The scaling up of small batches to larger batches to provide sufficient drug to conduct clinical trials and ultimately to full-scale commercial batches needs to be carefully thought out and co-ordinated to ensure that these items do not become part of the critical path. Manufacturing strategies are often complex and expensive; senior management therefore needs to be aware of all the ongoing issues.

Preclinical/toxicology. This section should outline the *in-vitro* and animal tests that will be required to ensure that regulatory requirements are met. It is important that such studies are initiated sufficiently early to provide adequate toxicological cover for human studies once they are initiated.

Clinical pharmacology. A Phase I/II clinical development strategy should be detailed in this section. The initial Phase I single- and multiple-dose studies may take place in healthy volunteers to provide data on safety and tolerability, together with data on the pharmacokinetic profile of the drug. Depending on the type of project, Phase I development may take about one year.

Further Phase II dose-ranging studies in patients will provide data on the dose selection and any possible drug interactions. Phase II dose-finding studies are of critical importance to a good development programme: it is a costly mistake if the wrong dose is taken forward into full Phase III clinical development. It is rare for full Phase III development to be initiated until dose selection has taken place and this is one of the major milestones in any development programme.

Clinical research. The major Phase III clinical development programme will be detailed in the clinical research section of the ICDP. These studies will form one of the major elements of the regulatory submission and it is vital to obtain regulatory buy-in to the development plan prior to initiating Phase III. Within the ICDP it may be appropriate make contingency plans in case one of the pivotal studies has a negative outcome; while obviously planning for success, it may be appropriate to ask: 'Is there a Plan B?'

The ICDP should set out and justify the following key elements:

- target populations;
- primary efficacy end-points; and
- safety parameters.

The regulatory submission plans and timelines should also be detailed in this section. It is imperative that those clinical studies pivotal to support regulatory approval are agreed from the outset, together with any that may form part of a Plan B strategy. Likewise, those clinical studies on the critical path should be clearly identified and monitored closely to ensure that key milestones are met, always remembering that if other studies are allowed to slip, they may also contribute to critical path activities or even end up on the critical path themselves!

Health economics. It has become increasingly important in today's commercial environment to be able to justify the need for and cost of additional therapeutic agents. Some regulatory agencies will not enter price negotiations without some supporting health economic data (*see Chapter 14*).

Outsourcing strategy (if required). If part or all of the clinical development is to be outsourced, then both the strategy and the operational steps that are required need to be addressed in the ICDP.

Commercial strategy. The commercial strategy should encompass the novel features of the drug under development and the possible positioning that could be achieved. This section should conclude with a commercial forecast (usually given with both an upside and a downside forecast), based on a number of clearly defined key assumptions.

The ICDP is a living document that requires updating on an ongoing basis as the various milestones are met, delayed or revised. Many companies now have ICDPs available on their own company intranet systems, thus allowing for easy access and updating. It is essential to revisit the ICDP continually to ensure that corrective action is taken, if required, to avoid timelines slipping. Likewise, at the project outset, it is important to ensure that the time-critical tasks are identified and that any activities on the critical path are well planned and resourced. The key to success is to ensure that all stakeholders have had input into the plan at the early stages. These same key stakeholders need to be involved in reviewing project milestone events, given that drug development is typically undertaken in a stepwise manner with incremental investment and resource only forthcoming after key milestones have been achieved. Key milestones will include:

- first dose in man;
- proof of principle in man;
- start of Phase II studies;
- dose selection;
- start of Phase III studies;
- last subject to complete Phase III; and
- new drug application/marketing authorisation application submission.

However, it is important to emphasise that to defer initiating a rate-limiting development activity until a particular milestone has been successfully passed could lead to unnecessary delays. For this reason most projects 'plan for success', highlighting where calculated risks may be worth taking. In the race to be the first to market, it is good planning that can make the difference and a well thought-out and up-to-date ICDP is one of the cornerstones of such planning. A typical simplified development plan with estimated timelines is shown in Figure 8.

EFFECTIVE USE OF PROJECT MANAGEMENT TOOLS

Many kinds of project management tools are available; this section will focus on project management software because it is now almost ubiquitous. Project management software is invaluable in trained hands but can be a hindrance if not used properly. Off-the-shelf software was not designed for clinical research. Although customised software has many advantages, it is almost always based on software that was designed for use in a manufacturing

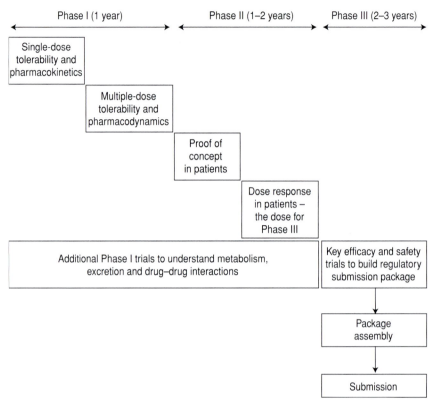

Figure 8. International clinical development plan.

context. The more sophisticated software requires extensive training to avoid pitfalls, and most users tend only to scratch the surface of the potential utility. With the exception of full-time planners, users have to re-learn the software every time a new plan is needed. Fortunately, most of the major companies have professional planning functions. Getting the right level of detail is imperative (Lewis, 2000); for instance, trying to track a 100-centre trial in detail at centre level requires almost as much effort as conducting the study. With project management software, it is easy for the plan to become mightier than the project itself, particularly if the attempt is made to track progress in detail. A key principle is to provide only useful information. Over the years, plans and templates have become more and more simplified by including less and less detail. Gantt charts have been referred to as 'confusograms'; this may appear flippant, but the name holds more than a grain of truth. Simplicity and clarity are the keys to effective communication and a useful general rule is: the more senior the manager, the less detail required. However, this does not mean that it is inappropriate to have a more detailed schedule at the individual trial level.

Basic software tools have no provision for tracking recruitment other than as a percentage total, and although bespoke software systems (O'Shea, 1998) allow tracking of recruitment and produce recruitment graphs, this is sometimes achieved at the expense of re-entering voluminous baseline tracking data. The ideal is to enter data only once and it is now possible to collect on-line recruitment data from monitoring tracking tools, central laboratories or central randomisation providers. The authors are unaware of any system that links project management software to an on-line database capable of providing on-line recruitment data. However, it is inevitable that software providers will claim to have done this already.

Bespoke software tends to be very expensive and although skeletal versions may be available off the shelf, additional customisation and maintenance will be needed. Even with a very sophisticated system, it may be necessary to cope with trials as diverse as anaesthetic trials that last one day, and oncology trials that continue over many years. A single system that copes with centre status, recruitment, trial supplies inventory, data flow and budgets is still some way off; most people will continue to cope with a marriage of spreadsheets for information management and project management software for planning and scheduling. Future trends in project management tool development are discussed in a later section under the heading 'The way forward'.

Commercial/clinical interface

Until the 1980s, companies tended to perform regulatory and commercial development separately, i.e. they were handled by different departments. The team responsible for delivering the regulatory package usually had little or no communication with the commercial department, or in the early stages, with the clinical/commercial group. This resulted in licences being granted for regulatory packages that fell well short of commercial needs and expectations. The launch support phases usually started too late to be included in the launch package and, from a commercial perspective, this was totally unsatisfactory. Peak year sales and time-to-peak year sales are largely determined by the quality and strength of the launch platform, especially in the case of 'me-too' products. The pattern started to change once the clinical and commercial teams began to merge so that one team managed the whole product life cycle.

The move towards project-led organisational structures further improved co-operation by putting commercial and clinical skill groups together in the same project team. Instead of perpetuating the clinical/commercial rivalries, both groups tended to focus on delivery of the project.

Commercial strategy

Better communications between clinical and commercial departments gave rise to the need for a clear strategy. Having a defined strategy and defined deliverables is the key to fulfilling commercial expectations. Before the regulatory and launch support packages are designed there should be a discussion about what is needed and why it is needed. This is the prelude to the operational phase that concentrates on how and when, rather than what and why. Most companies will devote much time and effort to collecting and interpreting commercial intelligence, qualitative and quantitative market research data and external advice. The project team will have to convince its internal sponsors that there will be an adequate pay-back on their investment. The sponsors may impose certain conditions on sponsorship – usually time limits. The project manager should be involved in the preparation of strategy to ensure that it is possible to do what is required to quality and to time. Strategy and operations are, by their very nature, iterative processes.

Product profile

A widely used vehicle for converting a commercial strategy into an operational plan is the product profile. This is a means whereby the commercial and clinical teams agree deliverables – usually labelling and promotional claims. The clinical team designs clinical trials in outline that will provide the deliverables. It may not be possible to deliver all the claims on the wish list, or it may be simpler to modify the wording slightly in order to improve operational feasibility. Once agreed, the study outlines define as a minimum the treatment, the population and the primary and secondary end-points. With this information it is possible to prepare a clinical development plan.

Life cycle management

Life cycle management covers the total life of the product from launch to patent expiry and usually refers to its commercial development. A current trend is for the regulatory Phase (IIIa) and launch support Phase (IIIb) to be merged. The focus has shifted from obtaining marketing approval to building effective launch platforms. This has had a major impact on project management by apparently making regulatory packages bigger. It is important to understand that it is not just regulatory requirements that are responsible for bigger packages. In order to be able to promote fully in the USA, a 'label claim' is required, and to have label claims at launch, it is necessary for the supporting data to be included in the regulatory submission package. However, the project management implications are independent of the reasons for increasing package size.

Project managers are expected to deliver bigger more complicated packages in shorter timescales and to increase the quality wherever possible. Although more activities can be performed in parallel to avoid delays, this immediately increases complexity and puts greater demand on resources. Manpower shortages have largely been resolved, either by contracting people in or by outsourcing. Project managers rapidly need to acquire new skills – e.g. how to negotiate with and manage external partners. Outsourcing itself is associated with a new set of issues which require additional management skills.

Strengthening the launch platform

The commercial success of a new drug is closely related to the success of the product launch. The ingredients of a successful launch are:

- sound clinical trial data in the public domain;
- a differentiated product;
- a clear marketing strategy; and
- solid opinion leader support.

All the above need to be underpinned by a sound clinical trial programme. There will be two major components to this: the Phase III package, aimed at getting regulatory approval, and the launch support package, sometimes referred to as Phase IIIb, which will not form part of the regulatory package. Ideally, launch support trials should start after the data cut-off for the regulatory package and their results should be available in time for launch, giving a period of approximately one year to collect the data.

Publications plan

One of the key deliverables from any clinical trial should be a publication. This exercise involves extensive planning insofar as it requires the integration of people inside and outside the organisation. Involvement of external authors makes it very difficult to adhere to any defined timetable. Further, it is very difficult to predict how long it will take a journal to accept and publish an article. Choice of author, choice of journal and timing of release into the public domain are important aspects of the overall commercial strategy.

Usually, separate publication or communications teams are set up. Key members of the publication/communication team include the doctors who have conducted the clinical trial and the project manager to provide progress reports. Contingency planning is vital in publication planning because the rejection rate of quality journals may exceed 80% (*see Chapter 18* for guidance on the publication of clinical research data).

Communications plan

Publications are but one aspect of communication in the context of drug development; a significant amount of effort goes into producing presentations, abstracts and posters for symposia (*see Chapter 18* for guidance). Since these activities are driven by the availability of clinical trial data, this is another key interface for the clinical team.

This team should be responsible both for internal and external communications. It is probably more straightforward to have a single communications plan, which includes publications, rather than different plans for each aspect. Ideally, the communications plan should be linked to the clinical development plan.

Life cycle management plan

After a successful launch, clinical research activity continues up to the time of patent expiry. For me-too products, initial sales come mostly by taking a share away from rival products. Market expansion tends not to be product-specific and benefits all products. The early phases of drug development are concerned with obtaining market approval and gaining a share of the market via product differentiation, whereas active comparator trials are mostly designed to demonstrate superiority over existing products.

New formulations will be developed to extend a drug's duration of action by altering the site of absorption. Slow-release formulations can give better efficacy/safety ratios and thus differentiate the product.

Market size can be expanded by researching new indications for the product. For example, angiotensin converting enzyme (ACE) inhibitors were developed initially to treat hypertension, but are now also used in heart failure and diabetes. Regulatory approval for new indications or new formulations will require submission of supplementary data packages which, although smaller, will necessitate the same project management techniques as those described above.

The early phase studies will involve end-points that are usually readily measurable in all study subjects, although some end-points will be surrogate markers (e.g. hypertension and cholesterol level as surrogate markers for cardiovascular events). Outcomes trials measure the benefit of the drug on a key 'outcome', e.g. prevention of cardiovascular events (such as stroke or heart attacks) or death. Since the frequency of these events tends to be relatively low, outcomes trials tend to be of long duration, possibly involving many thousands of patients, and are very costly. Companies are therefore reluctant to invest in outcomes packages until they are very confident of bringing the product to the market; in most cases they will wait until they have seen Phase IIIa data before making such a potentially huge financial commitment.

Current best practice

Most organisations attempt to define best practice from within. Ideally, companies should be open to the widest possible spectrum of ways of conducting clinical research well. Professional associations such as The Institute of Clinical Research provide networking opportunities, which are probably under-utilised. External meetings allow fellow professionals other opportunities to share best practice. Most of what we do is common knowledge or in the public domain; however, without a frame of reference it is difficult to judge how well the team or organisation is performing. Benchmarking data are available but are difficult to interpret because they tend to be an amalgam of different kinds and phases of trials. For a meaningful analysis, like should be compared with like. It is therefore important that companies have standard internal milestones that should be reviewed within projects. Project managers should be set performance improvement targets based on their own performance. Comparisons of overall drug development times are helpful, but the size and complexity of regulatory submissions vary considerably. The most meaningful comparisons are probably those from within one's own team or organisation.

As a rough guide, the aim should be to provide team and management structures that are conducive to rapid decision-making, and to providing appropriate resources to the project.

Processes and systems should be as simple as possible and designed to provide the information needed to facilitate decision-making. Contingency plans need to be in place to cope with pre-identified threats and weaknesses. Plans should provide appropriate levels of information and be structured to enable project managers to drill down to the detail when required. Links to a high-level global operational plan obviate the need for across-plan updates. The objective should be to organise information so as to facilitate identification of trouble spots and their underlying causes.

The way forward

As timelines for the delivery of clinical trial data become shorter, new parts of the process are brought on to the critical path; for instance, there is less time for drug manufacture and this can lead to shortages of clinical trial supplies and to a situation in which more data have to be gathered from less drug. This can be achieved by using randomisation at the trial level and interactive voice response systems (IVRS) to reduce drug wastage (Bishop, 1999).

With more and more information becoming available through IVRS (O'Shea, 1998), tracking tools, central laboratories and databases, the volume of information is potentially overwhelming and requires careful management. Project managers should be able to view high-level data on a website to look for potential slippages in problem areas. This should enable them to drill down to the detail and focus in on the problem. Access to on-line, up-to-date information should permit early identification of problems. Accurate identification of their root causes should promote faster and better decision-making. Since the essence of good project management is spotting and fixing issues quickly, this should make life a little easier. Project managers are faced with ever-increasing pressure: as the rate and quality of delivery goes up, so do the expectations.

However, sophisticated software coupled to on-line data and giving access to more and more information should not be accorded panacea status. Project managers will still have to learn to pick out the needles from the haystack.

CONCLUSION

The need to build effective launch platforms and the increasing stringency of regulatory authorities have tended to make drug development packages bigger and more complicated. As companies have simultaneously attempted to reduce development timelines, these factors have combined to create a demand for better and better project management. These pressures have forced the pharmaceutical industry to move away from line management organisations towards matrix management structures, thus giving projects greater autonomy.

Most companies use similar processes and international or global development teams that work to a predefined strategy. Timelines and budgets are determined by a series of integrated operational plans. This chapter has focused on the international or global clinical development plan to give guidance on typical team composition and plan structures, but these guidelines are equally valid for national or smaller organisations. Project management software has been successfully integrated into the drug development planning process and is almost ubiquitous.

Drug development is planned from cradle (entering formal development) to grave (end of patent life) and project management encompasses communications planning. Clinical and commercial departments now work increasingly closely to produce a more coherent overall development package.

Project management will continue to play a prominent role in the future. New web-based technologies will improve communications and access to information, but the fundamental skill of using the right information to detect and resolve issues quickly will not change and will, it is hoped, be facilitated by increasingly powerful project management tools. It is a reasonable assumption that skilled project managers of drug development will remain a very marketable commodity for the foreseeable future.

REFERENCES

Andersen, ES, Grude, KV and Haug, T (1998). *Goal Directed Project Management – Effective Techniques and Strategies*, Kogan Page, London.
Bishop, K (1999). Interactive voice response technology. *Clin Res Focus* **10**, 4–8.
Gwede, CK, Johnson, D and Troth, A (2000). Tools to study workload issues. *Appl Clin Trials* **9**, 40–44.
Kerzner, H (1998). *Project Management – A Systems Approach to Planning, Scheduling and Controlling (6th edn)*, John Wiley, Chichester.

Lewis, JP (2000). *Project Planning, Scheduling and Control – A Hands-On Guide to Bringing Projects in on Time and on Budget*, McGraw-Hill, New York.

Meredith, JR, Mantel, SJ Jnr (1999). *Project Management – A Managerial Approach (4th edn)*, John Wiley, Chichester.

Michael, N and Burton, C (1992). *A Practical Guide to Project Management – How to Make it Work in Your Organisation*, Kogan Page, London.

O'Shea, K (1998). Interactive voice response technology – as a management tool for clinical trials. *Appl Clin Trials* **7**, 30–34.

Posner, K and Applegarth, M (1998). *The Project Management Pocketbook*, Management Pocketbooks Limited, Alresford, Hampshire, UK

18

Communicating effectively

Helen Glenny and Brenda Mullinger

INTRODUCTION

In the hectic activity of initiating centres or achieving data lock by a target date, how best to present the study results can often become a minor consideration. However, unless the study data are communicated clearly to all who need to know, from regulators to marketeers, or from specialists to primary care physicians, effort will have been wasted. The potential value of the study will not have been fully realised.

The need for good communication within clinical research is ever more important with the globalisation of the pharmaceutical industry and the escalation of regulatory requirements. Fortunately, advances in technology have gone hand in hand with the increasing demands of modern industry, greatly facilitating the communication process.

It often falls to the clinical monitor to prepare either an interim or final study report for regulatory purposes, or to write a paper for publication to support marketing initiatives. Along the way monitors may also be called upon to present the data, often in a preliminary form, to investigators and colleagues, and they may even be responsible for organising or chairing some meetings. These tasks can seem particularly daunting, even though 'good communication skills' are often a key requirement for a clinical research position.

This chapter is therefore designed to help those faced with presenting study data. It provides practical guidance on the following topics:

- preparing clinical study reports,
- writing papers for publication in scientific and biomedical journals,
- giving a presentation; use of visual aids,
- designing a poster, and
- organising meetings.

In addition to the advice offered here, much can be learnt from extensive reading (see the References at the end of this chapter) and by observing others. To quote Henry Ford: 'Before anything else, getting ready is the secret of success'.

WRITING

Written communications remain an important facet of clinical research. Letters to investigators, protocols, study reports, meeting reports and papers for publication serve not only to inform the reader but also to document the conduct of a trial and as such may become components of an audit trail. The importance of clear, accurate writing is therefore all too apparent but often overlooked.

The great virtue of the written word is that it may be improved. Unfortunately, in these days of rapid communication there is often little opportunity for this. Managers are inclined to set very exacting timelines. Before starting to write any document, authors should think through what they want to say, and from the outset they should have a clear idea of the answers to these fundamental questions:

- Who is it for?
- What is it about?
- How long should it be?

Preparing clinical study reports

Since July 1996, clinical study reports have had to be written to International Conference on Harmonisation (ICH) guidelines so that they are acceptable to all regulatory authorities of the ICH region (ICH Guideline, 1995). It is part of a sponsor's responsibility under good clinical practice (GCP) to ensure that a final clinical study report is written, so most companies issue standard operating procedures (SOPs) and/or guidelines for clinical report writing, which should be consulted at the outset. Individual companies often require reports to be formatted according to a particular 'house style' and provide a template, available electronically and as a hard copy. Writing to ICH guidelines, and the use of templates, dispenses with the challenge of working out a report structure. The study report writer can concentrate on the wording of the text and how best to support that using tables and graphics. Easier said than done!

An 'integrated' clinical study report is a single report incorporating clinical and statistical descriptions, presentations and analyses, with appendices containing the protocol, sample case report forms, investigator-related information and so on. In the interests of saving time, report writing is usually done in parallel with the data management and statistical analysis, with close contact between the report writer and the biometrics group. It is usual practice for the writer to generate those sections of the report that can be based on the protocol and other information available, before the analyses are complete. Typically, a draft clinical report can be available within two to four weeks of completion of the statistical report.

Because the ICH guidelines are so comprehensive, there is little point in reiterating the details here. However, the following comments may be helpful.

List of missing information

While the report is being drafted, it is useful to keep a separate list of queries, usually about missing information, which may need to be chased from a variety of sources, e.g. colleagues in data management, the investigator(s), study monitor(s), clinical trial suppliers.

Protocol deviations

When describing the conduct of a study, it is particularly important to clarify features that were not well described in the protocol. Any deviations from the protocol and what (if anything) was done in the statistical analyses to account for them, need to be identified and discussed.

Synopsis

The reader should not have to refer to the main body of the report. The numerical data and overall tone of the summary should be the same as the rest of the report, especially with regard to the safety and efficacy data.

References

Because they are often cited incorrectly, it is advisable to read and check any bibliographic references quoted. It is very easy to perpetuate errors! References to unpublished materials should only be recorded as 'in press' if the paper has been accepted for publication; otherwise refer to 'unpublished work' in the text.

Getting the report to read well

Great literary style is not expected for a clinical study report, but it is essential that the report is free from ambiguity, is well-organised and easy to review. The text should be structured into well-ordered paragraphs to avoid the impenetrable appearance of solid blocks of print. Common mistakes of style and grammar, such as poor sentence construction, ambiguous sentences, and use of jargon, clichés and meaningless phrases, need to be avoided.

Paying attention to detail

Inconsistent use of spelling, headings, typefaces, hyphens, etc., errors in punctuation or word processing, and unexplained abbreviations, are also to be avoided. Such lack of attention to detail not only gives a poor impression, but also undermines the reader's confidence in the author's technical ability.

Editing for error

The completed draft report needs to be read, and corrected, then read and corrected at least once more. The author must take full responsibility for these two edits, the first looking for sense, logic and consistency, and the second for accuracy and syntax. A paper copy of the report should be used because what appears on the screen is not always what appears on paper. For instance, page breaks can be in the wrong place, the tabs out of alignment, etc. A spell check can pick up spelling errors but not the context of the word:

- *Easy for a spell check:*
  The test treatment was administered for three moonths.

- *Impossible for a spell check:*
  The test treatment was administered for tree moths.

Recommended margin formats to ensure that documents can be printed on either US or European size paper are:

- Left margin   = 1.5 in/3.8 cm
- Right margin   = 1 in/2.5 cm
- Top margin   = 1 in/2.5 cm
- Bottom margin = 2 in/5 cm

It is best to check a report in a series of short bursts, rather than at one sitting. Concentration is likely to wane after half an hour or so, and error-filled lines may be missed. Particular care is needed when information is repeated in different sections of a report. If some information is changed, as a result of a re-analysis perhaps, it must be checked that the data have been amended in all the relevant sections. For instance, if the number of serious adverse events occurring in a treatment group needs to be changed, it is essential to check not only the safety section, but also the synopsis, discussion, summary tables, listings and patient narratives.

Review and approval

Once the report has been written, it invariably goes through a review and approval process, the details of which are generally specified by a company SOP. A back-up copy must be kept of all the work to date, plus copies of earlier drafts, which must be clearly dated. A final version of the report is not issued until comments from reviewers (such as the project director, statistician, study monitor, investigator and Quality Assurance) have been addressed, and the report has been appropriately signed off.

Writing papers for publication

Every clinical trial should be written up in a study report but not all studies lead to a paper suitable for publication in a biomedical journal. Essentially, a paper must present the facts and discuss them as succinctly as possible. Achieving this is a very different task from that associated with producing a detailed and exacting clinical study report. The biggest difference is the length; the average paper stretches to no more than four or five printed pages. As a consequence, each paper has to be started from scratch; there is no opportunity to 'lift' text from other more wordy documents such as the protocol.

Before starting to write, the first priority is to decide whether the work warrants publication as a full-length paper and, if so, where? According to Albert (2000a), writers can be incurable optimists; they fail to understand that publishing is like any other commercial activity where supply outstrips demand. So finding the idea for a paper is only half the battle; the other half is finding a publisher.

A good recipe for a paper with market value is:

- an important, topical subject (if possible, adding to an ongoing debate),
- a definite message (including negative results),
- a defined target audience (the readership),
- obvious target journals, and
- clear, stylish writing.

Where to submit a paper

In identifying a target journal, consider whether the work is of general or specialised interest, and then assess its quality in relation to the prestige, popularity and circulation of the journal. Preferably, the journal will be one that is seen by the target audience all around the world, so advice should be sought from those working in the appropriate field (e.g. investigators). Rejection rates and publishing delays vary widely between journals. On the one hand, prestigious weekly publications such as the *British Medical Journal*, *The Lancet* or *The New England Journal of Medicine* have short delays between receipt, acceptance and publication but high rejection rates (over 80%). By contrast, specialist journals may accept 30–40% of the papers they receive but then take over a year to publish them. It is for these reasons that it may be advisable to approach one of the many journals that offer rapid publication of clinical trial results in return for a fee.

Once the target journal has been decided:

- obtain some back issues, peruse them for feel and suitability;
- identify the most appropriate journal section for the article; for example, is it an original paper, a review or a commentary?
- above all, read the *Instructions to Authors*; they are either printed in every issue or once per annum (and can also be obtained from the editorial office); and
- use these guidelines to note the recommended length for the paper and summary, the layout of main sections, how references should be cited, and policy on abbreviations or nomenclature.

Journals regularly receive papers that are incorrectly spaced, wrongly referenced, or inappropriate. Such carelessness does not put the journal editors on the author's side, however sound the science, and certainly does not expedite publication. Those new to the challenges of biomedical publishing should read the advice offered by Huth (1990), Apley (1993) and Hall (1998).

Electronic publishing

In an article published in 1987 entitled 'Has the medical journal a future?' Lock fancifully envisaged the demise of the whole system of medical communication by the year 2000 (Lock, 1987). He was concerned, among other things, with withdrawal of advertising revenue and declining library budgets – not the impact of the Internet!

At this stage it is difficult to predict how the availability of some journals either partially or solely through a web site will affect the publication of paper copies. It is likely that for some time to come the two forms of communication will co-exist, although probably with altered appearance. In the same way that cinema did not put an end to live theatre, so electronic journals may not sound the death-knell of the printed versions. However, there are likely to be some considerable changes, according to Albert (2000b), that may well have several benefits to authors. Undoubtedly, lack of publishing delays, wider accessibility, and more appealing format have their attractions. However, the need to communicate clearly in a standardised manner is likely to remain in one form or another.

Organising the paper

Most papers presenting clinical trial results are based around the well-known IMRAD structure (Introduction, Methods, Results and Discussion) and, with some minor modifications, this is a useful model, regardless of where the paper is to be published.

Title and abstract

Titles should be chosen with care; time spent on this vital part will be rewarded (Lilleyman, 1994). Not only is the title the first thing seen by a potential editor, but it is also used by casual readers to determine their level of interest in the paper. It should be short, informative (with at least one keyword) and as interesting as possible.

Most journals require an abstract of specified length (usually 150–200 words) and often of predefined structure. It should summarise the important points in a simple, straightforward manner and, because most companies use papers for marketing support, should present the message clearly. The abstract is the starting point for most readers; unless it is sufficiently interesting and informative, they will read no further.

Introduction and objectives

For most European journals, the shorter the introduction, the better. It should aim to place the study in context and be suitable for readers without detailed knowledge of the subject. More background information is acceptable in American journals. The objectives of the study must be clearly stated here and referred to again in the conclusion.

Materials and methods

It should be possible to repeat the study using the information in this section. If necessary, guidance may be sought on the write-up of statistical methods (and results) (Altman *et al.*, 1983). This section also describes the ethics review and consent processes.

Results

Time putting these in a logical order, either chronologically or in order of complexity, is time well spent. The careful writer will check for any discrepancies between numbers in the text and those in tables/figures and will resist the temptation in this section to discuss the data.

Discussion

The first three or four sentences should summarise the findings, after which they may be discussed one by one in the context of the disease under treatment or the clinical programme. Journal editors frequently complain that discussions are too long and muddled; proposals for a structured discussion seem to be spreading (Docherty and Smith, 1999). The discussion should close with a brief statement of the conclusions in the context of the study's objectives.

Acknowledgements

Acknowledgement of financial sponsorship is now standard practice; others who have made a significant contribution (scientific, typing, editorial) can also be listed.

References

References should be cited according to the policy of the target journal. It is essential to keep a copy of each reference cited, and to check every detail to ensure that the spelling and dates are correct and that punctuation, capitals and italics are in precisely the form the journal requires.

Authorship

Publishing the results of multicentre trials can cause no end of discussion concerning authorship (McLellan, 1995); this can often be pre-empted by agreement with the investigators at the protocol stage. The request to 'ghost' a paper on behalf of the investigators should be considered an honour. A high-quality first draft will make it easier for the 'official' authors to finalise the paper.

Authorship is just one of the issues addressed in the 'Uniform requirements for manuscripts submitted to biomedical journals': this document was drawn up by The International Committee of Medical Journal Editors (1991) – a group that met originally in Vancouver in 1968. More than 400 of the world's biomedical journals now follow this guidance; it can save authors a great deal of time when revising manuscripts. In particular the 'Vancouver' style of references, as found in the *British Medical Journal*, for example, has the advantages of minimising the space needed for references in the text, by using superscript numerals, and not interrupting the flow of words. However, the reader has no indication of the author's name or date of publication without referring to the numerical list at the end of the paper.

Tables, figures and photographs

Most journals have definite rules about the presentation of tables and illustrations. These are given in each journal's *Instructions to Authors*, but the following checklist will be helpful.

- Use tables or figures to present information in a clear, condensed fashion; avoid any temptation to repeat this information in the text.
- Ensure that each illustration is necessary – it should aid the reader.
- Check that the illustration is comprehensible on its own – is the point obvious?
- In tables, compare data across columns (e.g. between treatment groups) rather than down rows whenever possible.

- Keep units of measurement out of the body of a table.
- Provide a title (and key) for each illustration.
- Graphs are used to correlate data; independent variables (and, by convention, time) should be plotted on the horizontal axis and dependent variables on the vertical axis. Ensure the axes are labelled (including units) and calibrated.
- Use histograms for non-continuous variables; they can show trends that might be difficult to illustrate using other techniques.
- Include the standard deviation/standard error of the mean or confidence intervals where appropriate and clearly indicate which statistic is being used.
- Ensure that all lettering will still be readable after reduction to fit the journal page.

Style, presentation and review

An effective communication is one that is easy to read, easy to understand and easy to assimilate. All of these depend on clarity and flow of the writing, with care being taken over composition and grammar. Good style is hard to achieve when the writer is still sorting out the content of the paper. Early drafts should concentrate on getting the facts in the right place, leaving stylistic polishing until a later stage.

Style is probably the most contentious issue in writing, whether in medicine or any other area. In science and medicine, the object of writing is to impart facts and ideas. Writers should try to develop a style that is concise and clear, and to convey meaning without obscurity. A good style for writing can be defined as *the maximum amount of information in the minimum number of words written in a pleasing way*. However, in the words of Robert Seeley: 'Easy reading = hard writing'.

It is very difficult to give exact guidelines on good style, particularly as an element of individuality must be preserved. Here are a few general tips, culled from a variety of sources including standard texts, such as Fowler (1983) and Gowers (1986), coupled with more targeted material from Kirkman (1992), Gregory (1992), Pearce (1994) and Albert (2000b).

- Choose familiar words but be aware of jargon.
- Prefer short sentences (< 20 words on average) but vary the length for impact.
- Punctuation and paragraphing aid clarity; think how to use them most effectively.
- Focus on the flow of words and ideas; *listen* to what you have written.
- Never lose sight of your message; it is easy to get lost in superfluous detail.
- Last but not least, think international; remember that not all readers will be fluent in your language (Kirkman, 1996, Heath and Nilsson, 1996).

All pharmaceutical companies operate an approval process before a paper concerning one of their products may be submitted for publication. This generally involves the legal and patents departments, as well as medical and scientific colleagues, and will be specified in an SOP. In the case of multi-author papers, all must agree the final wording of the manuscript.

Submitting the paper

Once the internal approval process has been completed, it is best to pause before forwarding the manuscript to the chosen journal without further delay. The accompanying letter to the editor (usually signed by all authors) should not be dismissed lightly. It gives the opportunity to explain why the study is felt to be important and of interest to others. It also provides a means of explaining any deviations from expected practices.

A final check for compliance with all the instructions to authors should be made before transmitting the paper in the preferred format (on paper, on disc or by e-mail) and indicating to whom correspondence (including the proofs) should be addressed. As an insurance against unforeseen accidents, it is wise to store copies on disc and paper in separate places.

Any paper considered potentially suitable by the editor is usually sent to two or three specialists for review; the editor makes a decision based on the reviewers' comments. If on-line peer review for electronically available papers is found to be a success (Bradbury, 1996), this process could undergo a radical overhaul.

The editor's reply will state one of three decisions:

1. Acceptance without revision. This is unusual.
2. Revision requested. In this event, suggestions should be considered carefully, and the paper rewritten as necessary (if considered worthwhile) and returned to the editor. The covering letter will thank the reviewers for their comments and usefully state what has been changed.
3. Rejection. Rejection rates are between 80 and 85% for the principal general medical journals and between 35 and 65% for specialty journals (Scott, 1993).

Following receipt of a rejection letter, there are four possible courses of action (O'Connor and Woodford, 1976). A paper that is considered too specialised, not specialised enough or outside the scope of the journal for some other reason, may be sent, with or without amendment, to a more appropriate journal. If rejection is on the grounds of length or content, these may be modified according to the criticisms offered and the manuscript submitted elsewhere. If the editor thinks the findings as reported are unsound or the data incomplete, then the paper may be revised when further information becomes available. An industry author is unlikely to take the fourth course of action, namely to contest the editor's decision.

There are special notations for corrections in printing. If these are not supplied, all corrections must be explained in a covering letter to the editor when returning the proofs. Copies of a complete list of symbols for correcting proofs may be obtained from the British Standards Institution, 2 Park Street, London W1A 2BS. Alterations to the manuscript are not acceptable at the proof stage since they may affect the length of the paper or change the balance of arguments within it.

Letters and short communications

Traditionally, writing a letter or short communication to a journal has provided a means of publication with minimal delay. As might be expected, guidance on the length, number of references and format is provided by the journal. With the adoption of electronic publishing, these brief communications are likely to become almost instantaneous, allowing for a healthy debate on contentious issues.

SPEAKING AT MEETINGS

Most people in clinical research have little training in public speaking even though it is often an important part of their work. As with other art forms, it comes more easily to some than others; however, almost everyone can become competent with prior thought, some background reading (e.g. Dixon and Hills, 1981; Hornby, 1992; Hindle, 1998; Siddons, 1999) and plenty of practice.

Success depends, like so many things, on good planning. When planning a talk, whether it is a 10-minute scientific communication (Garson *et al.*, 1986), a lecture or an informal presentation to study site personnel, consider the nature of the event and the likely composition of the audience. Is the presentation intended to inform, to bring the audience up to date, to stimulate debate or to move a project forward? Will the audience be familiar with the subject and, if so, at what level? Will all audience members be fluent in the language?

With consideration of the following general principles concerning the structure and techniques for verbal presentations, even the most inexperienced can give a creditable presentation.

Talk preparation

'It usually takes me more than three weeks to prepare a good impromptu speech.'
Mark Twain

As a rule, the more work done in preparation, the clearer the final talk. It never works to try and save time by using a study report or draft paper as text for a presentation. The construction, content and style, as well as techniques for holding the audience's attention, are quite different; no one will want to hear a 'talking book'.

There are three separate stages involved in preparing a talk:

- collecting and selecting the data/information,
- organising the structure and content; choosing the most appropriate visual aids (see below), and
- refining, re-writing and rehearsing the delivery.

In any presentation the main problem is condensing important and interesting information or ideas into the allotted time. Hence it is important to identify the objectives at the outset and to have a crystal-clear idea of the message to be communicated. Selection of the key information to be presented should not digress from this message.

Whatever the length of the talk, it should follow a simple design – beginning, middle and end. A brief introduction, perhaps only a few sentences, must capture the attention of the audience. Some amusing insight or a slightly provocative statement can have the desired effect.

The next step is to outline the reasons for the presentation and, if relevant, the intended objectives of the meeting. The audience should be left in no doubt as to the purpose of the talk. The main points are then assembled in a coherent, logical sequence. A presentation of study results should start with the aims and then progress through the materials and methods fairly rapidly. The audience will be most interested in the results and conclusions. Results should be illustrated simply and aptly, and the conclusions, related to the study aims, should stem naturally from what has been said.

The talk will conclude with a summary of the main points and conclusions, followed by an indication of possible future developments. The overriding message must shine through. It does no harm to reiterate the important issues at the end if the presentation is designed to inform and thereby train the audience.

For formal presentations, or for those new to speaking, it is advisable to write out the talk in full. This can be used for rehearsal to check content, timing and delivery, and to invite constructive criticism from others. Once the script is satisfactory, the speaker should make notes on prompt cards while avoiding the temptation to read the script or learn it by heart. Once prompt cards and visual aids have been prepared, the presentation can be rehearsed in front of colleagues, family or friends.

Visual aids

'Hearing 100 times is not as good as seeing once.'
Japanese proverb

The nerves that lead from the eye to the brain are many times larger than those leading from the ear. Visual aids add impact and can turn a good presentation into a great one. They also offer structure, interest and are a useful means of leaving a summary of the findings.

There is a wide variety of support materials from which to choose – from the simple flip chart or overhead projector transparencies (acetates), to the more sophisticated computer-generated slides, to video and multimedia presentation software. The choice of visual aid often depends on the amount of preparation time available, the facilities at the presentation venue, the budget for such things, and the organisation's standards.

Flip charts and whiteboards

These aids have the major advantage of needing no power supply for them to work. Flip charts are particularly valuable for small audiences such as plenary sessions or facilitating creative/internal meetings. The writing on flip charts and boards, and the images on them, must be big enough, bold enough and neat enough to be read from the back of the audience. This is easier said than done. Broad-tipped, dark-inked (black, blue, green or red) pens that work are needed; the speaker must never stand in front of what has been written. To help reduce stress, flip charts can be prepared in advance by pencilling in notes or outlining figures, none of which will be noticeable to the audience.

Overhead projector transparencies (acetates)

Acetates are the most versatile of visual aids, and offer several advantages over 35 mm slides:

- they are cheap, and quick and easy to produce without professional technical assistance;
- overlays, prepared by hand or by photocopying techniques, can be used to allow a complex picture to be built up step by step;
- the overhead projector (OHP) does not require complete darkness, so that the audience is more likely to stay alert; people can take notes, and see the presenter or others in the audience; and
- a projectionist is not needed.

Professional-looking acetates can easily be prepared using a straightforward word processing package and appropriate font size. However, speakers not already *au fait* with one of the graphics software packages and wishing to include charts in their talk must be prepared to invest many hours acquiring the requisite skills – or delegate the task.

Practical tips: before the presentation:
- Any type of information can be conveyed using an OHP, including drawings, notes, photographs, letters, and so forth.

- Make sure that the information is readable when projected on a screen. No more than 50 words/6 lines per acetate is advisable. As the bottom third of an acetate often cannot be seen from the back of the room, use the top two-thirds only.
- Use large, bold, lower case lettering, in a simple sans serif font such as Helvetica: no smaller than 15 point for text typeface; 22 point works well for headings (Hague and Roberts, 1994).
- Blue or black lettering projects best; light reds, oranges and yellow lettering on a white background should be avoided in a large room as they cannot be seen from the back. Use of a colour background, such as dark blue with 'reverse' text in white, or a yellow background with text in black, is less tiring on the eyes than a white light screen.
- Clear transparent folders, with white 'wings' folding out from the sides, are handy for keeping acetates clean, separate and organised. They also eliminate unnecessary light. The 'wings' have a write-on, wipe-off surface for noting key points or examples, providing the speaker with convenient cues.
- When using pre-prepared acetates, remember to include a few blank acetates and pens to amplify points during the talk or the ensuing discussion.
- The precise talking time allocated for each acetate will vary. As a guideline, a typical 45–minute presentation requires 20 to 25 acetates, averaging out at two to three minutes each.

OHP acetates are suitable for presentations aimed at audiences of 20 to 40 people, in a small conference room. In a large room, the chances are that people will find a conventional screen hard to see. If the screen is directly behind the presentation area, finding a place to stand without blocking the screen can be a challenge! It is best if the screen (and projector) can be moved to one side of the presentation area where the audience can see it, leaving centre stage to the presenter. The projector should be positioned directly towards the screen, or angled screens can be used to avoid distortion.

Practical tips: during the presentation:

- Place the acetate on the projector only when referring to it.
- Ensure that the acetates are not askew.
- Point to the screen to draw attention to particular graphs or numbers without obscuring the audience's view of the image. Some presenters like to use a light pointer (laser pen) for this task. Others prefer to avoid turning their back to the audience and use a slim pen, placed appropriately on the acetate; a hand-held pen reveals any nervousness.
- If appropriate, cover parts of an acetate with a sheet of paper to reveal material, and focus the audience's attention on only one point at a time. (Note: the paper is less likely to fall off if it is placed *under* the acetate.)

- Place discarded acetates in a neat pile.
- Have a second copy of an acetate that may be referred to more than once. This avoids getting into a fluster, rummaging through discarded acetates.
- It is often a good idea to provide the audience with a copy of the visual aids, especially if the purpose of the presentation is to inform rather than persuade. These provide an *aide mémoire* and a place to make notes during the presentation. Speakers preferring to distribute their handouts at the end of the presentation will find it helpful to tell the audience in advance.

35 mm slides

35 mm slides are used for formal presentations to large audiences or for high-impact presentations. The overriding advantage of 35 mm slides, provided that they have been well designed, is their quality of reproduction, which is superior to that of acetates. This means that the presentation will appear very professional. Slides can be prepared by a graphics company which, with the appropriate cameras, processing facilities and software, can create three-dimensional effects and backgrounds of appropriate colour and hue. Alternatively, speakers with access to presentation graphics software, notably Microsoft® PowerPoint, can create their own slides and print out audience handouts and speaker's notes.

Practical tips: before the presentation:

- Fewer words should be used on a 35 mm slide than on an acetate, a handful of words being the ideal and 30 being the maximum. It is tempting to cram too much information on a slide with the inevitable consequence that the speaker reads from the slide to a bored and restless audience. It is much better to show summary slides or a greater number of slides containing less information. Key points can be built up, by adding text, as a series of short bullet points for maximum impact.
- Remember the general guidance of one slide per minute. As with all visual aids, slides should complement, not distract from, what the speaker is saying.
- No slide should be shown unless it can be read by the back row of the audience. To achieve this, the writing on a slide should be easily legible by the naked eye when the slide is viewed by hand with no magnification.
- Use double line spacing, preferably with double letter spacing between words. Tables should be limited to four columns and seven lines, while graphs should contain no more than three or four curves. Make sure that all lines and curves are thick enough to be easily seen by the audience.
- The layout of information is important: plan the content to fit the proportions of a slide (35 mm × 22 mm; 11:7.33). Slides should be uncluttered, well balanced and, if possible, designed to be shown horizontally

(landscape) rather than vertically (portrait). The latter often seems too cramped and there is a risk of losing the top and bottom of each slide.

- Colour should be used whenever possible. Colour in itself wakes the brain up; more specifically, it can highlight important parts of the slide, and it can link related topics. Use strong contrasts and bright colours for visual impact. Note that colour-blind people may experience problems distinguishing between some colours such as red and green. Also note that the sections on a pie diagram can be completely lost if the colours used are not sufficiently contrasting.

Slide production has been greatly simplified by the introduction of word processors with desktop publishing facilities. PowerPoint images can be e-mailed to an imaging bureau, many of which operate a next-day service. Once the slides are prepared, they must be checked carefully to ensure that they are accurate and show what is wanted. Slides are to be labelled using the international convention that calls for a small dot to be placed in the lower left-hand corner of the slide mount. This spot will be seen in the top right-hand corner away from the lens when the slide is inserted into a magazine. There are eight ways to load a slide and only one is correct; this responsibility should not be delegated to someone else. Slides should always be pre-loaded into the slide magazine and, once in the carousel, sealed with tape to avoid them falling out in transit. Finally, it is advisable always to keep slides in hand luggage; never entrust them to airline baggage facilities! Film is hygroscopic and can absorb a lot of moisture in a baggage hold, or if left in a car overnight, thus putting slides at risk of appearing foggy with condensation.

High tech audio-visual aids

35 mm slides and OHP acetates are the most commonly used visual aids; they achieve good effects without involving too much technical hardware. However, more complex audio-visual technology, including computer-based and multimedia presentation software, and video clips, is becoming increasingly available. Multimedia presentations use CD-ROM packages with moving images and an audio track on a large monitor with speakers. Videos may be appropriate to show short, live-action images, such as an investigator–patient interview, or a taped message from a speaker who is not able to attend the presentation.

Computer graphics software can be used to display graphs, charts or three-dimensional images on a computer screen. While this may be acceptable for a debrief to three or four people, a presentation to a larger audience requires the images to be projected through a small piece of electronic wizardry, a liquid crystal display (LCD) projector, on to a conventional screen. An LCD projector sits on an OHP light desk, connected to the computer (most conveniently a laptop), from which images are directed via the projector to a large screen. LCD projectors are available in various stages of sophistication depending on whether the speaker wishes to project in colour, or have moving images sourced from a video, CD-ROM or animation software. The more expensive models can present moving images, manipulate graphics, freeze the frame, insert blank screens, carry out automatic reveals, and so on (Levy, 1997). An 'air mouse' (a remote-control mouse that allows the presenter to change slides without having to touch the computer or a fixed mouse) will free the speaker to wander about the presentation area without being tethered to one spot. While special sound and visual effects (for instance, moving graphics showing how statistics will change over time) can be very effective, they can also be quite startling – so much so that they can actually detract from the message. It is best to choose a style for the whole presentation and to be consistent throughout.

Computerised presentations will almost certainly become more important in the future as they obviate the creation of 35 mm slides and offer advantages of speed and cost, once the technology has been acquired. However, because there is a risk of technical problems, presenters are advised to prepare a set of OHP acetates and/or handouts as a back up – or be prepared to go without any visual aids at all! Speakers without the requisite expertise to deal with any technical hitches that may arise should ensure that an expert will be present at the venue to help out.

Before the meeting

1. Check the exact venue, date and time of your talk.
2. Visit the room in which you will be speaking; allow enough time to check the equipment, re-arrange the furniture to your liking or set up your PowerPoint presentation.
3. Check that slide projectors, overhead transparency projectors, flip charts and whiteboards are in place as needed. Use a test slide/transparency to ensure that equipment is in working order; adjust focusing. Find the pointer and note how it works.
4. If you are not restricted by a stage and/or lectern, decide the best place to stand so that you do not obstruct the screen.
5. Check whether a microphone is provided; radio microphones with a tie or lapel clip are generally easiest to use. If you are provided with a fixed microphone, remember to speak into it at all times, using a normal speaking voice. When no microphone is provided, practise to ensure you will be audible to every member of the audience.
6. Acquaint yourself with any meeting 'courtesies' such as introductions, questions format, seating arrangements, remotely controlled audio-visual equipment, lighting, etc.

Giving the presentation

Everyone is nervous and apprehensive before a presentation, particularly to a large audience. A glance at the following tips may help direct that nervous energy into positive channels.

- Adopt a clear, lively style using short sentences.
- Remember that your enthusiasm will keep the audience receptive.
- Vary the rate of speaking to emphasise points; when nerves force you to speak too quickly, pause, then resume at a slower rate.
- Prevent monotony by varying the pitch and tone of your voice; prior practice will ensure that this happens naturally.
- Relax; try not to appear rooted to one spot.
- Minimise distracting mannerisms (e.g. fidgeting with prompt cards or telescopic pointers, folding and unfolding arms, jangling money in pockets).
- Above all, stick to the allotted time. A speaker who overruns is never popular.
- If humour comes naturally, use it to revive interest; avoid humour that is forced or artificial.

DESIGNING POSTER PRESENTATIONS

Poster sessions are now commonplace at all types of meetings. They allow greater numbers of research papers to be presented and allow participation in one-to-one discussions about specialised areas of interest.

A well-designed poster is usually regarded as the easiest way of communicating information at a meeting. However, producing a good poster that is both attractive and clear requires considerable thought and effort. Since the audience is not captive, as at an oral presentation, a poster that is not easy to read is likely to be passed by.

If they do not have support from an arts and media group, presenters asked to design a poster reporting the results of a clinical study should consider the following:

- *Title:* this should be short and informative.
- *Authors:* list the workers involved in the study, together with their affiliation, add a photograph of the author who is manning the poster, for later recognition.
- *Introduction:* give a brief background to the study and explain why the work was done.
- *Study design:* a basic outline of the methods and subjects used and treatment given is usually sufficient.
- *Results:* the results should be summarised using charts, figures, tables and, where appropriate, photographs; avoid including minutiae; tables, for instance, should ideally have less than 50 separate entries; colours can be used to relate groups of data.
- *Conclusion:* this should be a clear and concise summary of the evidence presented on the poster.

- *References and acknowledgements:* the same criteria should be used as in writing a paper; present them in a very small font, so that the information does not detract from the main message of the poster.

Practical tips for poster design

- To be effective, a poster must be attractive, clearly organised and legible to spectators standing up to two metres away. The information contained in the poster should be easily absorbed by the reader in no more than five minutes. The size of a poster is usually limited; check the size and orientation (whether vertical or horizontal) before starting.
- The need for impact and the restriction on space may seem to be irreconcilable, since impact is usually associated with large lettering. Lettering should be simple and its size determined by the overall design. Illustrations and photographs together with the judicious use of colour will also help the poster achieve impact.
- In deciding which information must be presented, keep in mind that a limit of 500 words per poster is recommended. Arrange the material in a logical sequence and aesthetically pleasing manner, with the introduction and conclusions highlighted for emphasis. If necessary, show links by using numbers, letters or keylines.
- A poster may be compiled by arranging several sheets of paper onto a larger backing sheet. Alternatively, if time and expense permit, a poster can be produced in the form of one large sheet. Useful information about the design and production of posters is provided by Davis (1997), Reynolds and Simmonds (1981), and Glickmann and Field (1983). The end product should be lightweight, easily packed and carried, and easily mounted and dismantled at the exhibition site.
- User-friendly software is readily available to produce electronic versions of posters; an electronic version has the advantage of being editable for both text and images, and therefore can be corrected or subsequently updated. The printing of A4 handouts is quite straightforward from this method of production. A large-scale electronic version can be printed in colour by large format printers (up to 145 cm wide), now sited at many imaging and reprographic bureaux, design companies and some universities.
- Before completion, check the contents of the poster meticulously for typographical errors; these can become enormously embarrassing and often undermine the effectiveness of the poster. Having prepared a paper/card poster, it may be worthwhile bringing scissors, glue, a ruler and a selection of pens for corrections on the day. In addition, adhesive tape and drawing pins may be needed for mounting the poster.
- To communicate your message effectively, provide a handout of the poster presentation for those who are interested.

ORGANISING MEETINGS

Progression and promotion within the pharmaceutical industry invariably lead to increasing amounts of time being spent running or attending meetings. Face-to-face meetings can offer opportunity for better communication, decision-making, brain-storming and problem-solving. Conversely, meetings can be time-wasting and frustrating and can provide scope for power games, dispute and hidden agendas. However, careful preparation in advance of each meeting will generally minimise or eliminate these negative aspects.

Within clinical research, meetings fall into two general categories. The first are 'internal' meetings, normally held to plan and manage projects. They occur at all levels within an organisation from section or unit to department, inter-departmental and corporate groups. Such meetings may be held on a regular basis – perhaps once a month – or may be *ad hoc* meetings, called for specific reasons.

'External' meetings, the second category, are normally organised on an *ad hoc* basis. They include investigator meetings, convened before the start of each multicentre clinical study and thereafter, as necessary, to maintain the smooth running of the trial. In addition there are meetings with consultants to discuss project strategy or an important issue or problem. External meetings are discussed in more detail later in this chapter. Useful advice is also provided by Spilker (1991) in Chapter 60, entitled 'Conducting a pretrial roundtable meeting' (pp. 418–422) and Chapter 125 on the 'Use of meetings and documents to assist in planning and managing clinical trials' (pp. 986–1005).

Objectives

All participants should be clear as to the purpose of any particular meeting.

An agenda must be prepared and distributed well in advance, once careful thought has been given to the individual agenda items and the order in which they should appear. Provision of additional background material prior to the meeting will often help to expedite discussion of a problem. However, the whole idea is sabotaged if the papers become too long; they should be brief or provide a short summary.

Administrative matters

Meetings may be broadly described as small (fewer than six people), medium (6 to 20 people) or large (more than 20 people). Inevitably, they tend to become more formal as their size increases. General discussion becomes difficult when the numbers exceed 20 and a question and answer session at the end of a lecture is the only practical arrangement. The type of discussion desired should determine the number of people invited to attend a meeting. The technical aspects of planning a meeting also change markedly as the meeting size increases.

Selection of an appropriate venue and convenient date and time for the meeting may prove to be no easy task. The layout of the table(s) and chairs can be an important consideration. For example, if everybody sits around a single table there appears to be better involvement and more active participation than in a classroom style layout. Further administrative points to consider beforehand:

- Audio-visual equipment and materials: which of the following will be required: a microphone, an overhead projector and pens, a slide projector, a laptop computer, LCD projector and screen, a video recorder and television, a flip chart and/or whiteboard?
- Remember to check that all items are working and that there is a spare bulb for projectors.
- Are you providing pens, paper and pre-prepared meeting paperwork?
- If the meeting is likely to exceed two hours, there should be an interval of 10 to 30 minutes to give everyone a break and the opportunity to partake of refreshments. These will need to be ordered in advance, as will the room and facilities.
- Arrange to have a suitably briefed secretary to keep notes/minutes and identify 'action' points to be pursued outside the meeting. Often this role is played by a clinical monitor. Minutes need to be distributed promptly to all attendees and other interested parties after the meeting.
- Choosing the right person to take the chair requires some thought. The task of chairman is not easy and, if badly performed, results in a valueless meeting that fails in its objective and wastes everyone's time. The chairman must be well briefed and should consider whether any agenda items are likely to be controversial. He or she should be prepared to provide a résumé of the meeting to ensure that everyone leaves on the same 'wavelength'.

All these administrative comments apply both to internal and external meetings. However, one subspecies of internal meeting, the teleconference, merits a brief section of its own.

Teleconferences

Use of satellites to conduct meetings of groups in different regions or continents is commonplace within the industry. Such conferences allow relatively small groups (up to 12 or so at each site) to meet without the expense, exhaustion and jet lag that accompany long-distance international travel. Teleconferences are particularly suitable and cost-effective for short meetings or meetings for which staff travel is undesirable. The ability to transmit documents simultaneously can be very useful. However, having two separate 'stages' can exacerbate an 'us and them' mentality, particularly if, for example, friction has been generated between the parties. Good chairing skills are needed at all sites involved and it is useful to have the agenda confirmed in advance. Recording teleconferences may be helpful for different language competencies.

It is not uncommon for a company's teleconference room to be booked weeks in advance during normal working hours, so it is essential to plan as far ahead as possible. Someone familiar with the technology should also be on hand in the event of technical hitches.

Consultants' meetings

It may become necessary to bring a group of external consultants together to provide expert input into management decision making. This is most often needed at the outset of a project when strategies are being developed or when an important issue or problem has arisen. It may also be valuable to acquaint groups associated with a drug's clinical development programme (e.g. colleagues from marketing, statistics and data processing, or project management) with the views of experts in the field.

The choice of specific consultants and their background will have a great influence on the type of advice they will offer. Consultants who understand the complexities of drug development often have a marked advantage over other experts who do not. Consider carefully the wording of specific questions to be posed to the consultants, as this may determine the nature of the advice offered. The purpose of the meeting and the issues to be discussed will need to be defined in advance to ensure that consultants have time to give them careful thought.

The agenda for the meeting should allow time for presentation of the background and statement of the issues; panel discussion; discussion between the consultants and company personnel; and lastly, recommendations. 'Internal' attendees would normally be chosen from among the project team and senior managers. Attendance at consultants' meetings is normally considered to be a privilege (unless one is taking the minutes!) so the choice of invitees may be politically sensitive. In any case, only those who are likely to contribute constructively to the agenda and discussion should be invited.

Generally, it is impractical to organise a meeting that lasts more than one day since almost all consultants are extremely busy. Selecting a venue close to an international airport can reduce travelling time. Consultants may expect to be reimbursed for the time spent travelling as well as that spent attending the meeting. Full travel and accommodation expenses and incidental costs should be covered as a matter of course.

Pre-trial investigators' meetings

Since problems in communication are usually the source of most major difficulties encountered in multicentre trials, bringing all the investigators together to review the protocol and discuss important points before the start of the trial will prevent misunderstandings and help achieve a uniform approach. At least one week before the meeting, all participants should receive copies of the agenda, CRF and protocol, with an indication of whether or not these have already been finalised and formally approved. The meeting should provide an opportunity for everyone to become acquainted and so, hopefully, generate a sense of teamwork and enthusiasm for the trial. If possible, allow for investigator input at the meeting and incorporate any agreed amendments into the final protocol prior to formal approval.

Investigators' meetings can provide a good opportunity for standardising techniques, by showing a video of a suitable interview between an investigator and a patient. Each participant will need an unobstructed and not-too-distant view of a video screen and a copy of any rating scale to be completed. It is very useful if the investigator who interviewed the patient on video can follow up by providing details of, and the rationale for, his/her own ratings. All completed rating sheets should be collected at the end of the inter-rater reliability session and the data collated and analysed. Such ratings are normally repeated at investigators' meetings held about halfway through the trial period, in order to check that inter-rater reliability is maintained within appropriate limits. These exercises are particularly relevant if the trial involves the use of rating scales that the investigator would not normally encounter in clinical practice.

Chairing investigators' meetings needs sophisticated skills and extra time should be allowed at meetings where many nationalities are attending. It is helpful if any investigators known to have limited fluency in the working language sit next to monitors with appropriate language skills. All investigators should have been visited by a monitor prior to the meeting so that the chairman can be thoroughly briefed and aware of what is negotiable.

One of the prime concerns for the meeting organiser will be the choice of venue. If the study is multinational then a central location, in a hotel near an airport, is likely to be the most effective. Should the investigators be based in Germany, Israel, Italy and the UK, then Istanbul could prove to be a convenient, interesting and cost-effective choice!

An investigators' meeting would normally be expected to last half a day; multicentre trials usually require a full day. Multinational trials will probably require more than one pre-study meeting and at least part of one of the meetings may need to be conducted in a language other than English, for example, in French for Swiss, Belgian or French investigators.

The agenda for the meeting may be as simple or as elaborate as necessary. A sample agenda is as follows:

1. Introductions
2. Current development status
3. Protocol review
4. CRF review
5. Study administration
6. Financial matters

The meeting is likely to be centred on discussion of the protocol; a very large number of topics may be discussed under the heading of 'Protocol review'. All practical aspects of the trial should be covered in detail, e.g. the recording of serious adverse events and dealing with medical emergencies, and the policy for patient discontinuation. Relevant aspects of GCP should be covered, including investigators' responsibilities, monitoring and audit activities. Technical details such as the procedures for obtaining, handling and shipping biological samples, or the staff and equipment required for specialised tests should also be discussed. If the trial is multinational, there may be a number of potential problems to consider: those relating to culture differences, availability of equipment, ability to perform necessary tests, health referral systems, import and export regulations, availability of drug comparators, regulatory requirements, ethics committee interactions and regulations, and transmittal of data collection forms – to name but a few.

This opportunity for face-to-face contact should be utilised to the full before the trial starts, when enthusiasm levels are high! In particular, arrangements should be made for a member of the pharmacy department to present details of the drug packaging, labelling, storage, dispensing and return of study drug. Also, if practicable, a colleague with a clinical audit function and the project statistician may be invited to discuss their respective involvement in the trial. After the meeting, all agreements should be confirmed in writing and expenses reimbursed promptly.

CONCLUDING REMARK

Since all clinical study reports, papers, presentations and meetings should come to a conclusion, the message of this chapter is: plan for success!

ACKNOWLEDGEMENTS

We would like to thank Rod Evans, Managing Director of Business Presentations, Ashwell, Hertfordshire (www.business-presentations.co.uk) for his constructive review of the section on visual aids, and also John Taylor, cartographer at the Open University, for his input to the section on poster presentations.

REFERENCES

Albert, T (2000a). Writing with purpose. In: *Short Words* **8** (3) (published by Tim Albert Training, Dorking, Surrey RH4 1QT).
Albert, T (2000b). *Winning the Publications Game. How to get Published Without Neglecting your Patients (2nd edn)*, Radcliffe Medical, Oxford.

Altman, DG, Gore, SM, Gardner, MJ and Pocock SJ (1983). Statistical guidelines for contributors to medical journals. *Br Med J* **286**, 1489–1493.

Apley, AG (1993). So you want to get it published. *J Roy Soc Med* **86**, 6–8.

Bradbury, J (1996). Interactive peer-review trial starts in Australia. *Lancet* **347**, 957.

Davis, M (1997). *Scientific Papers and Presentations,* Academic Press, London.

Dixon, D and Hills, P (1981). *Talking About Your Research,* Primary Communications Research Centre, Leicester University.

Docherty, M and Smith, R (1999). The case for structuring the discussion of scientific papers. *Br Med J* **318**, 1224–1225.

Fowler, HW (1983). *A Dictionary of Modern English Usage (2nd edn),* Oxford University Press, Oxford.

Garson, A, Gutgesell, HP, Pinksy, WW and McNamara, DG (1986). The 10–minute talk: organization, slides, writing and delivery. *Am Heart J* **111**, 193–203.

Glickmann, J and Field, T (1983). Design and production of poster sessions: a management system. *J Biocommun* **10**, 21–27

Gowers, E (1986). *The Complete Plain Words (3rd edn),* Her Majesty's Stationery Office, London.

Gregory, MW (1992). The infectiousness of pompous prose. *Nature* **360**, 11–12.

Heath, I and Nilsson, B (1996). Freedom of expression should be preserved. *Br Med J* **313**, 1323.

Hague, P and Roberts, K (1994). *Presentations and Report Writing*, Kogan Page, London.

Hall, GM (1998). *How to Write a Paper (2nd edn)*, BMJ Publishing Group, London.

Hindle, T (1998). *Making Presentations.* Dorling Kindersley, London, pp. 30–33.

Hornby, M (1992). How to give a presentation – and live to tell the tale. *Training and Development* (April issue), 19–24.

Huth, EG (1990). *How to Write and Publish Papers in the Medical Sciences (2nd edn)*, Williams and Wilkins, Baltimore.

ICH Guideline (1995). *Topic E3: Structure and Content of Clinical Study Reports*, International Federation of Pharmaceutical Manufacturers Associations, Geneva (Issued as CPMP/ICH/137/95).

International Committee of Medical Journal Editors (1991). Uniform requirements for manuscripts submitted to biomedical journals (4th edn). *Br Med J* **302**, 338–341.

Kirkman, J (1992). *Good Style: Writing for Science and Technology*, E & FN Spon, London.

Kirkman, J (1996). Confine yourself to forms of English that are easily understood. *Br Med J* **313**, 1321–1323.

Levy, M (1997). *Presentation Tips and Techniques*, Wyvern Crest Publications, Ely.

Lilleyman, JS (1994). Titles, abstract, and authors. In: Hall, GM (Ed), *How to Write a Paper,* BMJ Publishing Group, London, pp. 33–41.

Lock, S (1987). Has the medical journal a future? *Trans Med Soc Lond* **102**, 254–256.

McLellan, MF (1995). Authorship in biomedical publications: 'How many people can wield one pen?' *AMWA Journal* **10**, 11–13.

O'Connor, M and Woodford, FP (1976). *Writing Scientific Papers in English*, Elsevier, Amsterdam.

Pearce, N (1994). Style – what is it, and does it matter? In: Hall, GM (Ed), *How to Write a Paper,* BMJ Publishing Group, London, pp. 102–106.

Reynolds, L and Simmonds, D (1981). *Presentation of Data in Science*, Martinus Nijhoff, The Hague.

Scott, JT (1993). Rheumatology writing. Is it worth writing about? *J Roy Soc Med* **86**, 5–6.

Siddons, S (1999). *Presentation Skills (2nd edn)*, Institute of Personnel and Development, London.

Spilker, B (1991). *Guide to Clinical Trials*, Raven Press, New York.

19

Audits and inspections

Pamela Charnley Nickols

INTRODUCTION

New entrants to the pharmaceutical industry will encounter many new terms, familiar terms used in unfamiliar ways, and many baffling abbreviations. Clinical research staff moving to a new company later in their career will find that their new situation requires mastery of variations in the industry vocabulary. Terminology familiar from a former employment will assume new meanings and yet another set of abbreviations will provide early challenges.

Fortunately, within the quality system of good clinical practice (GCP), terms such as quality assurance (QA), quality control (QC), audit, audit trail, GCP itself, and source data verification (SDV) have a common interpretation. This interpretation should be applicable throughout the pharmaceutical industry, both nationally and internationally, and is set out in the glossary (section 1) of the International Conference on Harmonisation (ICH) GCP guideline (ICH Guideline, 1996). One of the most useful pieces of advice for anyone in doubt over a GCP issue is to consult this glossary and consider carefully the precise wording of the definitions presented there.

QUALITY

It will be helpful initially to consider why terms relating to quality, quality systems and audit are so important within the context of GCP.

1. *For public health and assurance.* In order to produce safe, effective and reliable medicines for use by the public, it is clearly essential to have standards that will ensure consistency in terms of their testing and manufacture. The growth in consumer power is reflected in public demand for quality systems to be in place and for compliance with those systems to be evident.

2. *To obtain marketing authorisation.* The assessors of marketing authorisation applications (MAAs) for new medicines have a duty of care to the public and therefore look for evidence of quality to be provided in all submissions.

3. *To avoid litigation.* Increasingly, when a medicine fails, public expectation is for investigation, compensation and increased control. Litigation is costly to the pharmaceutical industry both in financial terms and in terms of corporate and individual reputations. The application of sound quality systems can reduce the likelihood of failure and mitigate the effects of litigation.

4. *To make research efficient and cost-effective.* Where quality systems are absent, there is an increased likelihood that clinical research will follow false leads and fail to recognise unproductive or even dangerous directions in drug development. Clinical research is costly and time-consuming, and any reduction of unnecessary and unproductive activities will inevitably enhance efficiency.

5. *To increase pride in work.* Most people spend at least one third of their days in work-related activities and would prefer to enjoy that time rather than experience feelings of frustration and failure. It appears that individuals wish, at least initially, to do a good job. However, many of the problems arising at work serve to reduce the pleasure that was originally anticipated. These problems often arise because the system in which individuals are required to perform does not adequately support their performance. Application of quality standards such as those outlined in GCP provides a safe framework within which workers can take pride in their achievements and feed back suggestions to further enhance the quality of their work.

When does quality become an issue?

Quality is an issue at all stages of clinical research, and the only successful approach is to build in quality from the outset.

Recruitment and training of staff

Although the old adage that 'You get what you pay for' can be taken too far, it is a mistake for companies to try to conduct clinical research at the expense of their staff. Staff in all functions need to be appropriately qualified, experienced, trained and, most of all, motivated. Finance, however, is just one form of motivation. The feeling of being appreciated and valued comes from many sources and is nurtured when people are involved, respected and consulted. Management must therefore take time to recruit well, invest in ongoing training, establish a system of career development and foster a feeling of involvement in order to retain loyal staff and enhance their performance.

Establishment of quality systems for all activities

Quality is cited as Principle 13 in the ICH GCP guideline (section 2.13), but it could equally rank as Principle 1 because it should be inherent in every aspect of clinical research. What is required is a quality assurance system characterised by standard (high quality) procedures, quality control and audit, with appropriate feedback systems and a 'no blame' environment.

Commitment to quality: a pervading culture

Management commitment is fundamental to appropriate recruitment, training and systems maintenance. Regrettably, many companies' quality systems are led from below, with experienced and motivated staff trying to pull management into compliance with systems of which they have little awareness and in which they have had only the most rudimentary training. In the ideal corporate environment, commitment to GCP will be emphasised at recruitment and reinforced at induction. All staff in every function should understand the motivation behind the quality system, in terms of ethics, safety, data quality and ultimate job satisfaction. In a less-than-ideal environment, lip service may be the reality.

THE ESSENTIAL ELEMENTS OF A GCP QUALITY SYSTEM

Quality control

The ICH GCP guideline (section 1.47) defines QC as: 'The operational techniques and activities undertaken within the quality assurance system to verify that the requirements for quality of the trial-related activities have been fulfilled'. Section 5.1.3 emphasises that: 'Quality control should be applied to each stage of data handling to ensure that all data are reliable and have been processed correctly'. In other words, the data and documentation submitted should accurately reflect the conduct of the study and should be complete, unambiguous and easy to review.

The ICH GCP guideline further states that: 'Systems with procedures that assure the quality of every aspect of the trial should be implemented' (section 2.13) and that: 'The sponsor is responsible for implementing and maintaining ... quality control systems ... to ensure that trials are conducted and data are generated, documented (recorded) and reported in compliance with the protocol, GCP and the applicable regulatory requirement(s)' (section 5.1.1). Since quality control applies to every trial-related activity, every aspect should be double-checked. Auditors and inspectors look for evidence that this is happening.

Standard operating procedures (SOPs)

According to the ICH GCP guideline (section 1.55), SOPs are defined as: 'Detailed, written instructions to achieve uniformity of the performance of a specific function'. Once again, sections 2.13 and 5.1.1 are helpful and relevant. The sponsor is responsible for implementing and maintaining written SOPs and these must cover all systems relating to trial conduct, and the generation, documentation and reporting of data.

Audit and auditors

The ICH GCP guideline glossary definition of audit is: 'A systematic and independent examination of trial-related activities and documents to determine whether the evaluated trial-related activities were conducted, and the data were recorded, analysed and accurately reported according to the protocol, sponsor's standard operating procedures (SOPs), good clinical practice (GCP) and the applicable regulatory requirement(s)' (section 1.6). Most quality standards emphasise that audit (and therefore auditors) should be independent; typically, clinical auditors will not be members of the clinical research department, and they will have a separate reporting line to management. Their independent status is further confirmed in section 5.19.2 dealing with the selection and qualification of auditors.

Like ICH, the International Organization for Standardization (ISO) works towards international harmonisation; it developed in response to increasing international interest in quality management systems. The ISO has issued a series of standards dealing with the customer–supplier relationship and with contractually based relationships in a broad sense. The publication of the ISO 10011 series of guidelines for auditing quality systems demonstrates that organisation's perception of the importance of the auditing process (International Organization for Standardization, 1991). Section 4.2.1.4 of those guidelines also comments on the independence of the auditor: 'Auditors should be free from bias and influences which could affect objectivity. All persons, and organisations involved with an audit should respect and support the independence and integrity of the auditors'.

Finally, because audits themselves are to be systematic activities, auditors will have SOPs. When commenting on auditing procedures, section 5.19.3 of the ICH GCP guideline stipulates that: 'The sponsor should ensure that the auditing of clinical trials/systems is conducted in accordance with the sponsor's written procedures on what to audit, how to audit, the frequency of audits, and the form and content of audit reports'.

Quality assurance

The ICH GCP guideline defines QA as: 'All those planned and systematic actions that are established to ensure that the trial is performed and the data are generated, documented (recorded), and reported in compliance with good clinical practice (GCP) and the applicable regulatory requirement(s)' (section 1.46). From this it is apparent that QA is more than auditing, embracing as it does SOPs, QC and all other clinical research activities. QA should also be viewed in the context of section 5.1.1 which places a responsibility on the sponsor to implement and maintain QA in all clinical research-related activities. Importantly, this responsibility is extended to contract research organisations (CROs) in section 5.2.1.

Direct access

This aspect is covered in section 5.1.2 of the ICH GCP guideline: 'The sponsor is responsible for securing agreement from all involved parties to ensure direct access to all trial-related sites, source data/documents and reports for the purpose of monitoring and auditing by the sponsor, and inspection by domestic and foreign regulatory authorities.' Without direct access, regulatory authorities such as the US Food and Drug Administration (FDA) will not accept clinical data as valid support for a marketing application. In practice, this has led sponsor companies to insist on direct access and investigators and/or centres should not be recruited if this cannot be agreed.

Qualifications

According to the ICH GCP guideline, the sponsor should use (appropriately) qualified individuals (e.g. biostatisticians, clinical pharmacologists and physicians) throughout all stages of the trial process to supervise the overall conduct of the trial, design the protocol and case record forms (CRFs), plan the analyses, handle and verify the data, conduct the analyses, and prepare interim and final reports (cf. sections 5.4.1 and 5.5.1).

One of the ICH GCP principles (section 2.8) is that each individual involved in conducting a trial should be qualified by education, training and experience to perform his or her respective task(s). This theme pervades the guideline, and auditors and inspectors consequently place great emphasis on detailed, specific and up-to-date delegation lists and/or job descriptions, curricula vitae (CVs) and training records. These should be on file for current staff and archived securely for staff previously involved in clinical research.

Audit certificate

Section 1.7 of the ICH GCP guideline defines the audit certificate as: 'A declaration of confirmation by the auditor that an audit has taken place'. However, an audit certificate is not required in every situation (section 5.19.3: 'When required by applicable law or regulation, the sponsor should provide an audit certificate.'). Company practice will vary regarding the scope of such certificates. They may be issued for individual study or systems audits or an individual certificate may detail all relevant auditing activity during the entire course of a particular study or project. The certificate should make no statement about the degree of GCP compliance noted during the audit. There are several reasons for this. When filed in trial and site master files and as part of regulatory submissions, the audit certificate demonstrates quality assurance activity but without the full audit report, including context, any statement about GCP compliance or non-compliance would be open to serious misinterpretation. The neutral nature of the certificate also protects auditors from undue commercial influence to minimise findings in order to produce a favourable impression of standards. Thus, the independence of the audit is maintained.

Audit report

The audit report, a 'written evaluation by the sponsor's auditor of the results of the audit' (ICH GCP guideline, section 1.8), is a confidential document with very restricted circulation. This limited circulation minimises the opportunities for misinterpretation that might result in personal, professional and commercial disadvantage. Only those sufficiently informed to judge the report in context should be aware of its detailed findings. The report usually consists of a statement of the scope of the audit, a summary of the main findings and a detailed account of all findings. For some or all findings, responses may be requested from those who have been audited.

Audit trail

Defined in the ICH GCP guideline, section 1.9, as 'Documentation that allows reconstruction of the course of events', the audit trail's main components are detailed in Section 8 which lists the essential documents for the conduct of a clinical trial. These documents should be generated throughout the study, from the planning through to the reporting stage. Sponsor and CRO staff training records and job descriptions should also be included, and archived copies of all SOPs current during the course of the study should be available. It is helpful to include a list of relevant SOPs in each trial master file so that these can be readily identified for audit and inspection purposes.

CLINICAL QA DEPARTMENT

The growth of audit activity

The past five years have witnessed a rapid increase in the number of clinical auditors employed in the pharmaceutical industry to assess the GCP compliance of the conduct of clinical trials. Most companies now have established GCP compliance or quality assurance functions and the ICH GCP guideline, which came into effect in January 1997, requires implementation of quality assurance and quality control by both sponsor companies and CROs.

Initially greeted with some reservation by clinical research personnel, GCP auditors have had to work hard to establish an atmosphere of mutual trust and co-operation. However, auditors are now seen increasingly as part of the team and the very best provide a service that is based on extensive experience of clinical research processes coupled with in-depth knowledge and understanding of the principles underlying GCP.

Clinical monitors and clinical project managers or team leaders were the first to receive the attention of the auditors, but increasingly the audit focus has spread to include pharmacovigilance personnel, data managers, statisticians, investigational medicinal product units and pharmaceutical physicians.

In order to preserve auditor independence and to provide a consistent service to clinical research personnel, many companies have established separate clinical QA departments. Sometimes this department may be called GCP compliance or clinical audit, and sometimes a single QA department will also include specialist auditors in good laboratory practice (GLP) and good manufacturing practice (GMP). GCP does not specify the corporate structure required, except to stipulate independence from influence by those directly involved in the clinical research process.

AUDIT

According to section 5.19.3 of the ICH GCP guideline, the sponsor's audit plan and procedures for a trial audit should be guided by 'the importance of the trial to submissions to regulatory authorities, the number of subjects in the trial, the type and complexity of the trial, the level of risks to the trial subjects, and any identified problem(s)'. According to the same section, the auditor's findings are to be documented, the independence of the audit function should be preserved, and the circumstances are defined under which the regulatory authority may seek access to an audit report. GCP non-compliance, its implications and the action to be taken are covered in sections 5.20.1 and 5.20.2.

The ISO 10011 standard (Part 1) provides a useful framework for auditing GCP quality systems and studies (International Organization for Standardization, 1991). The section on responsibilities discusses the role of those who are being audited, the auditees. In the context of a GCP compliance audit, the auditees might be investigators, their staff, members of other departments in the investigator's institution, members of contract organisations such as archivists, clinical laboratory staff, clinical trial supplies unit staff, and sponsor company personnel, including monitors.

The responsibilities stated are that the auditee(s) should be informed about the objectives and scope of the audit; appoint responsible members of staff to accompany members of the audit team; provide all resources needed for the audit; provide access to the facilities and materials requested; co-operate with the auditors; and determine and initiate corrective actions based on the audit report.

Initiating the audit

Audit scope

In terms of the scope of the audit, ISO 10011 requires identification of the following (International Organization for Standardization, 1991):

- quality system elements, physical locations and organisational activities;
- scope and depth of the audit;
- the standards against which to audit;
- the objective evidence to be sought; and
- auditing resources to achieve the stated objectives.

Audit frequency

The ICH GCP guideline leaves it to sponsors to determine audit frequency, and there is the apparent suggestion in section 5.19 that auditing is optional ('If or when sponsors perform audits ...'). However, as noted, a number of specific factors will determine the sponsor's audit plan and procedures (section 5.19.3). A diligent company will therefore tailor its auditing activities in the light of any changes that have occurred since previous audits (changes in standards, staff, facilities and procedures; previous audit findings which may require follow-up; any other known problems). The company will then perform cyclical audits to provide insight into the full range of studies, monitors and systems over a specified period.

Preliminary review of auditee's quality system description

ISO 10011 suggests the advisability of reviewing various documents as a prelude to the audit visit itself. Auditors may ask to see the relevant SOPs, other work instructions and guidelines and any quality manual for the organisation to be audited. If a study-specific audit is to be undertaken, study documentation may be requested and, for a clinical study, this will usually consist of the protocol and any amendments, a blank CRF, samples of the informed consent documentation in use, the investigator's brochure, recruitment and serious adverse event information, and any available listings of the clinical database.

ISO 10011 even suggests that if these documents prove to be inadequate on preliminary review, it is not productive to proceed to the remaining audit procedures until the issues have been resolved. This may be appropriate for internal audits. However, there will be many cases where the audit will continue in order to assess other aspects, even though quite serious documentation deficiencies may be revealed on preliminary review.

Preparing for the audit

The auditors should have an audit plan, part of which will be to assign duties to the various members of the audit team. The tasks assigned will reflect the areas of expertise and the seniority of the various auditors as well as their individual workloads. The auditors may also prepare working documents for use during the audit. In some cases these will be standard documents used for all audits of a particular type. In other cases it will be necessary to generate audit-specific working documents, e.g. audit checklists for SDV and study-specific eligibility. Under these circumstances, the auditors may consult the research team for assistance in identifying key areas for review and assessment.

Executing the audit

Purpose of opening meeting

In audits of all types of quality system it is generally accepted that it is useful to hold an introductory meeting at each location where the audit is to take place. Monitors may be asked to assist in convening such meetings at their investigational sites and will probably be expected to attend. The introductory meeting has several functions:

- to provide an opportunity to introduce the members of the audit team;
- to allow the audit team to review the scope and the objectives of the audit with the auditee(s);
- to permit the auditee(s) to be briefed about the proposed methods for conducting the audit;
- to establish communication links between the audit team and the auditee(s);
- to allow confirmation that the resources and facilities required for the audit are available;
- to allow confirmation of the time and date for the closing meeting and any interim meetings;
- to permit clarification of any details of the audit plan that may be unclear.

Methods of collecting objective evidence

Although it may not be stated explicitly, the auditors will obtain information and evidence during the audit in a variety of ways. They are likely to conduct interviews with appropriate individuals, they will seek to review copies of documentary evidence, and they will use their senses to observe. They will probably seek agreement to make notes as they proceed with these activities and this should not be interpreted as an alarm signal. Auditors usually record many pieces of information – not necessarily negative findings. For example, they may make notes of conversations so that they can subsequently cross-check the spoken word against documentary and other evidence.

Although they will propose a plan and/or agenda at the opening meeting, it is not unusual for the auditors to deviate from this if something else unexpected or of interest emerges during the audit. Auditors may also sometimes stop the audit, usually because it has become impractical to continue or because a very significant finding requires immediate attention. Under these circumstances the auditors should explain their action to auditees and management.

Audit observations

For any type of good practice audit, auditors are trained that all observations should be documented. It is usual for the auditors to hold a formal or informal review meeting with the team to agree non-conformities and to resolve any misunderstandings. All non-conformities should be clearly documented and referenced with supporting evidence. Some auditors and inspectors will exercise their right to direct access by removing anonymised photocopies of evidence to be appended as exhibits to their reports. It is also useful for all concerned if the auditors indicate, for each non-conformity, the specific standard requirements that have been violated.

The closing meeting

The closing meeting is another very important feature of the well-conducted audit. It permits the hosts to be thanked, and affords an opportunity for the most serious findings to be discussed and for suggestions to be made for resolving findings and misunderstandings. The auditors should discuss the proposed arrangements and timelines for issuing their report. The auditees should also be congratulated on any points of good practice observed during the course of the audit.

After the audit

Most clinical auditors have procedures stating that audit reports should be issued promptly, often within 28 days of the final audit activity. The distribution of the audit report will usually be very restricted and, depending on a particular company's procedures, access will not necessarily be granted to the full text version. Whether individuals have full or only partial access to the contents of the report, preservation of its confidential nature is imperative. Personal and corporate reputations may be at stake and partial information can be very misleading.

However, all clinical research personnel should be made aware of findings relevant for their activities and for any study activities and locations with which they are involved. Monitors may be given responsibility for taking excerpts or summaries of the report to their investigational sites in order to obtain the responses requested during the audit. Responsibilities to follow up audit findings should be taken seriously, and planning and implementation of any action required should be performed as promptly as possible.

One of the greatest benefits arising from audit and from careful consideration of the audit report should be the insight this provides into training needs and opportunities. A series of audits of a single study will reveal patterns of compliance and non-compliance. These can be used to direct activity into the sharing of good practice and into analysing the causes of non-compliance, such as protocol or CRF design problems, impractical procedures and excessively tight eligibility criteria. Well-conducted systems audits are liberating in that they highlight strengths and permit discussion of obstacles in a blame-free environment. This important insight and the specific lessons learned should then inform the company's overall and individual training and development programmes.

THE STANDARD: WHAT IS THE SCOPE OF GCP?

GCP encompasses a number of different aspects that are represented in Europe, the USA and Japan by the ICH GCP guideline. ICH has made a major contribution to the harmonisation of pharmaceutical standards and regulatory requirements in these three major regions. However, the ICH document exists alongside other GCP guidelines, including those of the World Health Organization (1995). In addition, many nations have their own national laws requiring compliance with a specific set of GCP guidelines. In conducting multinational studies it is therefore essential to ensure that the individual requirements of the national laws for each participating country are observed in addition to the international guidelines. Moreover, GCP itself is predicated on compliance with the requirements for GMP and with the individual company's SOPs. Thus, the process of regulatory inspection for GCP compliance is a complex issue that extends far beyond the international GCP guidelines.

The ICH GCP guideline is numbered Topic E6 because it is the sixth set of guidelines in the ICH Efficacy (E) series (ICH Guideline, 1996). The GCP guideline cross-refers to Topic E2A: *Clinical Safety Data Management; Definitions and Standards for Expedited Reporting* (ICH Guideline, 1994) and Topic E3: *Structure and Content of Clinical Study Reports* (ICH Guideline, 1995). Any consideration of GCP compliance will therefore also extend to compliance with Topics E2A and E3.

The ICH Efficacy series has now reached E12 and provides a useful resource for many aspects of clinical research conduct. Familiarity with the following three Topics is particularly recommended:

- Topic E8: *General Considerations for Clinical Trials* (ICH Guideline, 1997);
- Topic E9: *Statistical Principles for Clinical Trials* (ICH Guideline, 1998);
- Topic E10: *Choice of Control Group in Clinical Trials* (ICH Guideline, 1999).

TYPES OF AUDIT

Systems audits

Systems audits may relate to GCP quality systems established by sponsor companies or to quality systems in operation by CROs. Consideration of quality systems is also a common feature of GCP inspections performed by the European regulatory authorities, and the FDA has recently begun to use this approach, with reviews of pharmacovigilance and monitoring systems.

SOP review

Because SOPs should reveal the intended quality procedures of the organisation (see ICH GCP guideline, sections 1.55 and 2.13), SOP review is one of the first activities in many audits. Each individual SOP must comply with national law and regulations, with GCP and any other applicable guidelines (e.g. GMP for investigational medicinal products or other ICH guidance notes), and with any statements of individual company policy. Auditors may seek information on SOP ease of use and how off-site access is gained in practice. For example, is an electronic set of SOPs available for monitors to take to investigational sites on a laptop, or do they have a small-format booklet of the most frequently used monitoring SOPs that can be carried easily with a pocket-sized copy of the ICH GCP guideline?

The responsibility to provide feedback on SOPs is a serious one. Auditors and inspectors will look for evidence of compliance with SOPs, and each company must have a mechanism for requesting review and modification of SOPs to ensure that they do not become out-of-date or impractical. To ensure that their requirements are met, clinical research personnel should ideally be consulted before new SOPs are finalised. Audits and inspections frequently find that lack of user input has resulted in SOPs that do not reflect practice.

Personnel

Auditors reviewing personnel records are looking for evidence that staff are sufficiently qualified, trained and experienced to perform the tasks allocated to them. Job descriptions and any study-specific delegation logs specifying these tasks should be up to date and accurate, as should all other personnel records. Although the ICH GCP guideline makes no specific requirement for CVs to be signed and dated, it does require them to be up to date and to provide evidence of the necessary qualifications. Signing and dating provide good evidence that the CV owner has taken responsibility for its accuracy on the date of signature and also indicate when the last review occurred. People moving from one employment to another may find that important training experiences are not included on their company-specific training record. If this is the case, it may be appropriate to include details in a general CV or some other document that can be produced as evidence. Auditors may interview staff to enquire more about their duties and their understanding of correct procedures. This is not intended as a detailed memory test, but simply as an indication of knowledge of the generalities and the appropriate sources of detail.

Specific functions

The scope of a systems audit will include one or more specific functions or activities: these will be examined in general terms and using examples and evidence of relevant duties performed across a number of clinical studies. Mainstream clinical research activities may be covered but QA itself, pharmacovigilance, data management and statistics may be considered because of their interaction with the areas of clinical research/medical advisor/monitoring. In general, the questions asked should reflect the GCP guidelines, other relevant ICH guidelines and Annex 13 of the Rules and Guidance for Pharmaceutical Manufacturers and Distributors (Medicines Control Agency, 1997).

Some systems audit findings may necessitate responses, and these will ideally involve both corrective and preventive action. They will address the particular instance of the problem observed, consider how to detect and deal with other similar instances, and examine the cause of the problem and whether any systematic action is required to prevent its recurrence.

Study-specific audits

In a study-specific audit the emphasis is on a single study rather than on the operation of a system across a number of studies.

Audit preparation

Audit preparation may involve review of the protocol, blank CRF, informed consent documents and the investigator's brochure. The auditor will seek to become familiar with the structure and detail of the study and will also check the documents themselves for GCP and SOP compliance and consistency.

Sponsor and CRO study files

The contents of the relevant sponsor and CRO study files will be reviewed to ensure that all the essential documents are present and in good order and that all approvals and appropriate actions occurred in the correct sequence.

Investigational site files

Similar documentary review may be undertaken at the investigational site, examining for the same issues and for congruity with the sponsor and CRO files seen previously.

At the investigational site, the data collected in the CRFs will be checked according to the auditor's planned sampling scheme against source documents residing solely at the site. The protocol statement indicating for which variables the CRF itself is the source document is important here because, by implication, any variables not so indicated should be supported by source documents. Auditors will not undertake 100% SDV; their remit is to review a sufficiently large sample to provide information on how well the routine monitoring and SDV processes are operating at the site. When planning routine SDV, it is advisable for the monitor to anticipate the possible future audit of this activity.

The auditors will also wish to ascertain that any laboratory tests have been performed correctly and in appropriate conditions and that any samples intended for laboratory analyses have been taken, handled, stored and transmitted to the laboratory in a manner which safeguards the integrity of the samples and maximises the probability of obtaining evaluable results. This may involve interviews with operational staff and review of records.

Both for laboratory samples and investigational medicinal products, documentation of handling and storage conditions will be considered and the auditors may wish to visit storage areas. All records concerning the disposition of investigational medicinal products will be examined carefully and investigational site staff will be asked about their roles in dispensing, administering or training subjects in administration, checking compliance and maintaining records.

Auditors will also wish to review the arrangements for the storage of the investigator's trial master file and any other relevant documents, as well as of source documents both during and after the study. Security, confidentiality, integrity during long-term storage and retrieval arrangements will be priority concerns.

Investigational products in clinical trials

The Recitals to the European Clinical Trials Directive (European Parliament and Council Directive, 2000) and section 2.12 of the ICH GCP guideline (ICH Guideline, 1996) both require that the standards of GMP should be applied to investigational medicinal products. Annex 13 of the *Rules and Guidance for Pharmaceutical Manufacturers and Distributors* (Medicines Control Agency, 1997), popularly known as the 'Orange Guide', defines the GMP requirements looked for by auditors and inspectors in relation to clinical trial supplies. It should be noted that packaging instructions are more complex than for marketed products and more liable to errors; when blinded labels are used, such errors are harder to detect than in marketed products.

One of the most relevant aspects for clinical research personnel concerns labelling and re-labelling procedures; these are regarded as manufacturing processes and are subject to the provisions of Annex 13. It is often necessary during a clinical study to re-label supplies with extension of expiry date information. This may be performed on site in accordance with specific SOPs but Annex 13 indicates that supervision procedures are also required. Label reconciliation, line clearance, independent checks by a second person present during the labelling process, and reconciliation at the end of the labelling process are all required. An additional label must be used, not simply an amendment of the existing label, and it should include the new expiry date and repeat the batch number. This label may be placed to cover the old date but not the original statement of batch number. If re-labelling has occurred during a study, auditors and inspectors may request documentary evidence of compliance with these requirements, and Annex 13 states that additional labelling must be documented in trial and batch records. Annex 13 further specifies in detail the requirements for the content of labels and distinguishes between outer packaging, immediate packaging, blister packs and small units. Recall procedures are also addressed in Annex 13; an SOP should cover recall issues and all staff involved should receive appropriate training.

Methods of transport and documentation of transport of investigational products to ensure their integrity are discussed, with Annex 13 confirming that transfer between trial sites should remain the exception and should only be considered for very expensive and scarce products or in an emergency. A procedure should exist for the transfer of products that have been outside the sponsor's control; this will usually cover re-labelling, full finished-product specification retesting and new release.

One of the more controversial aspects of Annex 13 (and one possibly subject to review or modification in the near future) requires retention of returned supplies until finalisation of the clinical trial and compilation of the final report. European GCP inspectors are prepared to sympathetically consider deviations from this requirement in respect of hazardous products, excessively bulky products, and studies with high recruitment and long treatment periods. However, they indicate that if destruction occurs prematurely, this must be fully documented and be justifiable on such grounds.

Clinical research personnel with responsibility for any GMP-related processes that they find to be challenging or unclear are advised to consult the GMP and GCP auditors in their company.

Clinical laboratories

Study monitors may be expected to interact with clinical laboratories, to negotiate contracts with them and to monitor their performance. Any clinical laboratory audit may involve a review of this interaction.

According to Chapter V, Article 12.1 of the European Clinical Trials Directive: 'Compliance with the provisions of good clinical practice shall be verified on behalf of the Community by inspection at *relevant* sites, including the trial site and manufacturing site, *at any laboratory used in the trial* and/or at the sponsor's premises, by inspectors appointed by Member States'. It is therefore important to establish standards for clinical laboratories and to monitor compliance with such standards in order to prepare for possible inspection and to provide confidence in the results produced.

Unfortunately, the issue of standards for the conduct and audit of clinical laboratories is one of the uncharted areas of GCP. The ICH GCP guideline says little specifically about laboratories, apart from a reference in Section 8 to '...current reference ranges, evidence of certification, accreditation or established quality control and/or external quality assessment or other validation to document competence of the facility to perform required test(s) and support reliability of results'. Sections 2.8, 2.10 and 2.13 are also relevant in this context but do not mention clinical laboratories specifically.

Audit of a clinical laboratory will involve assessment of: contracts, delegation and financial arrangements; personnel, training and experience, delegation and records; facilities and environmental conditions; equipment (particularly computerised systems); materials, labelling and storage; documentation maintenance, filing and archiving, and SOPs; methodology, specific tests, validation and quality control methods; reference ranges, highlighting, review and alerts for out-of-range values; reporting (both routine and urgent); and access for monitoring, audit and inspection. These points must be borne in mind when selecting and monitoring clinical laboratories. Finally, according to GCP, everything that is delegated should be stated in writing and agreed; conversely, anything not stated in writing and agreed is deemed not to have been delegated.

Clinical study reports

ICH Topic E3 provides information about the requirements for the structure and content of clinical study reports (ICH Guideline, 1995). It contains 16 sections and eight annexes and is intended to apply to integrated study reports, i.e. those integrating the clinical and statistical report. The detail in the report should be sufficient to allow replication of critical analyses, and the set of subjects from whom the data are generated should be clearly identified. User-friendly data listings and conspicuous identification of derived values are also required. Compliance with these points will certainly please auditors by reducing the detective work they need to perform in order to audit the final report.

The integrated study report should describe features that are not well described in the protocol and should highlight ways in which the study conduct and analysis differed from the protocol. A frequent audit and inspection finding is that the report does not reflect the true conduct of the study but merely the intentions of the protocol.

Auditors and inspectors will check for compliance with the ICH requirements for study reports, internal consistency, logical organisation, clarity of expression and accuracy. They will look for consistency by comparing the report synopsis with the main text; the main text with the statistics, tables and data summaries; the statistics and data summaries with the pre-processed data tabulations; and the data listings with the raw data, e.g. CRFs and source documents. They will also check for consistency with the study plan or protocol, the trial master file (*actual* study conduct), the regulations, guidelines and company SOPs, and standard formats and/or templates.

Audit of validation of computerised systems

Computerised systems are an increasingly prevalent feature of modern life in general and clinical research is no exception. Ideally, this development should reduce the opportunity for human error and enhance consistency and quality. However, in order for these improvements to occur, confidence must be established in the quality of the systems proposed for use. The ICH GCP guideline discusses the sponsor's responsibilities for trial management, data handling and record keeping and section 5.5.3 specifically covers the use of electronic trial data handling and/or remote electronic trial data systems. The sponsor is required to:

- Use validated systems that ensure complete, accurate, reliable and consistent performance in compliance with the sponsor's own standard procedures.
- Maintain SOPs for these systems.
- Document data changes, and maintain an audit trail, data trail and edit trail.
- Maintain security to prevent unauthorised access to the data.
- Maintain a list of individuals authorised to make data changes.
- Use systems that do not support unauthorised unblinding of study data.

In addition, the usual general requirements apply for personnel to be appropriately qualified, trained and experienced and for secure filing and archiving of data and documentation for the specified time periods.

Computer system validation is a subject that causes concern to many people. A variety of automated instruments may be held at an investigational site to perform study assessments and to record and transmit data. Auditors will expect evidence to show that these systems have been validated. However, it is not necessary for the study monitor to perform the validation procedures personally, merely to ensure that documentary evidence of such validation can be provided to the auditors. Like GMP, this is an area in which the inexperienced are well advised to seek help from experienced colleagues or a consultant.

Electronic signatures and records

As the use of computer-based systems has increased, the issue of electronic signatures and electronic records has become important. In response to public demand, the FDA has published rules for electronic records and electronic signatures in the *Federal Register* (Code of Federal Regulations, 1997). These rules set out the criteria under which the FDA considers electronic records and signatures to be 'trustworthy, reliable and generally equivalent to paper records and handwritten signatures executed on paper'. The rules also specify that relevant computer systems, controls and documentation should be readily available and subject to FDA inspection. The controls required include validation of systems, ability to produce human readable and electronic copies of records, retrievability, security, limitation of access, maintenance of audit trails, built-in checking of events and authorisations, checks of validity of source data and system operation, qualification of those involved with development, maintenance and use of systems, use of SOPs and controls on distribution, and changes to systems documentation and manuals.

When the issue of the proposed use of electronic records and electronic systems arises, it may be appropriate to seek expert assistance in order to ensure that the data and documentation will be acceptable to regulators as part of a submission.

INSPECTIONS BY REGULATORY AUTHORITIES

Inspections and audits compared

The process of inspection is essentially similar to that of audit. However, the inspectors are employed by government, through the agency of the regulatory or competent authority. The competent authority is that which is deemed by government to have the competence to issue and revoke licences and to regulate the conduct of clinical research.

The ICH GCP guideline (section 1.29) defines an inspection as 'the act by a regulatory authority(ies) of conducting an official review ...'. Sponsor companies take inspections very seriously because the consequences can have significant future implications at both a corporate and an individual level. Clinical research personnel who work in a company with an active clinical quality assurance (CQA) function or who have experience of a good, professionally executed audit should encounter few surprises when involved in a regulatory inspection. As with audit, the main features of an inspection usually include preparation by the inspectors and by those to be inspected, an introductory meeting, documentary review, interviews and observation, a closing meeting, production and issue of a report and possible requests for responses and action proposals.

Who decides to inspect?

Inspection is an activity conducted by regulators and assessors. These are the representatives of the regulatory authorities or competent authorities of national government or international governmental agencies. The development of such systems of regulatory inspection has included the history of the establishment of inspections by the FDA on behalf of the US government, by the regulatory authorities of individual Member States within the European Union and, most recently, by the Japanese Ministry of Health and Welfare (MHW). Internationally, the European Agency for the Evaluation of Medicinal Products (EMEA) has the remit of co-ordinating joint inspections performed by inspectors gathered from various Member States within the European Union.

Although harmonisation in the guidelines for GCP has been progressing well over the last decade, there is still a lack of consistency in the degree of legal provision within different national authorities. However, once the principle of inspection for GCP compliance has been established, it is interesting to consider who decides when an inspection is required. In general, this responsibility lies with the teams of GCP inspectors within each national authority. However, these teams are advised by experts who assess dossiers for potential marketing authorisations, by members of ethics committees, and by other groups within the regulatory authorities. They also welcome input from the pharmaceutical industry itself and from the public.

What triggers a request for an inspection?

In connection with a clinical study, an inspection may be required if there are concerns about its safety, data or ethics. The inspectors will seek to verify that ethical principles are being followed, to assess the validity and reliability of the data generated, and to examine the appropriateness of the scientific methods used. Inspections may be undertaken as part of a programme to monitor standards of clinical research on a routine or cyclical basis, or on an *ad hoc* or random sampling basis.

Inspections are also undertaken when there is suspicion of fraud or scientific misconduct (*see Chapter 24*) or where a serious quality systems breakdown has come to the notice of the regulatory authority. In these cases there are often major public health implications and inspection may result in legal action. Inspectors are trained in investigation techniques and in the collection of legally admissible evidence, and they may call upon specialist support services.

What should be inspected and when?

The ICH GCP guideline (section 1.29) continues its definition of inspection as '... an official review of documents, facilities, records and any other resources that are deemed by the authority(ies) to be related to the clinical trial and that may be located at the site of the trial, at the sponsor's and/or contract research organisation's (CRO's) facilities, or at other establishments deemed appropriate by the regulatory authority(ies)'.

In addition, the Recitals to the European Clinical Trials Directive state: 'Whereas verification of compliance with the standards of good clinical practice and the need to subject data, information and documents to inspection in order to confirm that they have been properly generated, recorded and reported is essential in order to justify the involvement of human subjects in clinical trials; whereas the person participating in a trial should be made aware of and consent to the scrutiny of personal information during inspection by competent authorities and properly authorized persons, provided that such personal information is treated as strictly confidential and is not made publicly available'.

For European regulatory submissions, all aspects of the clinical research process and all locations and staff involved in that process may be subject to inspection. This will therefore include the quality systems employed in the conduct of the clinical trial, the details of the performance and outcome of studies both during and after that performance, the study sites, the premises and personnel of the sponsor company, any pharmacies involved, clinical trial supplies units and manufacturers, and clinical laboratories involved in the analysis of samples generated during the course of the study. The inspection of European clinical studies by the FDA is already well established, and international companies should be aware that the growing force of European national GCP inspectors will inspect both within and outside Europe.

What are the results of inspection?

While they are necessarily interconnected, a number of different results can be identified:

- To provide evidence of official supervision by the governmental body in question.
- To raise international confidence in the standards of conduct of clinical research as verified by inspection.
- To assure both the subjects of clinical research and the potential recipients of new medicines that the methods employed in the generation of clinical trial data are scientifically valid and ethically appropriate and that they yield accurate and reproducible data.
- To encourage mutual recognition of clinical research data generated in different areas of the world. This will have the effect of reducing risk and unnecessary duplication of research.
- To accelerate the development and marketing of medicines internationally.
- To demonstrate that the process of verification and assessment frequently identifies a need for corrective and preventive follow-up action. The resulting quality improvements should be seen as a long-term and valued by-product of inspection.
- To present inspection as an educative process that aids harmonisation. This effect will be achieved in part by the publicity generated by the inspection process.

Who may inspect and where?

As a general rule, regulatory inspectors may request to inspect any location involved in the generation of clinical research data used to support an MAA in the territory of the inspectors. Within national boundaries, legislation may reinforce the powers of local inspectors. Outside their territories, they are unlikely at present to have powers of entry and seizure, but it would be unwise for a pharmaceutical company to deny access for inspection. Moreover, investigators are usually required to give contractual agreement to permit such access.

The European Clinical Trials Directive aims to establish a legal basis for GCP and GMP to be applied to investigational medicinal products. There appears to be a firm commitment to the inclusion of a requirement for Member States to verify compliance with GCP by inspection at relevant sites. Inspection is defined in Chapter I, Article 2 as: 'The act by a competent authority of conducting an official review of documents, facilities, records, arrangements for quality assurance, and any other resources that are deemed by the competent authority to be related to the clinical trial ...'.

In anticipation of the adoption of the Directive and its transposition into national legislation, most European Member States appointed teams of GCP inspectors who are already engaged in programmes of GCP inspection. Most of the Member States that have not yet appointed inspectors are planning to do so as soon as the necessary administrative arrangements can be completed.

Thus, the pharmaceutical industry in Europe faces a situation in the next two to three years when all Member States will have GCP inspectors actively reviewing all aspects of the clinical research process.

Inspection in the UK

In the UK, a system of voluntary inspections for GCP compliance is in operation pending implementation of national legislation. The scheme has proved very popular and the team of GCP inspectors is fully occupied in meeting demand. Volunteers from sponsor companies and CROs continue to request inspection and some companies are also turning to independent consultants to provide a 'mock' regulatory inspection experience, either in preparation for a voluntary MCA inspection or for its own sake in what they perceive as a lower-risk strategy.

Inspection in the rest of Europe

The teams of GCP inspectors established by European Member States since 1990 operate a variety of inspection schemes. Some, as in the Netherlands and Denmark, began with a voluntary scheme and then, with the support of national legislation, have moved on to a mandatory situation. Mandatory inspections may be cyclical or conducted to support a review of MAAs. As elsewhere, inspections may also be conducted on a 'for cause' basis in instances where there may have been a major or potential quality systems breakdown or some form of misconduct.

Some Member States (for example, Spain) have the legal powers to inspect ethics committees but this is not common practice. (In the USA, inspection of institutional review boards (IRBs) is routinely performed and has resulted in action against IRBs and, in some cases, suspension of their activities pending resolution of problems noted.)

An important feature of the approach to inspection adopted by the majority of the European inspectorates is their emphasis on quality systems, rather than focusing exclusively on a particular study. The combined systems and study-specific inspection encompasses study site, sponsor organisations, pharmacies, clinical laboratories and manufacturers of investigational medicinal products. In Sweden, however, for study-specific inspections, it has been customary only to inspect at the investigational site and to derive information on systems compliance from on-site evidence. This reflects the general practice of the FDA, until recently, when inspecting within the USA. Currently, the FDA is also undertaking systematic inspections of areas such as monitoring and pharmacovigilance.

Thus, like the auditors, the inspectors are establishing a relationship of education and consultancy rather than the traditionally perceived 'policing' approach. Informal discussions and suggestions for quality improvement are increasingly common during the inspection process. Inspectors continue to examine clinical data in very great detail, but they go beyond these findings to explore the systematic issues responsible for the observations.

Inspections by other regulators

Of all the world's regulatory authorities, the FDA in the USA has the longest history of inspection for GCP compliance, while the MHW in Japan is probably the most recent to conduct such inspections. The approach to inspection adopted by the MHW is similar to that of the FDA, from whom some of the Japanese inspectors have received training. Both these authorities inspect outside their own territories and may involve local national inspectors in joint inspections or as observers when inspecting in Europe. When the Committee for Proprietary Medicinal Products (CPMP) receives centralised applications for marketing authorisations, joint inspections by teams of inspectors from the European Member States may be requested.

In most cases, notice of inspection is given, varying from a few days to several weeks or months. The inspecting authority may request translations and re-analysis of data and may also issue questions to be answered in advance of the inspection itself.

IMPACT OF THE EUROPEAN CLINICAL TRIALS DIRECTIVE

Chapter I, Article 1 of the European Clinical Trials Directive states that its scope includes all clinical trials except non-interventional trials. The trials in question must involve human subjects and a medicinal product and may be single-centre or multicentre, single-state or multi-state. The most significant implication is that all those involved in the conduct of clinical trials (sponsors, investigators, CROs and ethics committees) will have their responsibilities, duties and functions governed by law. As we have noted, these responsibilities will include adherence to GCP principles. The Directive aims to promote harmonisation of the approaches to clinical research and offers clear advantages in the case of multinational studies. It also enshrines one of the highest priorities of GCP, the protection of the human subject.

In terms of its impact in the present context, auditors and inspectors will seek evidence of compliance with the detailed requirements of the Directive. Specifically, they will expect to find acceptable and documented standards and quality control systems to cover all stages of the clinical research process. In particular, the time taken for ethics committees to form an opinion about proposed research will be under scrutiny. So too will be the time taken to notify ethics committees and regulators of the normal conclusion or premature termination of a study, either at a specific site or overall.

Inspectors will have a legal mandate throughout the European Community to inspect any establishment deemed appropriate by the competent authority, and infringement procedures will be made available to them to handle cases where there are objective grounds for concern.

PREPARATION FOR AUDIT AND INSPECTION

There are differing views as to whether it is appropriate to prepare at all for audits and inspections. The opponents of preparation argue that the subsequent audit or inspection is devalued because it gives a false impression. Data and files have been tidied and made more complete and the people involved have rehearsed appropriate responses. However, if the outcome is important and has external repercussions, e.g. the placing of a contract or the grant of a marketing authorisation, then the potential cost of failing to prepare could be high, both for the organisation and for the individuals who may be held responsible. The preparation exercise itself can yield benefits. In a safe, blame-free environment it can highlight areas requiring attention and this can lead to improvements with implications far beyond the scope of the individual audit/inspection. Rehearsal also has the effect of reducing fear and misunderstanding and of helping individuals to demonstrate the quality of their work. In summary, there may be a case for conducting internal audits and external reviews of subcontractors on a 'surprise' basis in order to make an accurate assessment. However, if the outcome of the audit or inspection is likely to have significant future implications, preparation is recommended.

Preparation for audit or inspection requires knowledge of what these activities usually entail. Study of GCP auditing SOPs, attendance at conferences, discussions with colleagues, and a review of the literature are all fruitful methods of gaining this insight. The company QA group should be willing to contribute significantly to this information-gathering exercise, and experienced external consultants may be willing to offer preparation support and to conduct 'mock' audits and inspections with an independent eye.

It will be helpful to set up a folder containing all the information supplied to the auditors/inspectors. A duplicate folder is usually prepared so that the company has a complete record of the information submitted. These folders can be supplemented during the course of the audit/inspection and the duplicate folder can subsequently be related to the report and will be invaluable in preparing for subsequent audits/inspections. In addition to the information provided in the folder, auditors/inspectors may also request clarification on a number of other points. These may relate to the logistics of the audit/inspection and all arrangements should be confirmed in writing.

Preparation for audit and inspection is important. However, a company should have little to fear from the experience provided it displays genuine commitment to the principles of GCP, from senior management down to the most junior member of staff. Where that is the case, ethically and scientifically sound clinical practice will be routine and GCP-compliant, up-to-date procedures will already be in place. With its requirement for quality assurance by sponsor and contract research companies alike, GCP (its precise form yet to be defined) is about to become law: audit and inspection appear to be here to stay.

REFERENCES

European Parliament and Council Directive (2000). Common Position adopted by the Council with a view to the adoption of a Directive of the European Parliament and of the Council on the approximation of the laws, regulations and administrative provisions of the Member States relating to the implementation of good clinical practice in the conduct of clinical trials on medicinal products for human use. (Procedure number: COD 1997/0197. Common Position document date: 20 July 2000.)

Code of Federal Regulations (1997). 21 CFR Part 11: Electronic records; electronic signatures. *Federal Register* **62**, 13429–13466.

ICH Guideline (1994). *Topic E2A: Clinical Safety Data Management; Definitions and Standards for Expedited Reporting*, International Federation of Pharmaceutical Manufacturers Associations, Geneva (Issued as CPMP/ICH/377/95).

ICH Guideline (1995). *Topic E3: Structure and Content of Clinical Study Reports*, International Federation of Pharmaceutical Manufacturers Associations, Geneva (Issued as CPMP/ICH/137/95).

ICH Guideline (1996). *Topic E6: Good Clinical Practice – Consolidated Guideline*, International Federation of Pharmaceutical Manufacturers Associations, Geneva (Issued as CPMP/ICH/135/95).

ICH Guideline (1997). *Topic E8: General Considerations for Clinical Trials*, International Federation of Pharmaceutical Manufacturers Associations, Geneva (Issued as CPMP/ICH/291/96).

ICH Guideline (1998). *Topic E9: Statistical Principles for Clinical Trials*, International Federation of Pharmaceutical Manufacturers Associations, Geneva (Issued as CPMP/ICH/363/96).

ICH Guideline (1999). *Topic E10: Choice of Control Group in Clinical Trials*, International Federation of Pharmaceutical Manufacturers Associations, Geneva (Reached Step 4 in July 2000).

International Organization for Standardization (1991). *ISO 10011: Guidelines for Auditing Quality Systems*, International Organization for Standardization, Geneva.

Medicines Control Agency (1997). *Rules and Guidance for Pharmaceutical Manufacturers and Distributors 1997: Annex 13* (also known as the *Orange Guide*), The Stationery Office, London.

World Health Organization (1995). *Guidelines for Good Clinical Practice (GCP) for Trials on Pharmaceutical Products. Annex 3 of The Use of Essential Drugs*. Sixth Report of the WHO Expert Committee. World Health Organization, Geneva, pp. 97–137.

20

Trial master file

Nicola Goodwin

INTRODUCTION

The trial master file (TMF) is a hard copy of all the documentation relating to a clinical trial and, specifically, of the documentation held by the sponsor. In other words, it is the filing system containing the essential documents central to each individual clinical trial. According to the ICH GCP guideline, essential documents are defined in section 8.1 as '... those documents which individually and collectively permit evaluation of the conduct of a trial and the quality of the data produced' (ICH Guideline, 1996).

Typically, however, the TMF will include more documents than those defined as 'essential', with the result that retrospective analysis of a complete TMF should allow full reconstruction of the trial. The TMF exists to demonstrate the reproducibility of the data collected and it therefore has inherent scientific value. This fact immediately clarifies the importance of assembling an accurate and complete TMF that is open to scrutiny by sponsor auditing systems and by external review bodies. As a paper record of all the documents that were collected before, during and after the active phase of the clinical trial, the TMF will serve as a permanent record of what happened during a trial and thus reflect the professionalism and integrity of the clinical team.

RESPONSIBILITY FOR AND MANAGEMENT OF THE TRIAL MASTER FILE

The importance of the TMF as the central record for a clinical trial cannot be overstated. A clinical trial represents an enormous investment for any pharmaceutical company and the TMF will attest to the integrity of the data used by the company as it seeks to license a drug. It remains for inspection long after the study has been completed and it is a testimony to the conduct and success of that trial. Under such circumstances it would be unwise to allow the TMF to be undervalued within the clinical research team. The management of the TMF should be viewed as the responsibility of the whole team during the conduct of a trial, even though one individual may be formally designated to carry this responsibility. It is common nowadays for this individual responsibility to fall to the clinical trial administrator (CTA) or TMF coordinator. For the purposes of this chapter, this individual will be referred to as the CTA although the role title may vary from company to company, depending on size, location and structure. Designating one person to be responsible for the TMF has several advantages:

- the TMF becomes the highest priority for the CTA held accountable for it;
- missing documents are not 'overlooked' – the CTA will assume responsibility for ensuring that every document is complete;
- TMF management is provided from start to finish, with the expectation that the clinical team will have a complete and accurate record of the trial.

Confidence in the TMF is important for the morale of the team. A good CTA who is competent and enthusiastic about the TMF will make a good impression on those who require access to it. It is a great asset for the clinical team to have such a valuable member when audit or inspection is a possibility.

THE APPEARANCE OF THE TRIAL MASTER FILE

It is essential that the TMF is designed from the outset to be user-friendly and durable. There is no point in having a system that literally falls apart when a file is accessed or opened. Likewise, it is frustrating to encounter a complicated system in which reference must be made to multiple itemised lists before access to the subfile is possible. The key to a successful TMF is to have files that are easy to access and a system that is easy to follow. Labelling should be clear and the structure of the TMF system should be the same for every trial in the clinical programme for the product under investigation. A CTA (or auditor/inspector) assigned to one study should be able easily to locate TMF documents in another study. This offers the twin advantages of increasing team flexibility and efficiency within the department, and of smoothing the audit/inspection process when the time comes.

The clearer the information to allow ease of access for someone unfamiliar with the sponsor or clinical trial, the better the TMF. It is helpful to think of the TMF from the perspective of an auditor or inspector coming to it 'cold':

- Are the files tidy, up to date and clearly labelled? Have too many papers been crammed into each file?
- Is there a flow diagram indexing the location of all the documents in the TMF, with dates of filing?

- A tidy, organised and well-presented TMF literally 'speaks volumes' about the study team's perception of it. Conversely, a TMF consisting of battered files overflowing with documents that fall out the moment they are moved will create the negative impression it deserves.

The TMF should contain original documents, unless otherwise specified by local legal requirements that the original should be kept elsewhere (this applies especially in international multicentre studies). It should always be possible to identify the location of the original document. Units, subsidiaries or contract research organisations (CROs) participating in a clinical trial, but not responsible for the TMF, are recommended to maintain a file containing copies of their documents, preferably using a filing plan and rules similar to those set in place for the TMF.

ESSENTIAL DOCUMENTS IN THE TRIAL MASTER FILE

The essential documents that must be filed in the TMF are listed in section 8 of the ICH GCP guideline according to the different phases of a clinical trial: (1) before the clinical phase of the trial commences, (2) during the clinical conduct of the trial, and (3) after completion or termination of the trial.

Before the clinical phase of the trial commences

The start of the clinical phase of a trial is usually interpreted as the beginning of subject recruitment. However, the hardest work is usually done in setting up the study before recruitment begins. Indeed, the TMF reflects the work needed in this setting-up stage. The ICH GCP guideline (section 8.1) states: 'Trial Master Files should be established at the beginning of the trial ...'. The number of documents that should be available before the clinical phase of a study begins is considerable and these documents should be safely filed in the TMF from the outset.

Investigator's brochure

This is the document that contains all the background information about the investigational drug. The investigator's brochure (IB) is included in the TMF to demonstrate that the investigator has been fully informed about the medication under review on the basis of the information available at the time of study initiation. The IB should be updated whenever new information becomes available and should be fully revised at least annually. The number and dates of each IB version should be accurately filed and it is recommended that a record of receipt from investigators be kept to show which version of the IB they are currently using. Version control is an important element in many aspects of clinical development and the TMF is no exception.

Protocol and protocol amendments (if any)

The protocol specifies the study design and methodology and must be filed in the TMF, together with any subsequent amendments to the original protocol. It is essential that each edition of the protocol and any amendments should have a unique identifier (date and version number, at least). Failure to clearly number the protocol and its amendments is a recipe for confusion and unless proper version control is implemented, it is common to find file copies disagreeing with working copies. Without a paper record, it is impossible to establish the rationale for changes to the protocol after founder members of the study team have left the company or moved on to other projects. The TMF must arrange documents in a suitable and usable chronological order, again highlighting the absolute imperative to number and date documents.

Information sheets

The trial subjects' well-being and safety are at the heart of ICH GCP and, therefore, at the heart of the TMF. The information given to each subject in the trial must be clearly set out for each centre or site taking part in a study. Usually, the information given to the subject to read and digest (the patient information sheet) and the informed consent form are referenced in the protocol. However, when protocols are submitted to local ethics committees, these bodies may request a change to the information given to the subjects in their local centre. Although such changes are commonly minor, the TMF must contain every version of the patient information sheet and informed consent form for every centre participating in the study. These can be filed once the local ethics committee has formally approved the study, because information given to the subject is part of the ethics committee approval process. In fact, most ethics committees insist that the information given to the subject should be printed on the letterhead of the institution (hospital/clinic) where the subject will attend. This greatly facilitates the filing and tracking of informed consent by centre in the TMF.

Financial aspects of the trial

All signed financial agreements should be filed in the TMF before the study starts. As a minimum, the agreements with the investigator, hospital, laboratories and any CROs involved in the study should be in the TMF before recruitment starts. However, certain agreements (for example, with data management groups commissioned to process the data at some time in the future) may not become available until later in the study. All financial agreements must be worded very specifically, in order to avoid confusion later. It can be very difficult to sort out ambiguous financial agreements after the study has begun. Failure to agree and document the financial arrangements in detail from the outset can generate ill feeling and thus affect the progress of the study.

Insurance statement

Every subject participating in a clinical trial is protected under law. As a self-regulating standard for the pharmaceutical industry, the ICH GCP guideline takes further account of the subject's safety by specifying that the clinical trial should have an insurance statement, where required. This statement (section 8.2.5) documents that compensation will be available to subjects for any trial-related injury and that such compensation will be paid if the subjects are in any way endangered through their participation in the trial. The pharmaceutical company issues the insurance statement at the start of a clinical trial to reassure all those taking part that the sponsor has fully considered the subjects' welfare during the course of the trial.

Signed agreements

Without signed agreements, founded on ICH GCP principles, any investigator who unilaterally decides to re-interpret the protocol while a clinical trial is in progress (e.g. by adding an extra blood sample, missing out a study visit, or using the data collected to publish a scientific paper before trial completion) is effectively 'out of control'. The investigator and related responsible signatories must sign an agreement to abide by the protocol that has been approved by the ethics committee. It will further be agreed that data are only to be published after the study has been completed and that any alterations to the protocol are to be formalised and documented in official protocol amendments. This agreement is fundamental to the principles of GCP and is a major element determining the quality of the TMF.

Ethics committee approvals and composition

Ethics committees were introduced following the original Declaration of Helsinki in 1964 to protect the rights of the individual. Before recruitment begins in the centre in question, an ethics committee must give full approval for the clinical trial to be conducted. Such approval must have been received in writing and be filed in the TMF. To ensure that no-one can be recruited to a trial without ethics committee approval, pharmaceutical companies and trial sponsors will not release the shipment of study medication until the approval letter has been seen by an office-based member of the study team (usually a study monitor or the CTA).

Curricula vitae

The curricula vitae (CVs) of the investigator and any sub-investigators must be held in the TMF. While many pharmaceutical companies file the CVs of everyone involved in a particular clinical trial, the priority is to ensure that a subject's progress through the trial is under the supervision of an individual

with appropriate medical qualifications. Apart from evidencing suitable qualifications, the information on an investigator's CV must be recent.
Investigators must not simply regurgitate for pharmaceutical companies an
ancient CV that has been photocopied dozens of times and is brought out
every time a new clinical trial starts in their department. Company or sponsor
SOPs will dictate a definition of 'recent'. Typically, the CV should be no more
than 2 years old and must always contain information to demonstrate that the
investigator is suitably qualified to perform the study in question.

Laboratory procedures and normal values

In the context of a multicentre clinical trial, methods of laboratory measurement and analysis will differ from one hospital or site to another.
Standardisation between centres cannot be assumed, and even a seemingly
straightforward measurement (e.g. height) may be recorded differently from
clinic to clinic. Normal values and related documentation (e.g. accreditation
certificates) should be collected in the TMF for all tests under review, whether
they are conducted by a number of different laboratories or by one central
laboratory.

Investigational product (drug accountability)

Accurate and complete drug accountability is one of the best illustrations of
a high-quality clinical trial. The TMF must contain a full a record of the
manufacture, labelling and handling of the investigational product (trial
medication). The file must hold a detailed log of how the investigational
products were made, how they were dispatched to and received by the study
centres, how the subjects complied with the relevant regimens, and how the
investigational products were finally destroyed.

Master randomisation list and decoding procedures

The TMF contains the detailed procedure for dispensing study medication to
ensure that each subject receives the treatment that has been allocated to
him/her. The master randomisation list specifies which study drug has been
allocated to each subject. It lists the treatment that the subject is going to
receive against the subject number that identifies the drug package. The list
remains 'sealed' in the TMF with instructions for breaking the randomisation
code under rigorously defined circumstances. Details of each treatment should
be placed individually into a random code envelope so that breaking the code
for one subject does not 'unblind' the person opening the envelope to the
treatments received by other subjects. The study statistician (or delegate) will
open the master randomisation list to analyse the study data after the database
has been locked at the end of the trial.

Pre-trial monitoring report and trial initiation monitoring report

It is essential that the pre-trial monitoring report (investigator selection) and trial initiation monitoring report (on-site study set-up) are filed in the TMF immediately they are written. This will enable effective and informed review of performance metrics in cases where the study monitor originally involved in investigator selection or study set-up has moved on to other projects or another company.

During the clinical conduct of the trial

The start of subject recruitment into the clinical trial ushers in a phase of hectic activity when responsibility for keeping the TMF up to date and tracking all the documents becomes a major undertaking. Subjects are recruited at differing rates in different centres, and the maelstrom of incoming documentation would be unmanageable without the CTA to coordinate the TMF.

Updating documents in the TMF

The TMF forfeits its *raison d'être* if it contains documents that are out of date. Those that may require updating during a clinical trial are the protocol (and any amendments), the investigator's brochure, the information given to the trial subjects, regulatory and ethics committee submissions, laboratory procedures/normal ranges, and details of changes in study staff (with CVs). As an exercise in document tracking, TMF management is a skill that is acquired with training and experience.

Monitoring visit reports

Monitoring visit reports are a diary record of trial-related events recorded during visits to the investigator sites. Each visit to each site during the clinical trial must be written up by the site monitor and filed in the TMF; the clinical study manager should aim to review monitoring visit reports in a timely manner. Those from any site that is causing particular concern should be kept under close scrutiny. The monitoring visit reports also provide valuable information about the history of a centre and can be a powerful aid to future investigator selection.

Communications (other than site visits)

To run a clinical trial efficiently demands effective communication. Many people are involved in setting up and running a clinical trial and it is sometimes difficult to remember what was said and in what circumstances. The TMF should therefore contain a record of all communication relevant to the trial: file notes of all telephone calls, copies of letters, and minutes of study meetings.

When writing a letter, taking a fax, or simply confirming a monitoring visit date by telephone, each member of the clinical team must consider the importance and relevance of that communication. Does the information need to be retained and filed? Does anyone else need to be informed? Recent technological advances and a growing reliance on e-mail communication have blurred understanding of what should be held in the TMF. At the start of the trial the CTA, clinical study manager and study monitor must together agree the procedure for printing off, signing and filing e-mail communications. Company or sponsor SOPs may support this agreement. Whether they involve the investigators or simply the study team, all meetings should have agendas and their minutes should be retained. Because meetings are forums for critical discussions that can affect study procedures, timely production of minutes is strongly recommended.

Signed CRFs

In clinical research the 'product' is the data in the case record forms (CRFs). To be certain that the CRF is an accurate record of what happened to the subject during the trial, the site is routinely visited at predetermined intervals and checks are made to ensure that the data are accurate and complete. Each CRF collected and returned to the TMF (following data management processing) must have the appropriate designated signature (typically the investigator). This testifies that the subject has participated in the trial in accordance with the instructions given and under relevant supervision. The TMF will contain a CRF for every subject who gave informed consent.

CRF corrections

Even with the best intentions, mistakes may occur; this simply reflects the fact that the collection of clinical data on subjects participating in a clinical trial is a hugely complex process. CRF data have to be checked meticulously before they are collected from the investigator centre. If mistakes are not corrected before the CRF pages are collected from the investigator site, the TMF must include details of any CRF corrections made at a later time. The corrections are usually filed with the CRFs as data correction forms or data query forms.

Serious adverse event reports and safety information

The occurrence of serious adverse events (SAEs) and any relevant safety information that becomes evident during a clinical trial must be documented in the TMF – not only to ensure that the information is available immediately to anyone accessing the TMF but also to ensure that such information was recorded accurately and was available immediately following the event. Both the regulatory authorities and internal company/sponsor SOPs strictly define the timelines for SAE reporting.

Interim reports to ethics committees

Clinical trials usually begin with high levels of enthusiasm and excitement. Everyone works hard to set the study in motion and the ethics committees give approval for the study to start in a particular hospital or clinic. However, this early enthusiasm may dwindle for any of a variety of reasons: the study may be slow to get going, the principal investigator/study manager may leave, the company may no longer feel that the drug is as good as it once appeared, or recruitment may simply be poor. In the past when this happened, some studies 'disappeared' forever. To avoid the situation in which a study is conveniently forgotten, ethics committees now expect to receive an annual update on the progress of a clinical trial, focusing on safety reporting and details of any interim analysis performed. It is again the role of the CTA to ensure that these updates are filed in the TMF so that study progress reports are not overlooked.

Record of retained body fluids/tissue samples

The location of samples of body fluids or tissues taken during the clinical trial must be documented in the TMF. This applies particularly when samples (usually frozen) are 'batched' for analysis later – perhaps for a drug plasma assay or for a histological technique. Such record keeping is essential, especially now that the pharmaceutical industry is entering the growing area of genome experimentation and development.

After completion or termination of the trial

The end of recruitment in a trial often triggers the strange but predictable 'itchy feet syndrome' in the sponsor's clinical team. People want to move on to another project with all the excitement of a new venture. However, it is very important that the TMF is completed and this is not achieved until the clinical study report has been written and all the centres have been closed. The enthusiasm and excitement seen at the start of a clinical trial should be maintained until the project has been completed. The clinical team should put the champagne on ice until the TMF is ready for archiving, the activity that marks the true finishing-line. Other than those mentioned earlier, the following are the key activities that must be accomplished before the celebrations can begin.

Audit certificate

If the trial was audited, then an audit certificate should be filed in the TMF. The audit report need not be filed in the TMF (in fact, SOPs usually insist that it be filed elsewhere) but it should be available if requested by the regulatory authorities.

Final close-out report

Every investigator site should receive a final visit from the monitor to close the centre. This is not only an opportunity to collect any documents still outstanding for the TMF but also to complete the study with enthusiasm.

Clinical study report

The TMF is complete when the clinical study report (CSR) is filed. Some company or sponsor SOPs may allow the TMF to be archived prior to the completion and incorporation of the CSR. This should not be necessary because the trial metrics should support prompt completion of the CSR following study close; inevitably, however, this does not always happen. In such cases, archiving methodology should allow appropriate reuniting of the CSR and TMF in the archive.

Troubleshooting

From the discussion so far, it might appear that the management and filing activities required to produce the TMF are simply a case of following the instructions and keeping all documentation up to date. However, because clinical trials do not take place in a perfect world, there are certain pitfalls to TMF management. These are usually only discovered when the TMF is reviewed after the study has been in progress for some time or, even worse, after the study has been completed. In general, as discussed below, the three categories of defect are non-compliance with ICH GCP, missing documents, and wrongly dated documents.

- The essence of ICH GCP is to protect the rights and safety of the subject. The TMF must be organised from the outset to reflect this philosophy. ICH GCP compliance can be achieved if the TMF is reviewed periodically during the course of a study. The CTA will ensure that the essential documents are reviewed in the TMF on a regular basis. An in-house audit of the TMF should be part of the CTA's role and responsibilities.
- Often, even with regular review, the TMF may be found to lack some documents. In general, honesty is the best policy because the TMF is a reflection of how the study *actually was* conducted, not how it *should have been* conducted. In many cases, 'missing documents' turn out to be in the TMF but have been misfiled in some other volume. A file note to explain the omission or the late collection of the required document is acceptable as long as a clear explanation is given to account for chronological order inconsistencies.
- It is easy to question clinical trial conduct when the TMF contains documents that have been signed and dated but are in the wrong chronological order, e.g. the data correction form was dated *before* the investi-

gator signed the CRF; the protocol amendment was agreed by the investigator *before* the approval signatures from the sponsor company; or the subject gave informed consent *before* ethics committee approval had been granted. Many such errors are purely administrative and are simply due to human error in the process of filing: incorrectly typed numbers, confused dates, and dates that reflect that the TMF document was collected after the event. In most cases, these errors can be avoided by good TMF management throughout the course of a clinical trial. Where the chronological order of documents is not clear or indeed erroneous, it is important that this is explained in the TMF. It is better to have an explanation for errors that have occurred rather than to try to correct errors after the event.

It can be very rewarding and satisfying to review and set straight the TMF. With the help and support of the clinical research team, the CTA should have the experience and training for such a task.

CONCLUSION

Good TMF management is central to the success of every clinical trial. A well-ordered TMF, complete and accurate, reflects the way in which the trial was conducted. It mirrors the professionalism and ethical conduct of the clinical research team. It is therefore vital that responsibility for the TMF be given to one member of the team, the CTA, who will be accountable for TMF organisation and filing, among other study administration tasks. This individual will have the skills to organise the TMF so that it is easy to access, clearly labelled and user-friendly. The appearance of the TMF should create confidence in the system and in the conduct of the trial.

The TMF contains the essential documents required under ICH GCP to ensure that, in line with the Declaration of Helsinki: '... the interests of the subject must always prevail over the interests of science and society'. These essential documents fall naturally into three categories, depending on whether they are collected before, during or after completion of the clinical phase of a trial.

However, there are difficulties in TMF management and every clinical team must guard against complacency and incompetence. Careful and regular review of the TMF and diligence in collecting study documents throughout the trial will ensure that the TMF is a filing system of which the clinical team can be proud. The clinical trial is truly complete when the TMF is eventually archived. It should be the aim of every clinical team member to support and contribute to the success of the TMF: after all, as a record of the team's concerted effort, it will remain open to scrutiny for many years to come.

REFERENCE

ICH Guideline (1996). *Topic E6: Good Clinical Practice – Consolidated Guideline*, International Federation of Pharmaceutical Manufacturers Associations, Geneva (Issued as CPMP/ICH/135/95).

21

Archiving

Elizabeth Hooper

INTRODUCTION

The clinical trial process has become increasingly complex over time: as ever larger numbers of patients are recruited into clinical trials for longer periods, the accompanying volume of data and paperwork has undergone exponential growth. As clinical research costs have risen, so sponsors have become aware of the 'value' of the documents generated during the trial. Consequently, extensive archiving or document control units have been established within companies sponsoring or involved in clinical research.

Having conducted the clinical trial in accordance with appropriate good clinical practice (GCP) standards, it is essential that the sponsor is able to produce all the documentation generated during the trial in the event of inspection by the regulatory authority. Based on this documentation, it must be possible to reconstruct the clinical trial, from the clinical study protocol to first patient enrolment through to the final clinical study report, showing that the GCP guidelines and the company's own standard operating procedures (SOPs) have been adhered to, and thus providing assurance of the integrity of the data. In the event of a full audit, it may be necessary to produce all the data, or to track one specific patient's entry into and progress through the study.

While the International Conference on Harmonisation (ICH) GCP guideline (section 5.5.11) indicates that regulatory compliance is the principal reason why pharmaceutical companies archive all their data (ICH Guideline, 1996), other considerations also underlie this expensive exercise. First, the sponsor needs to retain its documentation in the event of further research with the product into different dosage regimens, or into use in other indications or other therapeutic areas. Secondly, the data may be needed to support licence applications in other parts of the world. Thirdly, it may become necessary to re-analyse the data to assist marketing departments, or to answer any questions that may arise subsequently. Finally, in cases of suspected medical fraud or other litigation, it is vital that the sponsor is able to produce all the relevant documentation.

The ICH GCP guideline (section 5.5.11) requires that the sponsor should retain essential documents for at least 2 years after the last approval of a marketing application. If the clinical development of a product is discontinued, the essential documentation needs to be retained for only 2 years. However, many companies retain this information for much longer periods, as there have been occasions when a product that was judged to have been a failure suddenly becomes the focus of a new area of research. The 'old' data then become the basis for new clinical trials. Section 8 of the ICH GCP guideline provides detailed guidance on the essential documentation that must be retained in the trial master file (TMF), together with the stipulated time periods for data retention. However, no guidance is given concerning the conditions under which and the location where this documentation should be stored. In contrast to good laboratory practice (GLP), no compulsory system yet exists for GCP inspection. The archiving of the clinical trial is therefore open to very different interpretations concerning the precise standards to be applied regarding the long-term retention of the data. It would appear that a locked cupboard controlled by a secretary might comply with the regulations equally as well as a purpose-built archive controlled by qualified staff. Many archivists believe that the regulations should be more specific about the standards to be applied to the running of the archive. As the practice of 'voluntary' GCP inspections becomes more widespread, a clearer picture will emerge concerning the archive itself and the facilities and systems deemed to constitute a secure archive. The ICH GCP guideline states that when the clinical trial is conducted by a pharmaceutical company, the sponsor is responsible for retaining all essential documentation and investigators are responsible for retaining their copies. When the pharmaceutical company uses a contract research organisation (CRO) to conduct the trial, the situation may not be so clear. The CRO may either store the data for the pharmaceutical company at the end of the trial, or arrange for all the data to be transferred to the sponsor. Demarcation of responsibilities for data retention should be defined before the contract is agreed and the contract itself should clearly state what will happen to the data at the end of the study. Since the sponsor owns the data and will have to produce the required documents for any inspection, it is customary for the sponsor to assume responsibility for the data at the end of the trial. If the CRO has suitable staffing and storage facilities, it is acceptable for the CRO to retain the data and charge the sponsor for this service.

Regardless of whether the study is conducted by the sponsor directly or via a CRO, the archiving of the study documentation must be planned from the inception of the trial. Ideally, the archivist should be a member of the study team and thus be aware of the volume of data to be deposited in the archive and of the relevant timelines. In reality, however, the archivist's first involvement in the study is often signalled by the arrival of numerous boxes in the archive. This lack of foresight complicates the planning of space allocation and staff resources. An archivist who is a full member of the study team can plan for the documentation to be processed into the archive system. The benefits of this are four-fold in that the archivist is familiar with the protocol and study plan (e.g. required patient populations, number of participating centres); informed concerning the idiosyncrasies of the case record form (CRF); aware of regional variations for document requirements overseas where local GCP guidelines may differ; and able to advise investigators on storage and archiving systems, thus ensuring compliance.

THE ARCHIVE

Typically, guidelines and SOPs do not stipulate the conditions under which essential documents should be stored. However, since it would be futile to keep the data for long periods of time if they can no longer be read when the documents are needed, the archive must provide the best possible conditions for paper preservation. Two separate aspects are involved here: one relates to the environmental conditions most conducive to the long-term storage of the data and the other to the security of the data whilst in the archive.

Paper is usually considered to be readable for 25 years but, if kept under unsuitable conditions, this period is much reduced. An archived faint bottom copy of a no-carbon-required (NCR) CRF will not retain its legibility as long as a high-quality printed original. A document that is illegible when deposited in the archive will still be illegible when it is retrieved.

The size of the archive to be provided depends very much on the number and size of the clinical trials being sponsored by the company. For a very small company running single-centre studies that recruit only a few patients, it may well be acceptable to provide lockable fire-retardant cupboards under the control of a nominated individual (e.g. the librarian). These may provide all the long-term storage that is necessary. However, for larger sponsor companies and CROs, a dedicated room or rooms will be necessary. For a pharmaceutical company storing all its own data on site, the archive can range from a couple of rooms, through a dedicated Portakabin® specially adapted as an archive, to a separate, purpose-built archive, with suitable accommodation for staff and space for many years' documentation.

The areas designated for use as archive space are frequently chosen because of the erroneous perception of an archive as a damp 'black hole' where data are dumped into oblivion. The archive must provide an environment that is secure from the threat of water. A basement location, for example, has a number of disadvantages. The presence of water (e.g. ornamental lake, river or canal) on or near the site will expose the basement to a potential risk of flooding. Basements usually accommodate water and central heating pipes that service the whole building, and again there is the inherent danger of leakage and flooding. Conversely, an archive located in the basement can solve the problem of floor loadings – paper is heavy, and compact storage racking often produces weight levels that exceed the load-bearing capabilities of the flooring. An archive housed on an upper floor requires reinforced flooring, which is an expensive structural modification. If the building has no lift, it is preferable for the archive to be located on the ground floor, thus eliminating the need for large numbers of boxes of data to be carried up and down stairs.

One of the most important considerations concerns the size of the archive. It needs to be sufficiently large for the data it currently has to store, and there must be vacant space so that data from future trials can be added. Although no firm recommendations exist as to the spare capacity of an archive to accommodate future holdings, it is generally felt that space for 5 years' growth is optimal.

To ensure the long-term preservation of paper, it is important that certain conditions are maintained in the archive. The British Standards Institution (BSI) has produced a set of recommendations detailing the ideal environmental conditions for the storage and exhibition of archival documents (British Standards Institution, 2000). First, extremes and large variations of temperature must be avoided: ideally, paper should be stored at between 13°C and 18°C. It is also important that humidity, which leads to the formation of mould, is kept low (preferably between 55 and 65%). A thermometer and a hygrometer should be placed in the archive to allow temperature and humidity to be monitored on a weekly basis. However, if the temperature or humidity rises outside these normal ranges, this should be recorded along with the reasons for the changes. Air should circulate around the archive and be filtered to remove dust particles.

Adherence to these environmental conditions will also help to deter the varieties of pests that find archives to be desirable residences. Mice, cockroaches, book lice and their ilk essentially look for warmth and a supply of food. Paper or cardboard provide a gourmet feast. In addition, mice tend to chew at electrical cabling, with the attendant danger of fire. Regular inspections of archived documentation should be made to check for signs of pest activity.

Documents are conventionally stored on some form of racking in boxes clear of the ground to allow air to circulate. Boxes of a uniform size should be used to ensure the most economical use of storage space. Several companies produce archiving boxes and racking for libraries and archives (see list of suppliers at the end of this chapter). Racking systems may range from relatively basic designs to mobile racking that allows for the largest volume of data to be stored in the most compact area. The latest forms of mobile racking are motorised (a benefit much appreciated by staff who would otherwise have to crank the shelving by hand) and can incorporate systems to assist retrievals. Whichever type of racking is chosen, a system of identifiers must be used so that a box or a file has one specific location within the archive.

To minimise the risk of injuries and accidents, all staff should receive training in correct techniques for lifting and moving archive boxes. Boxes should not have to be lifted above shoulder height. Steps must be provided for access to higher shelves. Helpful information is available in the UK from the Health & Safety Executive (1993), and the International Organization for Standardization (ISO) (1998) has issued a guide to manual handling.

The security of the archive and the documents held there is of paramount importance. Only the archive staff should have access to the archive and all entry into the archive should be logged. The archiving SOP should clearly state who is authorised to enter the archive, who may recall documents, and whether originals or photocopies only will be provided. If original documentation is loaned out, the loan period should be defined and systems should be in place for chasing overdue material.

The storage conditions best suited for the preservation of paper do not provide comfortable working conditions for archive staff. Therefore, another room, preferably adjoining or adjacent to the archive, needs to be provided where the archive staff can prepare the documents for archiving. Ideally, all paper clips, staples or other metallic means of attaching paper together should be removed, to prevent rusting or other chemical deterioration. Rubber bands perish and should not be used and plastic wallets should be avoided because they encourage condensation and hence mould growth. Any documentation on thermal paper must be copied before archiving.

Within this same area the staff can service requests for information or for retrievals from the archive. In addition to keeping records of what material has been requested and by whom, most archives keep a statistical record of archive usage. If the company microfilms its documents, microfilm readers can be sited in this area, along with a desk for inquirers to refer to archive material that is not available for loan. Some companies have an in-house facility for making microform back-ups of paper documentation. The archive staff area should be used to house such a unit and for cataloguing and indexing newly deposited material.

When to archive

The ICH GCP guideline makes no reference as to the most appropriate time to archive the clinical trial. Two different schools of thought exist. Either the documents are not sent to the archive until the end of the study, when all trial-related activity has finished; or a central document unit collects all the essential documentation as the trial progresses.

Under the first system, the TMF remains with the clinical team until the end of the trial. The clinical team will be responsible for maintaining the file and for checking its completeness before transferring the TMF to the archive. When this system is adopted, data managers and statisticians will usually send their data to archive separately and often at a later date than the clinical team.

This is not necessarily a problem but misunderstandings and oversights may arise. With this system, the archive staff may well be actively involved in chasing documentation and in ensuring that the clinical and biometric teams do not duplicate effort when providing material to be archived.

With the alternative approach, all documentation pertaining to the trial is first sent to the central document (or pre-archive) unit where it is identified and filed in the TMF. The document can either be scanned, so it is available to monitors and statisticians via their personal computer, or a photocopy can be supplied. This system has the advantage that all original documents are kept safely on file from the outset. The documents should not become damaged or lost during the trial, filing is undertaken by specialist staff (thus minimising the possibility of incorrect filing), and any missing documentation is flagged before the end of the trial. Monitors and statisticians know at the end of the trial that any documents in their own personal files are only copies and can be safely destroyed. The TMF is already logged into the archive and only has to be moved from a pre-archive, i.e. current filing system, over to the 'deep' archive, i.e. the inactive section. The only real disadvantage with collating all the data under this system is the resource required to implement the scheme, thus making it the more expensive alternative. The pre-archiving stage requires specialist staff to maintain and log the files, and to provide the copies requested by the clinical team.

The system to be followed must be clearly specified within an SOP. A written procedure must state precisely who is responsible for the documentation at each stage of its life. The SOP should also define responsibilities for checking the files for completeness and for acquiring any missing essential documents. The SOP must also clearly stipulate the point in the process at which the TMF becomes the responsibility of the archivist. This is particularly important in multinational trials where potential problems may arise over which documents are to be retained centrally and which documents need to be retained in the country of origin to comply with local regulatory requirements.

INDEXING AND CATALOGUING

The sheer volume of paperwork to be stored demands that meticulous attention is paid to the logging, indexing and tracking of the data. Data retention is pointless if a particular document cannot be located precisely and within a reasonable time period when requested. Most archives will have a service agreement with other departments stating what is considered to be a reasonable amount of time for retrieval of data. Depending upon the type and complexity of the request, this might vary from 2 hours for the simple retrieval of one sheet of paper from an on-site archive to a week for the research and retrieval of an item stored off-site.

The procedure for depositing data in the archive will cover all aspects of checking, logging and indexing of the documents. When the archive boxes are packed, a detailed list of the boxed contents must be produced. If the archive staff have not packed the boxes, then their first task is to check the contents of the box against the listing provided. Any discrepancies must be noted, investigated and corrected. Each box is assigned a number to enable it to be distinguished from all other boxes. Sometimes this number is purely an acquisition number (i.e. the one-hundredth box deposited in the archive is box number 100). Sometimes the numbering also includes a location code, so that the location of the box in the archive is fixed at the same time. Many archives incorporate bar-coding into their labelling system to help with the tracking of boxes. A very small archive can manage with less complex systems.

Most indexing systems incorporate details of drug number, generic name, trade name if applicable, study number, investigator name and centre number, clinical monitor name, the therapeutic indication, and other drugs used in the trial. Numerous computerised systems are available for controlling the archive, either using an off-the-shelf software package, or using a purpose-built database. Many companies compromise by adapting a standard system (e.g. Oracle or Microsoft® Access) and tailoring it to suit their particular requirements.

MICROFORMS

The vast amount of paperwork generated during the course of a clinical trial has led some pharmaceutical companies to turn to alternative methods of data storage, the most widely used being microfilm or microfiche. A roll of microfilm can hold 2500 A4 pages of information, filmed as one page per frame. This is equivalent to the contents of a standard archive box ($12 \times 12 \times 17$ in or $30 \times 30 \times 42$ cm) or approximately 1 m of shelving. Microfiche consists of cards approximately 6×4 in (15×10 cm) containing 24 pages of information. This medium is commonly used for archiving journals and published articles. Although microfilming technology has been available since the 1950s, microform use became particularly popular in the 1970s. Data stored in this way may be accessed simply with a microform reader incorporating a light source and a form of magnification. Unlike computer technology, where early systems are now completely obsolete, microfilming has stood the test of time. If kept under correct conditions, microforms have a much longer life span than paper, with claims (as yet unverifiable!) that they remain readable for 100 years. Microform is legally acceptable in court proceedings and has been used by financial institutions and the legal profession for many years.

Although the current ICH GCP guideline contains no specific reference to microforms, the earlier Committee for Proprietary Medicinal Products (CPMP) note for guidance on GCP states in section 3.17 that archived data may be held on microfiche or electronic record, provided that a back-up exists and that hard copy can be obtained from it if required (Committee for Proprietary Medicinal Products, 1991). This statement implies that while data may be microfilmed, the original paper copy needs to be retained. In practice, pharmaceutical companies with a policy of microfilming still retain the original paper copies, usually in a secure deep archive. This reduces the volume of storage space needed on site, and the original hard copies can be retrieved from the deep archive if needed for an inspection. For added security, some companies make a working copy of the microfilm, while retaining the master film in a fire-proof safe, often at a remote location. Paper copies are easily produced from either microfilm or microfiche, but the process is very time-consuming if large volumes are printed.

The decision in favour of microfilm or microfiche depends on the purpose to which the copies are to be put. Specific references can be accessed more rapidly with microfiche and, if used simply to consult written or printed information, this may be the better option. Since many medical journals have long been available in this form, companies may already possess a microfiche reader. However, if the purpose is to retain a copy that is legally acceptable in court, then microfilm is the preferred medium. Whereas with microfiche, for example, another card may be substituted within a set of CRF pages, with microfilm it would be immediately apparent that tampering had occurred. The roll of film has running frame numbers along its edge, making any editing very obvious because frames cannot be removed or inserted without being detected. The edge numbers on the roll of microfilm can also form the basis of an indexing system. This can range from a very simple listing of which document starts at which particular frame number, which is then located manually, to computer-assisted viewers that will locate the required document.

If the microfilm is to be used as a legally acceptable copy, then an SOP will be required to ensure that the documents are properly prepared and to guarantee the authenticity of the film. Prior to microfilming, the paperwork must be free of paperclips and staples and checked for completeness: missing documents cannot be added later. The producer of the microfilm, either an in-house unit or, more commonly, a specialist contractor, will issue a certificate of authenticity stating that all paperwork submitted has been copied without amendment or omission. After microfilming, the film should be quality-checked for legibility and completeness. Any edits or camera problems (e.g. fogging) must be noted by the camera operator. A certificate of acceptance is then produced, and this should be retained together with the certificate of authenticity.

Many larger pharmaceutical companies have their own microfilming units. This ensures the confidentiality and security of the data, as the documentation does not have to be transported off-site to a bureau for filming. However, this advantage is offset by the considerable costs of purchasing and maintaining specialist filming equipment and of employing permanent staff, particularly if the flow of documents to be filmed is not constant. Microfilming bureaux are able to guarantee work that conforms to legally admissible standards (International Organization for Standardization, 1990; British Standards Institution, 1991), they use the latest equipment and their staff are experienced in the production of microforms. It is usually more cost-effective to take out a contract with a microfilming bureau than to set up an in-house unit. For the pharmaceutical company, as hinted above, the biggest disadvantage of the contract bureaux can be the perceived lack of control over the documentation while it is *en route* to the microfilming company and during the filming process itself. However, because these companies are experienced in handling confidential and valuable data, they have evolved their own stringent security procedures.

Microfilming can be particularly appropriate when research into an investigational drug is abandoned. According to the ICH GCP guideline (section 5.5.8), the sponsor should maintain all sponsor-specific essential documents for at least 2 years after formal discontinuation. Companies are often reluctant to discard all the information that has accumulated, and yet paper storage is expensive. Under these circumstances, a microfilmed copy provides an excellent solution. No data are lost, but storage space is minimised. If all paper copies are destroyed, a certificate of destruction must be issued, and this is to be retained together with the certificates of authenticity and acceptance. Retention schedules specific to the company's needs must be prepared, indicating how long microform and electronic records should be kept.

ELECTRONIC ARCHIVING

While most pharmaceutical companies have systems in place to retain their paper archives, not all have extended these systems to include electronic data. With increasing use of computers by staff at every stage of the clinical trial process, vast databases and files are now produced during the conduct of the trial. With the acceptance of electronic signatures and the growing practice of faxing CRF pages directly into a personal computer, there are times when the sponsor will not have a paper copy. In such cases, the raw data will be the electronic file. Many companies, particularly those with US markets, are considering ways of addressing the issues surrounding electronic signatures and electronic GCP-compliant records (Code of Federal Regulations, 1997).

Electronic archiving has remained relatively under-utilised for two main reasons. First, the organisation of the electronic archive does not usually fall within the remit of the GCP archivist, but is more often seen as the responsibility of the information technology (IT) department. Secondly, as computer hardware has evolved so rapidly, major problems have arisen in identifying a data preservation format that will be readable even in 5 years' time. As the provision of server memory space has become much less expensive, many companies have simply added another server to support the system instead of addressing the root of the problem.

The larger volumes of data that can be stored on a CD-ROM (compact disc – read-only memory) have made this the ideal medium for the storage of archive data. A CD-ROM can hold 650 megabytes of memory; this is equivalent to 400 floppy disks. The equipment is relatively inexpensive, CD writers are easy to use and can be added to any modern computer, and the CD itself is relatively inexpensive. However, the major question about the lifetime of a CD has still to be answered. Also, even if the hardware that allows them to be read survives, will CDs themselves stand the test of time? The latest development is the digital versatile disc (DVD): the discs hold four times as much information as a CD, and a DVD writer can also be added to any modern personal computer. With so much uncertainty over formats and the rapidly evolving technology, many companies prefer to rely on the tried and tested format of microfilm. The BSI has produced a code of practice regarding the legal admissibility of information stored on electronic document management systems (British Standards Institution, 1996).

OFF-SITE STORAGE

With such large volumes of data having to be retained for long periods, many companies have come to utilise the services of specialist contract storage depots. These contract depots offer economical rates for storage, with guaranteed retrieval times, and are usually able to return data within 24 hours. While provision may also exist for emergency retrievals within 2 hours and for retrievals at weekends and bank holidays, these special services can be very expensive.

Before a storage company is selected, the warehouse should be visited and checked for suitability by the archivist and, ideally, by a member of the Clinical Quality Assurance (CQA) department. It is important that the off-site storage facility offers the same environmental conditions as those necessary for a company archive, i.e. temperature and humidity control, racking clear of the ground, no water pipes, etc. Security guards should provide 24-hour cover, with closed-circuit TV and fire prevention/detection systems in place. The facility must be equipped with a gaseous extinguishing system: water-based systems are to be avoided. Any authorised visitors to the storage facility should be accompanied at all times. The storage company should also only allow previously nominated staff from the pharmaceutical company to have access to the data. Since the larger storage companies may have warehouses at several different locations, it is important to inspect the particular site where the data are to be stored. Concerns have been expressed that although the pharmaceutical archivist may have inspected a particular site, another site may be substituted if the first site becomes full. This can sometimes be without the knowledge or approval of the pharmaceutical company.

Most storage companies bar-code boxes to reduce the chances of incorrect filing. They also offer on-line access to their database of archive holdings, allowing for direct retrievals by their clients. While most companies will return a whole box when requested, some will remove files from boxes and fax individual pages to the client. Where appropriate, review dates can be incorporated into the database to facilitate recognition of time-expired boxes.

In addition to storing paper copies, most storage companies can accommodate CDs or back-up tapes/disks. They will also arrange for the secure disposal of confidential data and issue certificates of destruction.

INVESTIGATOR ARCHIVES

According to the ICH GCP guideline (section 4.9.5), investigators are required to retain all documentation pertaining to the clinical trial for 2 years after the last marketing application in an ICH region. With the burgeoning paperwork generated by a clinical trial, and especially as CRFs grow larger, often running to three or four hardbound volumes, investigators find it difficult to store the documentation for the required period of time. The archiving of data by investigators should be to the same standard as that applied by the sponsor company. This means the provision of a secure, hazard-free environment with documents adequately indexed to facilitate retrieval.

If an essential document cannot be found during an audit or regulatory inspection, it is the sponsor's expensive clinical trial that is in jeopardy. It is therefore in the sponsor company's interests to assist investigators in fulfilling their obligations regarding the long-term storage of data. Particular problems may arise with continued storage of documentation when an investigator leaves a hospital or retires. It is also difficult for the sponsor to be certain that the investigator site is still fulfilling its archiving obligations many years after completion of the clinical trial. However, if investigators only have to store the patient identifiers and consent forms, archiving is more likely to be successful than if they have to store all the documentation. As to the problem of storing the bulky CRFs, one solution is for them to be microfilmed, either by the investigator or by the sponsor company. The investigator retains a cartridge of microfilm or microfiche and the paper copies can then be destroyed, although there is no published evidence that this is acceptable to the GCP inspectors. Alternatively, the sponsor company can arrange for the CRFs to be stored, either in an archive specifically designated for this purpose or at a document storage centre. If this method of storage is chosen, the boxes should be packed and listed by the study site personnel, and sealed and signed by the investigator to ensure the integrity of the data. The investigator's copies must be stored separately and independently from the sponsor company's copies. It is vital that there is no suggestion that the sponsor might be able to alter or amend the information on the CRFs or in the files.

Investigators should be informed about the location of their data and the recall procedure. If the study documentation is required for an inspection or audit, then the sealed box should be returned to the investigator. Only the investigator or study site personnel are authorised to open the box. It is the sponsor's responsibility to inform the investigator in writing as to when the documents no longer need to be retained and may therefore be destroyed.

CONCLUSION

The increasing costs of running clinical trials, together with the requirement to implement the ICH GCP guideline, have made pharmaceutical companies more aware of the importance of archiving. Most companies now employ an archivist. The larger pharmaceutical companies often have large document centres, with in-house facilities for scanning and microfilming. Ideally, the archivist should be regarded as a full member of the clinical study team.

As more and more companies appointed members of staff to have specific responsibility for their archives, either on a full- or part-time basis, it became apparent that there was a need for these individuals to meet, share knowledge, and discuss common issues and problems. The Scientific Archivists Group (SAG) was formed in 1981 by a small group of archivists working in the pharmaceutical industry. Most of the original members came from the GLP side of the industry, that being the area most closely regulated in the early 1980s. Now, however, the membership is drawn from GLP, GMP and GCP disciplines. The aims of the group are to develop the professional status of its members, to improve the status of archiving, and to ensure that archives meet business, scientific and regulatory needs. The programme of regular meetings and training sessions is particularly beneficial for archivists working in isolation and provides ample opportunity for networking. Further information about SAG is available on: http://website.lineone.net/~sagroup.

LIST OF SUPPLIERS AND STORAGE PROVIDERS

The following companies supply archiving stationery, shelving and storage facilities. Inclusion on (or exclusion from) this list does not constitute a recommendation (or otherwise).

Archiving stationery and shelving

Rackline Systems Storage Ltd (tel. 01782 777666; http://www.rackline.co.uk)
Norfolk Storage Equipment Ltd (tel. 01953 458800; http://www.nsel.co.uk)
Kardex Systems (UK) Ltd (tel. 020 8885 5588; http://www.kardex.com)
Index Storage Systems Ltd (tel. 01425 656991; http://www.indexss.co.uk)

Nord-Plan Storage Systems (tel. 01293 776795; http://www.nord-plan.com)

Cave Tab plc (tel. 0800 616347; http://www.cavetab.plc.uk)

Southern Business Systems Inc. (tel. (+1) 770 416 6515;
  http://www.sbssolutions.com)

Storage facilities

Arkheion Storage (tel. 01480 8616881)

Iron Mountain (tel. 020 7633 9053; http://www.ironmountain.com)

Hays Information Management (tel. 020 8848 0226;
  http://www.hays-energy.com)

Box-It (tel. 01962 774536; http://www.boxit.co.uk)

Datacare Records Management Ltd (tel. 01869 233055;
  http://www.datacareltd.com)

Southern File and Data Management (tel. 01189 759200;
  http://www.sfdm.co.uk)

MJF Data Management (tel. 01895 909050; http://www.mjfdata.co.uk)

REFERENCES

British Standards Institution (1991). *British Standard 6498:1991 – Guide to Preparation of Microfilm and other Microforms that may be Required as Evidence*, British Standards Institution, London.

British Standards Institution (1996). *Code of Practice for Legal Admissibility of Information Stored on Electronic Document Management Systems*, British Standards Institution, London.

British Standards Institution (2000). *British Standard 5454: 2000 – Recommendations for the Storage and Exhibition of Archival Documents*, British Standards Institution, London.

Code of Federal Regulations (1997). 21 CFR Part 11: Electronic records; electronic signatures. *Federal Register* **62**, 13429–13466.

Committee for Proprietary Medicinal Products (CPMP) Working Party on Efficacy of Medicinal Products (1991). *Good Clinical Practice for Trials on Medicinal Products in the European Community* [111/3976/88–EN Final], European Commission, Brussels.

Health and Safety Executive (1993). *Lighten the Load. Guidance for Employers on Musculoskeletal Disorders*, HSE pamphlet IND(G)109L(rev), Sheffield.

ICH Guideline (1996). *Topic E6: Good Clinical Practice – Consolidated Guideline*, International Federation of Pharmaceutical Manufacturers Associations, Geneva, (Issued as CPMP/ICH/135/95).

International Organization for Standardization (1990). *ISO/TR 10200: Legal Admissibility of Microforms*, International Organization for Standardization, Geneva.

International Organization for Standardization (1998). *ISO/DIS 11228–1: Ergonomics – Manual Handling. Part 1: Lifting and Carrying*, International Organization for Standardization, Geneva.

22

Outsourcing clinical research projects

Wolfgang Schaub

UNDERSTANDING THE REASONS FOR OUTSOURCING

Response to external and internal pressures

Increasing requirements in terms of study complexity, human resources and material, as well as tighter than ever competition, and the restructuring of research and development (R&D) away from classical chemistry towards molecular modelling and other modern and more productive technologies, have made it necessary for the pharmaceutical industry and, more specifically, clinical development to focus on those areas that can best be carried out with internally available resources, and to contract out or 'outsource' the rest (*outsourcing* = outside resource utilisation).

The nature of outsourcing in clinical development

In this respect, the pharmaceutical industry is following the historical example of other (primarily commodity-based) industries where defined sections of the value chain have been *permanently* transferred externally, or economically independent companies have been separated and linked to the parent organisation through a *continuous* support contract. In clinical development, outsourcing has currently only reached the form of *case-by-case* contracting (Schaub, 1999). Individual activity packages that cannot be moved around swiftly in-house are identified on an *ad hoc* basis and are contracted out to contract research organisations (CROs). Once this activity has been completed, the next contract may be with a different CRO, and so on (Macarthur, 1994).

Worldwide, clinical trial services are provided by some 1000 CROs with varying capabilities, ranging from two-employee local companies to global enterprises with up to 20 000 employees. The individual, highly diversified nature of clinical trials makes *contracting* the preferred option over rigorous outsourcing in the classical sense.

Recognising and overcoming barriers to the outsourcing idea

In scenarios where, in principle, every clinical trial is carried out in-house, the only candidates considered for contracting out are those that go beyond available resource requirements (Figure 1). Seen in these terms, outsourcing remains purely reactive: only projects causing resource constraints are contracted out, whether or not they are suitable for a CRO to handle. This is the accidental, unplanned, *tactical* form of outsourcing.

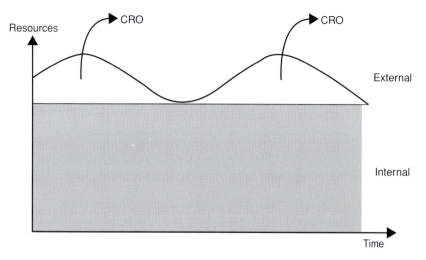

Figure 1. Tactical outsourcing.

Historically, tactical outsourcing was the prevailing form in the 1980s and early 1990s, especially in the larger sponsor companies. Outsourcing was often unpopular because it took work away from project teams and generated existential worries. In addition, working with a partner required skills other than those dictated by good clinical practice (GCP) and achieved by common training on a specific project. Many project managers found it difficult to relinquish direct hands-on involvement and move to hands-off management of an external partner. And unfortunately, CROs that should have assumed a partnership role often failed to come up to performance expectations.

Costing a fully overheaded project

Most sponsor companies faced with the need to contract out were initially surprised when they saw the seemingly high charges made by CROs. They had to learn how to calculate their in-house costs correctly, i.e. by adding in all overheads and management costs, before they could compare them with a CRO's cost estimates. Basically, they also had to learn how to calculate costs in an area whose prime direction was spending rather than earning money, since earnings come through the company's sales. Even if all cost contributors were known, the sensitivity of internal costing usually remained imprecise because these calculations were made top-down. In contrast, CROs have been accustomed from the outset to costing all sorts of items, and since they earned their living directly from what they did, their costing was bottom-up and therefore more accurate.

Moreover, sponsors had to learn and appreciate that CROs had to make a profit and that the very act of contracting out costs something: selecting the CRO, negotiating the project, preparing a contract, managing the project remotely – all these tie up resources and are therefore cost factors.

When in-house costs were then compared with the range of prices quoted by CROs, the two often turned out to be quite similar (Hill and Hubbard, 1996). The range of CRO price quotations, however, appeared wide at first glance, thus inducing sponsors to choose the lowest bidder, regardless of other selection criteria that would often speak in favour of a more expensive option. This has often been an important source of frustration, leading to uneasiness and lack of trust between sponsors and CROs.

Understanding internal/external cost comparisons and tactical outsourcing

Sponsors do not often realise their lack of freedom: once they are in a competitive situation and once the task considered for contracting out is on the critical path, there is no alternative other than to outsource. In such a situation, CROs can create immense value because they are ready to start work immediately. If this value is expressed in terms of time saved to market, its cash equivalents can be higher by many factors than the price charged by the CRO. For example, a study may cost USD 5 million; if time-critical, contracting out this study may save one year of development time for the product. Over the entire product life cycle, being on the market one year earlier than the competition may generate USD 100 million of additional profits. Seen in this light, it is of little importance whether the study costs USD 5 or 6 million (Schaub, 2000). Moreover, differences in the prices quoted by competing CROs pale into insignificance when compared with the potential value of working with a CRO. A sponsor who has received offers from two CROs and takes 2 weeks to evaluate them, will lose more than the price difference between CRO 1 and CRO 2. In conclusion, the CRO selected should be the one that offers the best technical, scientific and geographical capability to carry out the project and that has the best possible people to handle the task. Price is a relatively minor factor among the selection criteria, and sponsors should not spend more time than absolutely necessary in analysing prices charged by CROs. Analysis should focus instead on the activities that make up the price. A first-class service inevitably costs more, but high-quality products (data) make their way through the regulatory channels more easily than dubious, possibly deficient material.

The lesson is that tactical outsourcing saves time (while the CRO is working, in-house staff can address other issues) and generates value.

INTRODUCING STRATEGIC CONCEPTS TO OUTSOURCING

The benefits of tactical outsourcing can be increased even further if consideration is given to using CROs continuously instead of only occasionally (Colburn *et al.*, 1997). In this way, CROs will come on to the scene not only as an emergency rescue team; instead they will be actively sought *in advance* of a contracting event. Outsourcing will thus not only function as a safety valve to relieve the sponsor, but the sponsor will seek the CRO's assistance to create a business opportunity and invite them to be partners in the venture (Wyse and Hughes, 1993).

Piecemeal contracting v. outsourcing of larger packages

The act of contracting out requires the same processes, regardless of whether one small activity or an entire development programme is involved: definition of project specifications, searching for the best CRO, requesting and evaluating proposals, awarding and managing the project. These activities cost time and money although they are not directly productive; they merely mediate the generation of clinical trial data. Costs of this nature are called *transactional costs* and include an element of basic cost that is independent of the size of the contract. Therefore, what can be gained by simply increasing the size of the outsourced work packages? Clearly, it makes little sense to break a project down into many individual items and to contract these out one by one. It is far more sensible to contract out packages that are so large that the cost of the contracting process as such remains negligible. In other words, the ratio between transactional and productive costs should remain as small as possible.

Casual contracting v. outsourcing strings of similar work

Clinical development can be expressed in terms of activities, processes, studies, entire development projects (i.e. the total of all studies leading to a marketed product), development phases (I, II, III and IV), and therapeutic areas. In each of these categories there are elements that are more or less similar or adjacent (Schaub, 1998a). Those similar/adjacent elements should

Table 1. Casual contracting v. outsourcing similar/adjacent elements.

Instead of contracting out only:	Contract out:
Investigator identification	Investigator identification *plus* prequalification, collection of critical documents, ethics approval procedures because all these activities involve the study sites
Monitoring	Monitoring *plus* data management and statistics: this will leave data generation and work-up in one place
A single study	All studies in a project because the CRO will become familiar with the project
Phase II	Phase II *plus* Phases III and IV because all phases may be in the same kind of patients
A single project	All projects within the entire therapeutic area if the best expertise is available outside

therefore be combined to form a string and the whole string should be contracted out rather than its individual elements (see Table 1).

Setting criteria for outsourcing policies

In a pharmaceutical company the setting of such criteria requires management direction (Hadfield *et al.*, 1998). The issue can be approached on many levels and the optimum is probably a mix of all levels; decisions taken for one therapeutic area may not apply for another. Dermatology, for example, may be regarded as less important to the strategic interests of the company. The company does not have in-house dermatology experts and dermatology studies are comparatively straightforward: the best decision may then be to outsource the entire therapeutic area. Cardiovascular disease, however, may be a core competency of the company, experts are available in-house, and the studies are complex: the most appropriate decision in this case may be to outsource individual study activities only. Company management should structure its attitude towards outsourcing and cast this into a transparent, enforceable policy. If management ignores this and leaves outsourcing decisions to individual project teams, the company may not be able to progress beyond tactical outsourcing.

IDENTIFYING WHAT IS BEST TO CONTRACT OUT

As a matter of principle (not of constraint), the search for a strategic concept to outsourcing must also identify what CROs can do as well as, or better than, the pharmaceutical company and *vice versa* (Schaub, 1998b). The strategy must also seek to minimise transaction costs and to render the outsourcing process as smooth as possible.

The general rule calls for the separation of all those items that are best kept in-house: this will be everything that is highly complex, highly specific, rarely encountered, non-standard, highly uncertain in its development, highly relevant strategically, and with an unfavourable legal and/or technological framework. In contrast, everything that is of minimal complexity or specificity, occurs repeatedly, is highly standardised, straightforward and of little strategic relevance, and has a favourable legal and/or technological framework can be considered for outsourcing. In short, core competencies should be retained but all generic work should be outsourced.

Again, the solution may be sought at various levels: individual activities within studies v. entire studies v. individual processes across all studies v. entire projects v. development phases across all projects v. therapeutic areas (see Table 2).

Table 2. Examples to illustrate insourcing v. outsourcing decisions.

	May be kept in-house:	May be outsourced:
Individual activities within studies	Protocol development Writing the investigator's brochure Writing expert reports	Monitoring Data management Medical report writing to templates
Entire studies	Short Intensive care Involving treatment decision trees	Long-term General practice Unidirectional treatments
Individual processes across all studies	Project planning Obtaining product-related expert advice	Travel Transport Transformation of data into information
Entire projects	New chemical entities (NCEs) Novel indications	Line extensions Follow-up indications
Development phases across all projects	Phase I first dose in man Pharmacodynamics Phase II/early Phase III	Phase I kinetics/bioavailability Late Phase III/Phase IV
Therapeutic areas	Oncology	Dermatology

DETERMINING THE OVERALL PROPORTION TO BE OUTSOURCED

Unfortunately, the examples given above cannot be generalised. The dividing line between in-house and external work depends on company size, history, current status and degree of self-confidence. Small and start-up companies tend to outsource more than large, established R&D-oriented ones; companies that have done everything in-house in the past will approach CROs more hesitantly than open, co-operative organisations; companies in a transitional and restructuring phase will outsource more than settled ones; and finally, management that is prepared to take a conscious risk will promote outsourcing more enthusiastically than anxious or less experienced management.

Linking outsourced packages to form a continuous stream

Once any outsourced project approaches completion, it is a good idea to consider using the same CRO again for a similar follow-up project, even if the performance of the CRO did not appear optimal. In most cases, careful analysis will reveal that the reasons for performance complaints have their roots in both partners, and not in the CRO alone. Both partners have to go through a process of getting acquainted and learning to co-operate with one another before they come up to speed. Using the same team again reduces the next learning curve and gives a morale boost to the team members. The optimum is a sponsor thoughtful enough to appreciate that the assignment of a continuous stream of similar work packages to the same CRO may support the business better than causing disruptions between one project and the next by changing CROs in mid-stream.

Assessing the risks and benefits of strategic outsourcing

How much a company decides to outsource in relation to what remains in-house also depends on the risk that the company is prepared to take. In assessing core competencies, there will usually be narrow zones for which the decision is clear, and a broad middle zone for which the decision will be difficult. Managers have to weigh the potential benefits of advanced strategic outsourcing against the danger that outsourcing too much may erode the company's competency platform. In any event, the company should retain a minimum level of highly experienced resource for each competency field, so that rescue operations can be conducted if the CRO unexpectedly fails to deliver. Core competencies should also reside in more than one person so that continuity is guaranteed if one individual leaves the organisation.

Putting all your eggs in one basket

Devising and applying outsourcing policies based on core competencies is commendable as long as the company views itself as a closed entity. In reality, however, companies compete with others and are thus exposed to situations beyond their control. Companies sometimes therefore have to react swiftly in response to fierce competitive pressures. At such times, the best policy may be to 'put all your eggs in one basket', i.e. the critical project has to be developed with *all* available capacity. Even if it falls into the category of 'best kept in-house', the overriding priority of the project may mean that as many external resources as possible need to be taken on board.

Leveraging the maximum cost efficiency in strategic sourcing

Applying a strategy to outsourcing means reducing the prevalence of tactical scenarios (although they will never disappear completely) in favour of a more strategic use of resources. Whether these resources are internal or external no longer plays a fundamental role. Resources optimal for the efficient conduct of the desired project mix are then taken from whatever source. Hence, it is fair to abandon the prefix 'out' and to speak instead of strategic sourcing. Strategic sourcing may seem at first sight to imply that fewer resources than before may be required to carry out the remaining in-house tasks (see Figure 2 and compare with Figure 1).

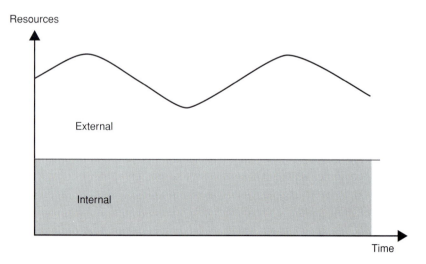

Figure 2. Strategic sourcing.

However, it would be more accurate to say that with strategic sourcing more projects than before can be carried out with the same internal staff levels. The only shift is in the ratio between internal and external, not in the absolute headcount.

In order for this to work, two conditions have to be fulfilled:

- Staff with functions that are no longer required have to be converted into staff with core competencies. This is not always easily achievable, and sufficient time must be allowed for the change process to be accepted by all involved.
- Developing more projects than before requires an initial investment that has to pay off in the medium term. For example, strategic sourcing with considerable CRO involvement opens up the possibility of developing multiple products at the same time (not just one), and multiple indications and line extensions for one product simultaneously (rather than consecutively). This brings the possibility that more products will reach the market faster.

While the investment in strategic sourcing should remain small (e.g. of the order of millions of USD/GBP), the medium-term return on that investment may be many times higher (e.g. of the order of hundreds of millions).

DEFINING ROLES AND PERSONS INVOLVED

When two partners have to find each other, one usually takes the initiative. In the sponsor – CRO relationship, the initiator is the sponsor when a specific project is to be contracted out and it is the business development manager of the CRO who 'markets' the service profile. Unfortunately, the relationship is complex and requires more than just two people in dialogue.

Enforcing strategic sourcing across the organisation

In the past, the sponsor company management alone decided when and what to outsource. The sponsor's project managers, each one often acting in isolation, were in charge (often reluctantly) of selecting the CRO. Over time, this situation produced a chaotic network of connections between various project managers and CROs, particularly in large companies. Conflicting opinions prevailed about which CRO to choose and 'old-boy networks' were not unusual. The situation became clearer when management carried out a structured analysis of its development portfolios, defined how much and what needed to be outsourced (possibly this became the role of a specific portfolio manager), and established CRO contract managers (Figure 3) (Schaub, 1998a, b).

Empowering portfolio and contract managers and establishing their roles

On a case-by-case basis, the portfolio manager determines and reviews the optimal ratio between in-house and external work, and identifies the type and

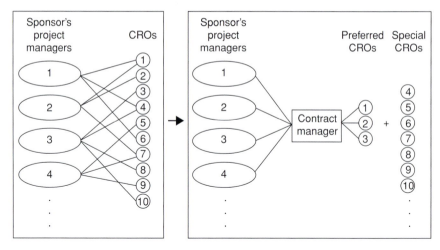

Figure 3. Moving from a chaotic network of CRO relationships to a structured pattern with a CRO contract manager.

volume of packages to be outsourced, with the aim of maximising cost-efficiency. The portfolio manager is fully empowered *vis-à-vis* project teams.

The contract manager has a more operative role: setting criteria for the evaluation of CROs, conducting pre-qualification assessments and categorising CROs into candidates for preferred providerships and second-line/specialised CROs, requesting and evaluating proposals, negotiating and contracting, overseeing the progress of outsourced projects, and possibly even managing day-to-day communication with CROs during ongoing projects. The contract manager is sometimes independent of specific project teams in a consultative capacity, and sometimes a temporary team member and mediator/integrator with the CRO, as long as the team has an ongoing project with that CRO. It is primarily the contract manager, in co-ordination with the project manager, who decides which CRO is to be awarded a particular project.

The contract manager must be acquainted with and keep abreast of the service patterns and track records of all CROs in his/her sphere, and act as a focal contact point to filter CRO marketing materials for those items that are of prime interest to the project teams in the organisation. The contract manager will acquire the broadest overview of the CRO scene and of clinical service providers in general (this may encompass central laboratories, couriers, electronic data acquisition, evaluation agencies, etc.).

Moreover, contract managers should retrospectively analyse CRO performance and the quality of co-operation with each CRO, enter this information into internal databases and thus act as the 'corporate memory' (although this latter role is being diluted by the current string of mergers occurring within the pharmaceutical industry, and including the CROs themselves). It is important to remember that assessments of CROs lose their value as staff come and go, and are only reasonably justified if the same CRO is used repeatedly in rapid succession.

Portfolio and contract managers serve to support the strategic objective of working with CROs. Although the cost of funding these two functions adds to the transaction costs, the money would appear to be well spent.

GEOGRAPHICAL ATTRACTIONS OF OUTSOURCING

Pharmaceutical companies tend to establish affiliates in a given country only if that country represents an interesting market for the foreseeable future; this decision is driven by marketing considerations and may even involve investment in a production plant. Sponsor companies, therefore, are often slow to penetrate new territories because all departments need to move in a co-ordinated manner; CROs tend to be faster because they focus only on clinical trials.

Use of CROs in virgin investigational territories

A strategic opportunity presents itself when the geographical zone covered by a sponsor does not match the geographical reach of CROs. Sponsor companies wishing to expand their development activities into regions which are not (yet) attractive in marketing terms, but which offer the necessary infrastructure for conducting clinical trials, may then be well advised to resort to CROs that are already established locally. Typical examples of such regions include Eastern Europe (Hughes, 1994), South East Asia, Latin America and South Africa.

The appeal of this construct is the strategic anticipation of economic progress in the region concerned: clinical trials carried out today lead to marketable products years later and by that time the region may be ripe for marketing.

In addition to the classic regions considered for clinical trials (North America, Europe and Japan), several countries offer 'virgin' patients for a particular treatment, centralised hospital structures, reverse seasons, 'attractive' ethnic patient populations, or simply lower prices and a political climate that invites R&D. These are all reasons for considering locally-based CROs if the sponsor company itself does not have a physical presence there.

CHOOSING THE OPTIMAL CRO PORTFOLIO

Starting from a total of some 1000 CROs worldwide, this section will illustrate how a manageable set of CROs can be distilled, from which to make a final choice (Spilker, 1990).

Benefits and limitations of commercial CRO databases

CRO databases are commercially available (e.g. CROCAS® from DataEdge, Inc., Fort Washington, PA 19034; Technomark Register, Technomark Consulting Services Ltd, London W2 4UA), in addition to directories that are free of charge (PharmaBusiness, Engel Publishing Partners, West Trenton, NJ 08628; and others). Whereas the directories list CROs by name and country with details of address, number of employees, claimed therapeutic experience, languages spoken, names of senior staff and annual turnover, the more comprehensive databases provide more detailed technical information, but there is an access fee. A simple directory will be sufficient to identify and eliminate those CROs that are too remote, located in undesirable regions, too small to handle the foreseeable tasks, or unversed in the therapeutic area of interest. Screening a directory will quickly bring down the number of potential candidates to some 30 or so CROs.

The detailed information in CRO databases would appear to provide the basis for an even narrower choice. However, the author does not recommend selecting CROs solely on this basis: database information is presented in such accurate detail that it will be outdated by the time the database is consulted. The apparent value of CRO databases is therefore artificial. They are no substitute for the need to make personal visits to a reasonable number of CRO candidates in order to form a first-hand impression (Wise, 1994).

Preparing for a CRO prequalification cycle

Going out and visiting CROs requires yet more decisions. Will a specific project be discussed at this stage or not? (The author recommends that CRO prequalification should not be biased by the requirements of a particular project.) Who will make up the prequalification team? It is wise to consider around three people for the team, e.g. the contract manager, a quality assurance (QA) auditor, and a senior staff member with a good knowledge of human nature and the ability to distinguish marketing talk from factual information. It is important too that the prequalification team composition should remain stable throughout the prequalification exercise.

Working towards objective CRO evaluation criteria

The team members have then to agree on the criteria by which they intend to rate CROs (see Table 3). The criteria will be both objective and subjective, verifiable and 'soft', and thought should be given to formulating a series of 'trick' questions to check the credibility of 'soft' information presented (Vogel and Linzmayer, 1993).

Table 3. Non-exhaustive list of CRO evaluation criteria.

Category	Individual criteria
Technical	Location of offices Are staff office-based, field-based or mixed? Number of years CRO in business Business development since foundation Number and breakdown of staff Organisational chart Ownership
Scope	Geographical area covered Range of services offered Experience in therapeutic areas (is this simply exposure or experience/expertise?) Experience in IND studies Experience in preparing regulatory documentation/applications/NDAs Special methodologies available? Which?
Business structure	Business volume Current number of projects, status, size Number of clients: current v. cumulative Share of most important clients Percentage of repeat business
Staff	Time monitors have been with CRO Time monitors have worked in current role Educational background of monitors Extent of fluctuation; reasons
Adaptability	SOPs compatible? Data management procedures compatible? Adverse event reporting procedures compatible? Able to start with new project soon? Methods of speeding recruitment and counteracting delays?
Finances	Chartered economic assessment available? Ratio number of staff/number of ongoing projects (gearing) Pricing policy preferred Fixed-unit or decoupled pricing possible?
Interest in co-operation	Readiness to name referees Value attributed to preferred providership
Interpersonal climate	Easy, friendly, or hectic, tense?
Result of a systems audit	Acceptable, curable/non-curable deficiencies?
Quotation on a fictitious study	Format, style, content of mock proposal

Attributing proper importance to subjective feelings

In business life today a high value is placed on everything that is solid, objective, reproducible and verifiable. While the prequalification of CROs yields a large volume of evidence that is presented in this way, there is usually also a hidden truth that is based more on impressions formed. For example: What is the state of the CRO building? Are you received as a guest or as an intruder? Is the meeting held in a stressful or relaxed atmosphere? How does the CRO management speak about other clients?

As with partnerships in private life, so it is with a CRO partnership: alongside 'hard evidence', it is important to follow intuition and 'gut feelings'. A high value should also be placed on the 'soft' aspects because ultimately the chemistry between the sponsor and the CRO will determine the influence the sponsor will have in critical situations.

Categorising and weighting the criteria

Senior managers within the sponsor company will wish to see a transparent evaluation of the group of CROs visited, and the prequalification team will have to cast its evidence into a presentable form. Unbiased preparations for this have to be made before embarking on the prequalification visits. The team must ask itself two questions right at the outset:

- Is the plan to use the CRO once only or repeatedly? If once only, then criteria such as technical and scientific capability will have a higher weighting than if the CRO is to be used repeatedly, in which case the location of CRO offices may be a prime factor.
- Is the plan to outsource a wide and fluctuating variety of tasks or streams of projects that are similar in size and nature? The former option will yield a wider choice of CROs than the latter.

The next step is to draft a list of evaluation criteria (using Table 3 as a guide). The prequalification team must agree on the individual scores assigned to each criterion (e.g. ranging from 1 to 3) as a measure of its importance. The specific opinion of each team member may also be weighted (e.g. senior members' opinions may be given a higher weighting). This method is known as *conjoint analysis*. The more comprehensive the analysis, the more convinced management will be of its integrity.

A different analysis method (*trade-off analysis*) may yield a more balanced final set of CROs: one by one, the CRO with the lowest score is eliminated, and the influence of this elimination on the scores of the remaining CROs is taken into account in the next step. This procedure avoids eliminating CROs with some unique features that are a 'must' in the final set.

Prequalifying CROs

Once all in-house preparations are complete, contact with CROs can begin: to rush and omit any or all of the previous considerations is to prepare for failure (Vogel and Resnick, 1996).

All the CROs on the short-list (maybe 12 to 15) should be contacted at once and in a uniform fashion, proposing an agenda for each visit that should extend over a full day. It should be made clear to every CRO contacted that the sponsor company will conduct a systems audit and discuss preferable forms of contracting and pricing, and that the visit may be the starting point for a long-term relationship. The visits should be planned so that the entire prequalification process can be concluded within a short period of time. If the visit schedule is too protracted, there is a danger that team members will lose interest, and that they will not fully remember the result of the first visit by the time the last visit is made.

After each visit, the team should meet and conclude the evaluation of the CRO visited, noting the score assigned. Allowances should be made for criteria emerging during the prequalification round that were not envisaged originally. A small set of CROs (e.g. three) should be defined as candidates to be awarded large, reasonably non-specific studies, plus another, slightly larger set of CROs (e.g. eight) that qualifies for small, unique, highly specific studies.

Management approval must then be obtained for the selection made and management support enlisted to enforce this choice across the entire company. The aim is to become acquainted with a small number of CROs, to contract out streams of studies, and to reap the benefit from this strategy, as described above. Having too many CROs on the list will merely serve to dilute the effect.

The final step before the process becomes project-specific is to consider appointing the chosen CRO candidates as preferred providers. Conferral of preferred provider status will increase the CRO's readiness to enter into co-operation, and may favourably influence the later quality of the relationship.

SPECIFYING WHAT IS TO BE DONE (REQUEST FOR PROPOSAL)

Breaking the work down into meaningful process steps

Every work package contracted out must be described so that the recipient (the CRO) understands what is to be done. It is important that these specifications are clearly arranged, unambiguous and complete and that they convey a clear message (Vogel and Nelson, 1993). It is essential to stipulate which activities are to be handled by the sponsor and which will be the responsibility of the CRO, and to define the start and end-points of CRO involvement. The document thus created will include the request to the CRO to prepare a proposal and is therefore known as the *Request for Proposal* (RFP).

For example, if a clinical study is to be contracted out, the CRO might be expected to become involved first with prequalifying the investigational sites while all previous planning and preparation is still done by the sponsor. Likewise, the CRO might be expected to deliver a database at the end of the study, or an integrated clinical/statistical report. The division of responsibilities must be defined in unambiguous terms.

The RFP must also provide clear information about timelines, indicating when the work is to start and finish, how important it is to meet the timeline, and whether it is of additional value to the sponsor if the timeline is beaten. In terms of where the work is to be carried out, the sponsor should state whether this is relevant at all, or whether only certain countries should participate, and if so, to what level of intensity. Information should be provided to the CRO concerning patient requirements (hospitalised or outpatient; number per site; number to be screened, enrolled and complete treatment; duration of treatment and follow-up). If already available, the full study protocol should accompany the RFP. (In this context, many sponsors pay great attention to confidentiality. A simple confidentiality agreement form should be included for the CRO to sign, especially if elements of the study are to be kept confidential from investigators. In most cases, however, this safeguard is not needed because CROs necessarily adhere to an unwritten code of conduct that forces them to confidentiality.)

If CRF design and/or data management are involved, the RFP should specify the number of CRF pages, breaking this down into unique and repetitive pages, and (if possible) the average number of data items on a CRF page.

The sponsor should also clarify the overall relevance of cost versus time. Fast may cost more than slow. This forms a natural link to the question: what type of personnel does the sponsor expect to be costed on the study? The project manager, monitors and other specialist functions should be listed in the correct number and proportion. Especially where monitoring is involved (and this will usually be the largest cost item), it is helpful to provide a precise definition of monitoring (extent of source data verification, duration and frequency of monitoring visits, etc.).

Designing a specification sheet, identifying roles and responsibilities

If a clinical study is to be contracted out, a checklist of all necessary activities should be prepared, arranged chronologically, and grouped in blocks, for example, 'pre-study', 'within-study', 'post-study', or 'preparation', 'clinical', 'data management', 'statistical evaluation', 'reporting'. The responsibility for all items listed should be assigned either to the sponsor or to the CRO. Joint responsibilities are meaningless and should be avoided; in cases where it is difficult to assign responsibilities clearly, the activity must be broken down further until accountabilities become clear.

RFPs: other formal aspects

A *reasonable* deadline (between 1 and 3 weeks) should be set for when the sponsor expects to receive a response from the CRO. The RFP should name contacts so that the CRO can obtain additional information from the sponsor, if required (it is very much in the sponsor's interest to ensure open communication at all stages). Intimating the number (but not the names) of other CROs competing on the same RFP will help to keep prices low.

All CROs approached must receive the same information in the same format, otherwise the resulting responses cannot be fairly compared. Although irrelevant information should be avoided, hypothetical assumptions may be included if the information provided to the CRO is still preliminary; in this event, all CROs must receive the same hypothetical assumptions.

At the RFP stage, it is fair and saves time if every CRO involved is allowed to use the pricing scheme that it is familiar with: the sponsor's primary interest is the *total* that each CRO believes the contract will cost. However, it should be ensured that all pricings are calculated according to the pre-defined *gross* process steps. The overly narrow definition of processes may cause a CRO to make arbitrary breakdown assumptions, and the prices shown in the response will reflect an accuracy that is in fact not there.

CONDUCTING THE TENDER PROCESS

The size of the project will usually determine the number of CROs involved in the tender, but the number should never be greater than five.

The sponsor's contact persons should be available during the period when the CROs are working on their responses, to answer questions arising and to clarify misunderstandings. Just because a CRO asks a large number of questions does not mean that it is not capable of correctly interpreting the information already provided. CROs are simply interested in making as few assumptions as possible when responding to the RFP: consequently, every uncertainty clarified in advance (especially if cost-relevant) helps to limit unnecessary degrees of freedom and makes pricing more accurate. In fact, if a CRO asks intelligent questions or raises points not previously thought of, this could be taken as a good indication of its experience, expertise and awareness of the project's requirements.

If justified, CROs should be permitted to carry out a feasibility study, usually in the form of a detailed interview with some representative investigators. Again, the small amount of extra time invested pays off once the CRO comes back with a solid prediction of its own and its investigators' capabilities and patient availability. The feasibility study should not last longer than another week or two, and the extra effort should be free of charge to the sponsor (although the CRO which is awarded the project may later be able to recover this small cost).

EVALUATING TIME AND COST ESTIMATES

In response to an RFP, CROs return time and cost estimates (also called bids, or proposals). These have to be evaluated and, naturally, the reviewer is tempted to look first at the total price proposed for the work to be done. While no other information appears to be more solid and factual, other important aspects demand careful consideration.

Appreciating which information is important and which is not

As a first step, the serious evaluator will check whether the instructions of the RFP are mirrored by the bid. Any deviations from the RFP instructions should have been highlighted, otherwise it is likely that the discrepancy occurred through oversight. In cases where the RFP was unrealistic, deviations from the RFP instructions may be well worth considering (Vogel and Schober, 1993).

The second step is to search for creative proposals volunteered by the CRO, or for alternatives going beyond the RFP instructions that have been offered for discussion (sponsor companies should always be ready to accept free lessons from a CRO). Such proposals indicate that the bid has been prepared intelligently and not simply following a standard scheme. On the other hand, the reviewer is well advised to be wary of unrealistic proposals in a bid that cannot be kept later.

The third step is to ensure that there are no hidden contradictions and that the text is presented in a logical and coherent manner.

The accuracy of additions, totals, and currency exchange rates should now be checked, and the overall price compared with the other offers received. Prices outside a certain credibility range will give cause for concern (some CROs use dumping prices when they submit a first bid to a sponsor; others do not wish to be awarded the project in question and use extraordinarily high prices as a deterrent). The bid price should also be compared with the size of the company making the bid; a small company with fewer overheads would be expected to submit a lower bid.

The following step is the most time-consuming and important: analysis of the fine pricing structure. As part of the RFP, the sponsor will have presented a bid grid (a chart requesting subtotal prices to be entered for activity or process blocks). Ideally, the figures in the CRO's bid document should be well comparable with the corresponding figures of competitor CROs. Very often, however, this is not the case, even though the sponsor specifications were set out in great detail. Where subtotals are virtually identical across all bids, there is no reason to inquire; where there are major discrepancies, however, the CROs should be requested to explain the precise breakdown of that price. It may be that personnel and material have been allocated to one or other activity block with different intensities. This is the most rewarding item for negotiation. The sponsor should not automatically demand the lowest possible price, but should consider buying a more expensive package, thus removing all the potential pitfalls inherent in the cheaper solution. Bid negotiation should not be equated with driving prices down, but with recognising and appreciating the services that stand behind a price, and then deciding in favour of the preferred option.

The least important and most disruptive information in a bid is often marketing-related. This should be excluded and covered elsewhere.

Removing difficulties with interpretation

CROs often present approaches that are not easily understood. Sponsor companies should not be deterred from asking for additional explanations out of fear of 'losing face' for not being an expert. After all, this may have been the original reason for seeking CRO assistance.

Introducing the preferred pricing scheme

Three price categories will invariably show up in the bid document: CRO fees, out-of-pocket costs (covering expenses for material, fees, tickets, etc.), and investigator grants. The latter two are often referred to as 'pass-through' elements. The earnings and profit are in the CRO fees.

Unless instructed otherwise, CROs will suggest the pricing scheme that they prefer and in most cases this will be material- and time-based ('*fee for service*', '*open pricing*'). This offers the greatest advantage to the CRO because, as it suggests, every activity performed by the CRO must be paid for, whether or not it yields a result. Almost by definition, fee-for-service policies tempt the CRO to run its business inefficiently. As long as sponsors tolerate contracts based on fee-for-service pricing, most CROs will not deliberately abstain from them.

Fee-for-activity pricing schemes (also referred to as 'unbundled' pricing) are a step forward as far as the sponsor is concerned. They define prices for distinct activities and introduce transparency in the sense that they provide sponsors with a steering instrument to keep the CRO from performing unproductive activities during the project. Otherwise, fee-for-activity pricing shares the disadvantage of the fee-for-service scheme: sponsors pay for activities without being certain that they will create value.

Under a *fixed total pricing* policy, the entire project is arranged on a price that is fixed for a defined scope. Regardless of how the project develops, the price remains non-renegotiable provided that the scope does not change. Although there is a high risk that a CRO may run into negative cash situations under this policy, it offers manifold advantages if the project is straightforward and/or not under time pressures. It allows the CRO to run the project at its own pace, and if it completes ahead of the original target, the profit may be immense. There is also the complementary attraction that the sponsor has to negotiate only once and enjoys budget security.

Milestone payments link payment to the successful attainment of certain steps in the course of the project at a given time. This makes CROs dependent upon steady efficiency. The downside is that this is not easy to guarantee, and progress during a project may not always keep pace with the suggested timeline. Thus, while the CRO may miss out several milestones along the way, the end-point may well be achieved on time, and all instalments thus accumulate in a final, massive payment. It is this negative cash flow scenario that makes CROs wary of milestone payments.

Fixed-unit pricing (Winkler *et al.*, 1995, 1996a, b) bypasses these drawbacks and offers the optimal model for both CRO and sponsor: payments are only for activities representing deliverables, i.e. added-value items. Each unit carries a distinct price so that simple arithmetic allows extensions from the originally agreed scope to a broader scope in an ongoing project, without the need to re-negotiate.

A fixed-unit pricing schedule will specify, for example, the payments due:

- for each investigator qualified;
- for each ethics committee approval obtained;
- for each site initiated;
- for each CRF page in house with data complete, legible, plausible and consistent; or
- for data double-entered and inconsistencies removed.

Items not qualifying for fixed-unit pricing are those that do not necessarily imply added value, for example:

- site visited;
- meeting held; or
- patients treated.

Fixed-unit pricing stimulates CROs to achievement while leaving the timeline open. The result is a combination of discipline coupled with flexibility towards the course of project development. If, for example, enrolment is slower than expected, the model provides for less CRO income from 'CRFs collected', while at the same time stimulating the CRO to initiate more sites. Fixed-unit prices drive the CRO towards the desired end-point without rigidly prescribing the course to be taken (Winkler *et al.*, 1997).

'*Decoupled*' prices may also be negotiated: this term describes the independence of an item's price from the scenario under which it becomes due. For example, a site initiated should always cost the same, regardless of whether it occurred early or later during the study. This rules out the possibility of prices escalating during the life of the contract and the CRO recouping lost profits by arguing that late site initiation is more expensive than early initiation. The exception here would be if the scope of the study were to change significantly during the intervening period, e.g. increased number of assessments due to a protocol amendment and necessitating further investigator training.

One very modern but generally impracticable arrangement is *risk sharing*: both partners agree that payment will be in the form of equities or royalties, to be paid only when the product investigated reaches the market place. By definition, there is an inherent risk that the product will not; however, assuming that it does, income for the CRO can massively exceed the earnings that would have been due under a conventional pricing scheme. As a result, risk sharing may only be considered by small start-up sponsors (financially thin) working with relatively powerful CROs (financially strong): this, however, is a rare combination.

If necessary, those CROs that still stand a chance of being awarded the project will now have to cast their proposals into a new format involving the sponsor-desired pricing scheme. Nevertheless, the resultant delay is worthwhile.

Project meeting with CROs

By this stage some of the CROs originally invited to bid will have been dismissed from the reckoning. It is highly recommended that meetings should now take place with the remaining serious candidates and that all facets of the project be discussed person to person. The CRO should present its chosen project manager and/or lead monitor who will begin communication on detailed project requirements. The sponsor will have the opportunity to test the project manager's indication-specific experience.

Applying conjoint (trade-off) analysis to identify the optimal CRO

If doubts still remain as to which CRO should be awarded the project, there may again be recourse to conjoint or trade-off analysis, as explained earlier. On the other hand, no matter how elaborate it may be, no avenue can completely eliminate uncertainty: the sponsor and the CRO will work together as partners, and neither will be completely autonomous any longer.

AWARDING THE PROJECT (LETTER OF INTENT)

Appointing the CRO and issuing a letter of intent

The decision in favour of one CRO over all the other candidates involved in the tender should be communicated clearly, giving reasons for the decision. All CROs deserve this, and it is even in the long-term interests of the sponsor to help CROs to improve those areas that had given the sponsor reason to reject their proposal.

Outsourced projects often evolve over time and, at the point when it is awarded to a CRO, it is sometimes not clear what the precise scope of the project will be. If total clarification will take longer than a few days, the contract should be postponed, but work can and should already begin in specifically defined areas. To reassure the CRO that all premature endeavours of this nature will not be in vain, a letter of intent (LoI) should be issued. The LoI documents in brief (one or two pages) the fact that the project has been awarded, that work should go ahead in given areas, that the sponsor will supply all necessary materials, that a start-up payment will be made (up to 10% of the total anticipated), and that a full contract will follow in no more than a few weeks' time.

Recognising the transient nature and limited legal power of LoIs

The LoI merely expresses the parties' intention to enter a contract later. It should make clear that all further arrangements necessary to secure the complete delivery of the intended service are 'subject to contract'. In this way the contractual intention is formally negated, and the parties are not bound until formal contracts are exchanged. The LoI should never be considered as a substitute for a contract and it is essential that the time until the final contract is kept as short as possible (a few weeks at maximum).

Installing long run-in periods

A wise sponsor will complete the tender and LoI steps as early as possible. This will provide the CRO with ample time to become familiar with the requirements, form a team and carry out all preparatory work without stress, so that once the project requires full resources, these are readily available. This can result in a wide gap between issue of the LoI and provision of full specifications, and is inconsistent with the intentions set out in the previous paragraph.

An intelligent solution to this problem (especially in the case of complex projects that are difficult to oversee) is to write up all specifications, as they become definite, in the form of a preliminary contract, and to identify those areas that still require definitive specifications. These draft documents serve as an intermediate step between the LoI and final contract: legally they are nothing more than 'developed' LoIs, but technically they help both partners to approach the final contract in a disciplined manner.

Thus, the longer the run-in period, the better prepared the partners will be to co-operate, the more chances there will be to eliminate friction early and pro-actively, and the easier it will be to start the project at full speed once everything is specified and ready.

Identifying and assembling the 'dream team'

A sufficiently long run-in period also allows the sponsor to have input into the optimal make-up of the CRO team: not only will the CRO make the desired number of team members available, but the sponsor may exercise the right to assess the suitability of individuals in the team.

WORKING TOWARDS THE MOST BENEFICIAL CONTRACT AND PRICING MODEL

Part of the above strategic measures should include devising a contract template that serves the sponsor's purpose. Reliance on the contract model offered by CROs may save the sponsor time and effort initially, but in the long term the sponsor may lose out on a variety of strategic options, as follows (Schaub, 1998a, b).

Standardising contract formats and separating generic from specific issues

A survey of the contracts prepared by CROs quickly reveals that they are all very similar to each other: they include a number of generic, recurring items, as well as project-specific items. By collecting a few CRO contract templates, the sponsor's contract manager will rapidly be able to compile a sponsor contract template. All CRO contracts used to form the basis for the sponsor template have already had legal input from the CRO's lawyers, thus making it unnecessary to re-invent the wheel.

Ensuring generic issues and project specifications are separated into connectable documents

If a sponsor intends to use a CRO for a number of projects, the contract manager's task is now to collect and assemble all generic items (paragraphs addressing general scope, term, definitions, legal standards, confidentiality, ownership of results, liability and indemnification, insurance, procedures for amendments, early termination, extension, relationship to sub-contractors, *force majeure*, miscellaneous 'boiler plate' text, governing law, and rules of arbitration/court of jurisdiction, etc.) to build a template for a master (umbrella) contract that can be used for all CROs and all outsourced projects.

These master contracts (one for each favoured CRO) should be designed so that they do not bind sponsors to specific contract volumes or monetary commitments toward the CRO. They remain void as stand-alone documents, i.e. as long as no project specifications are added. They are issued on a specific date and remain in effect until one of the partners decides to terminate. In fact, there is no need for the sponsor company to terminate because it can step out simply by no longer contracting out to the CRO in question.

As they come up, all project specifications are attached and interconnected to the master contract. All items intentionally left unspecific in the master contract have to be referenced to specific statements in the attachment. Only the conjunct master contract and project specification attachment form a valid legal entity, and thus it becomes clear that the sponsor and CRO are bound to each other only during ongoing projects. In the remaining 'void' periods, only the intention to co-operate prevails.

Project specifications include the precise project scope, contract start and end dates, verbatim and detailed descriptions of mutual responsibilities (as summarised in the specification checklist), timelines, and payment procedures, as well as contingencies (see below) (Vogel *et al.*, 1995).

This contract model serves two purposes:

- It invites repeat use, implicitly conveying the message that the sponsor may wish to pursue a long-term objective with the CRO. This may enhance co-operativeness and quality.
- It saves on transaction costs. The master contract has to be negotiated with the CRO once only, with future negotiations able to focus simply on project-specific issues.

Finally, any contract with a CRO should ensure that the CRO has adequate Professional Indemnity/Errors and Omissions cover in place.

Introducing modern contractual features and pricing schemes

Master contracts can be enriched with features that secure sponsor interests and usually do not come from the prototype contracts offered by CROs. For example, both partners can *mutually guarantee* well-defined standards of care (such as educational and training standards for staff, exclusion of the CRO's right to substitute personnel without the sponsor's consent, agreement on appropriate overlap periods, procedures in the event of staff substitutions, and security of data files). It is important to specify these guarantees in such detail that they can be legally enforced.

Furthermore, agreement can be reached on certain *metrics* by which the partner's performance can be measured. Metrics can be time-, cost- and quality-related (for example: How long does the CRO take from first application to final ethics committee approval? Will the CRO be able to recruit investigators at a given per-patient cost level or below? How many data correction loops have to be made per site?). If linked to payments, these metrics can become powerful instruments to ensure minimum performance standards.

Master contracts can lay down the conditions under which both partners would consider mutual *preferential treatment*, e.g. contract volume over time as a measure to induce step-wise higher flexibility levels from the CRO.

Advanced pricing schemes, such as fixed-unit pricing and milestone payments, have been discussed above. Regardless of which pricing scheme is applied, *incentives* (Vogel, 1993) can be agreed upon, expressed as bonus systems. Once again, these can be time-, cost- and quality-driven or mixtures of all three. However, if a tight timeline is fixed from the outset, or the project is run on a low budget, or high quality levels are demanded, it will be almost impossible for the CRO to surpass these marks, and it is more likely that they will not be met at all. Therefore, a CRO agreeing on an incentive system may seek short-cuts to earn the desired bonus or may seek ways of blaming the sponsor in order to avoid accusations of poor performance. In conclusion, incentive systems may bring new hassles rather than helping to clear the air, and they can disturb rather than promote stable equilibrium.

The prime purpose of a contract is to safeguard against the negative: if projects always unfolded positively, agreement would be required on very little. Every contract should therefore include a section on *contingencies* that defines the steps to be taken in the event of unexpected disasters. A variety of scenarios may be imagined in which one or other partner suddenly wishes to terminate the agreement, and fair compensation has to be paid for the damage that this causes to the other. Reasons for early termination of the contract may include:

- cancellation of the product's development for commercial, regulatory or medical reasons, or due to the product being licensed away, following which the new licensee has no interest in continuing the project;
- one partner approaching/suffering bankruptcy or being acquired by another firm;
- the partners being unable/unwilling to co-operate; or
- *force majeure* (war, strike, riot, fire, floods, earthquake, etc.).

In other less extreme situations, escape routes may be found, such as interrupting and postponing the rest of the project, redesigning the project to adapt it to the new circumstances, or transferring the project to another CRO or back to the sponsor. Whatever the situation, discussions and agreements on contract amendments when the unthinkable happens are inevitably hampered by the stress under which the partners are having to operate. It is a much better solution to have appropriate *exit scenarios* fixed beforehand: this keeps minds clear so that they can focus on other fronts.

MANAGING PROJECT AND CRO TOGETHER

True co-operation is possible only in an environment characterised by free and open exchange of opinions, trust, mutual respect, shared values, no fear, rewards, visions of short- and long-term goals, continuity, interpersonal fit, and compatible systems and processes. These values can be facilitated, developed and reinforced, for example, by frequent face-to-face meetings, encouragement of feedback and contribution, one-to-one project teams on both sides, regular status reports, efficient spread of instructions across the organisation(s), and a proper balance between hands-on and hands-off management. It would be unwise for the sponsor's project manager to run the project as if it had been kept in-house. Unless a great deal of responsibility is shifted to the CRO and the CRO is empowered to a defined extent, there is little reason or benefit in employing the CRO at all.

Sponsors should be aware that while they manage the CRO, they also are being managed by the CRO. Mature CROs scrutinise the performance of their sponsors, and the submissive attitudes of the past have now been replaced by sound self-assertion. Successful modern CROs are in the fortunate position of being able to refuse contracts when sponsors behave unprofessionally or have unrealistic expectations, project timelines and/or objectives.

ASSESSING PARTNERSHIPS

As human beings, we compensate for our own deficiencies through relationships with partners who have complementary expertise. Partnerships are driven by a longing for experience, efficiency, stability, peace and trust.

Understanding various degrees of partnership

In the context of this chapter, the lowest level of partnership is the *preferred provider/preferred vendor*. Typically, in this setting, similar assignments are continually awarded to the same CRO. In return, the CRO may give preference to that sponsor in terms of team composition and other aspects. A master contract may be applied in the sense described above, but there is no contractual commitment binding the parties if there is no ongoing project, making exit by either party unproblematic should it ever become necessary. The partnership is more a form of mutual exploitation, a mental or physical barter that is terminated when one or both parties is no longer able or willing to supply.

The desire to increase economies of scale and reduce transaction costs even further may drive the parties to the next highest level, a *preferred partnership*. Mutual commitments are made (e.g. a minimum annual contract volume is guaranteed in return for the sponsor's right to unlimited access and re-use of the same team at any time and location; discounts may be granted). Sponsors will treat such CROs as 'one-stop shops'.

The highest level of a partnership is the *strategic alliance*. In this case, the CRO becomes an autonomous part of the sponsor: both parties will invest in each other's future, both are committed to each other's success, and both will share the risk of development.

Assessing the benefits and drawbacks of partnerships

Partnerships bring a number of attractive benefits. The list includes probable or guaranteed stable cash flow, smooth production flow, predictable resource availability at predictable quality, improved communication, no contract hassle, and higher emotional empathy. The drawbacks include danger of sudden break-up with substantial cash flow losses, the need to form a broader than usual platform for co-operation (perhaps in parts of the organisations that do not have so much in common), reduced profit margin for the CRO, some dependence on the partner, some loss of freedom of choice, reduced ability to compete, and the risk that both parties may become complacent if the engagement is too cosy.

Appreciating the unequal nature of sponsor–CRO partnerships

Too often, partnerships do not really flourish because both partners have not made it clear to themselves that they cling to divergent patterns of interest with minimal overlap. To illustrate this in black and white: sponsors remain masters, CROs servants; sponsors have funds, CROs earn them; sponsors are primarily interested in the progress of their projects, CROs primarily in making money; sponsors regard investigators as clients, CROs view them as suppliers of data. As a consequence, CRO–sponsor partnerships do not generally survive longer than one project before they are dissolved. Nevertheless, the drive towards partnerships continues to be fuelled by timid managers.

Looking at ownership when considering a CRO partner

Large public CROs in the hands of anonymous shareholders will not be able to sustain partnerships for long because, given their size and structure, they have lost their focal point of interest. Management will change too often, and along with these changes will come new attitudes and preferences. In contrast, there is a much greater chance of forming gratifying, rewarding partnerships with small CROs that are still in the hands of their founders who take a personal interest in ensuring that the CRO–sponsor relationship flourishes to mutual benefit. The reverse also holds true: a CRO will never find a true partner in a huge multinational sponsor organisation, but rather in a small, 'smart' start-up company.

A GLANCE AT CONCEPTS RELATED TO OUTSOURCING

The concept of outsourcing aims at increasing cost-efficiency. At first glance, it is surprising that three similar concepts – insourcing, contracting-in and virtuality – have found only minimal use in the pharmaceutical industry.

As the word suggests, *insourcing* is the opposite of outsourcing. Insourcing attracts work from external sources provided that this work falls into the realm of core competency. To illustrate this, a strong development department of a pharmaceutical company might invite competitors to use its own facilities to carry out clinical studies, thus levelling off its occasional resource troughs. The value-adding chain would become broader (rather than thinner as in outsourcing). The obvious shortcoming of this concept relates to confidentiality/secrecy problems that would prevent companies from handing their projects out to the competition. However, the concept appears to work well in commodity-based industries, so perhaps it only needs to be discovered by the pharmaceutical industry, and might ultimately work there too.

Contracting-in is a special form of insourcing. Individuals (freelancers and CRO staff) are leased for specified periods of time to sponsors and are integrated into the sponsors' teams. In that sense, contracting-in may also be regarded as a special form of outsourcing, only the individual's work location is different; otherwise, contractual agreements resemble those in outsourcing. Contracting-in is enjoying increasing popularity. Not only are communication and control easier if a person is physically part of the sponsor organisation, but people contracted in are believed to be more flexible by nature than the employees of a CRO, their speed of response is said to be higher, and they have a closer association with the sponsor's development process and project. Contracting-in is widely regulated by governments and the ease or difficulty with which it can be implemented varies from country to country.

Virtuality is a modern form of self-centration and self-determination. A virtual company draws from a small managerial and administrative nucleus and operative work is either purchased externally or provided through decentral, self-reliant associates (Steiner, 1994). The 'virtual' part is the integration of these external providers into a corporate entity that has no legal existence but that works in practice. The strength of virtual companies lies in their extreme flexibility to respond to oscillating needs, and in the complete absence of overheads and corporate barriers. In all probability, the people embarking on virtual enterprises of this type are the more creative individuals in our community (Byrne, 1993).

Recently, large numbers of *virtual companies* have sprung into being. They may be sponsor-type groups of a few individuals (who, for example, carry on the development of projects that have been abandoned by the classic pharmaceutical industry; once these projects yield attractive results, the virtual company tries to sell them back to the original owner) or CRO-type networks of freelancers, managed in a form of franchise.

THE WAY AHEAD FOR OUTSOURCING

The race for greater efficiencies within the pharmaceutical industry will continue into the years ahead, and outsourcing and other forms of organisational decentralisation will benefit. Outsourcing will continue to grow but the rate of increase will plateau in the face of divergent responses from CROs.

Valuing growth against more intelligent business strategies

Some CROs will attempt to grow using any means available; if they do not acquire sufficient business, they will grow through acquisition. This will produce a small number of very large, global CROs. As they grow, these CROs will witness the growth of their internal overhead costs, and this will make them very similar to sponsor companies. Somewhere along the line they will most likely become sponsor organisations themselves, with their own product developments. This will be one way for the large CROs to survive.

Smaller CROs, especially those in a 'niche', will develop instead into deep specialisation. Their business objective will be to secure a non-competitive environment in their niche for as long as possible. Although there is a constant risk that their niche may be lost, the ever-increasing complexity of clinical development and novel methodologies in the fields of information technology, electronic data acquisition, and patient recruitment via the Internet are factors that militate in favour of this kind of CRO. Indeed, sponsors may feel increasingly that it is safer to use small CROs because they are less likely to become competitor sponsor organisations (see above).

The medium-sized CROs will find themselves increasingly in trouble. They are neither large enough to compete successfully with the major players, nor do they have a specialised business niche. More and more medium-sized CROs will become eroded and swallowed up by ravenous 'big fish'.

At the same time, the pharmaceutical industry will be able to finance only a reduced number of developments, and it is foreseeable that the number of development projects will shrink until new methodologies (combinatorial chemistry, biotechnology, molecular modelling, high-throughput screening, etc.) wash sufficient new revenue into its coffers again.

Outsourcing: a passing fashion?

From time to time, naïve analysts voice assured opinions about the potential that outsourcing may still have in clinical development. Statements such as '70% of R&D is outsourceable' suggest that 70% of R&D *should* be outsourced, and help to drive the outsourcing wave into the stratosphere (Lightfoot *et al.*, 1998). A rational look at outsourcing does indeed indicate that the proportion of projects outsourced versus in-house must be highest in start-up companies and less in established pharmaceutical companies.

It appears highly likely that at some time in the future the pendulum will swing back, and companies will remember that it was so much more comfortable to rely on their own resources, provided that these are as flexible, productive and motivated as CRO staff are today. There is nothing to prevent pharmaceutical companies from aiming for this: it simply requires management who are determined to achieve and staff who are willing to follow.

REFERENCES

Byrne, JA (1993). The virtual corporation. *Business Week* (8 February), 103.

Colburn, WA, McClurg, JE and Cichoracki, JR (1997). The strategic role of outsourcing. *Appl Clin Trials* **6**, 68–75.

Hadfield, SG, Findlay, G, Hughes, RG and Lumley, CE (1998). *Current and Future Strategies for Outsourcing by International Pharmaceutical and Biotechnology Companies*. Report of the Centre for Medicines Research International Ltd, Carshalton, Surrey SM5 4DS.

Hill, TJ and Hubbard, J (1996). Is outsourcing clinical trials really more expensive? *Scrip Magazine* **44** (March), 19–20.

Hughes, G (1994). Contract clinical research in Central and Eastern Europe. *Appl Clin Trials* **3**(6), 52–59.

Lightfoot, GD, Getz, KA, Harwood, F *et al.* (1998). Faster time to market. *The Monitor* **12**, 13–26.

Macarthur, D (1994). *Optimising the Use of Contract Services by the Pharmaceutical Industry*. Scrip Report, PJB Publications Ltd, Richmond.

Schaub, W (1998a). Strategies that work in CRO relationships. *Appl Clin Trials* **7**(10), 28–36.

Schaub, W (1998b). The role of CROs in the development of new drugs: A sponsor's view. In: Witte, PU and Mutschler, E (Eds), *Clinical Research in the Border Regions of Germany, the Czech Republic and Poland*, Pharma Industrie Serie Dokumentation, Editio Cantor, Aulendorf, pp. 91–99.

Schaub, W (1999). *Good Outsourcing Practices in Clinical Development*. Published and distributed by Vision in Business Ltd., First Floor, 30 City Road, London EC1Y 2AY. This volume (ISBN 1 902967 02 X) includes a more comprehensive list of references.

Schaub, W (2000). Comparing outsourcing costs. *Appl Clin Trials* **9**(6), 56–60.

Spilker, B (1990). Roles of medical contractors in drug development. *Drug News Perspect* **3**, 148–152.

Steiner, J (1994). Virtual integration – a solution for biotechnology? *Scrip Magazine* **28** (October), 23–24.

Vogel, JR (1993). Achieving results with Contract Research Organizations: pharmaceutical industry views. *Appl Clin Trials* **2**(1), 44–49.

Vogel, JR and Linzmayer, MI (1993). Achieving results with Contract Research Organizations: evaluating and selecting CROs. *Appl Clin Trials* **2**(8), 36–41.

Vogel, JR and Nelson, SR (1993). Achieving results with Contract Research Organizations: determining the study specifications. *Appl Clin Trials* **2**(5), 70–79.

Vogel, JR and Resnick, N (1996). Achieving results with Contract Research Organizations: a case study in evaluating and selecting a CRO. *Appl Clin Trials* **5**(6), 30–36.

Vogel, JR and Schober, RA (1993). Achieving results with Contract Research Organizations: requesting and evaluating proposals from CROs. *Appl Clin Trials* **2**(12), 32–41.

Vogel, JR, Schober, RA. and Brent Olson, R (1995). Achieving results with Contract Research Organizations: contracting with CROs. *Appl Clin Trials* **4**(2), 20–28.

Winkler, G, Williams, KA and Marsh, R (1995). Using fixed-unit price contracts to simplify sponsor-CRO negotiations. *Appl Clin Trials* **4**(6), 56–59.

Winkler, G, Williams, KA and Marsh, R (1996a). Creating win–win situations with fixed-unit price sponsor–CRO contracts. *Appl Clin Trials* **5**(3), 36–40.

Winkler, G, Williams, KA and Marsh, R (1996b). Easy contracting with CROs: the fixed-unit price contract. *The Monitor* (Summer), 26–28.

Winkler, G, Randall, M and Marsh, R (1997). Closing the gap between project and contract management. *Appl Clin Trials* **6**(11), 25–30.

Wise, AH (1994). Merck's experience in prequalifying CROs. *Appl Clin Trials* **3**, 32–39.

Wyse, RKH and Hughes, RG (1993). *Contract Research in the 1990s*. Report of Technomark Consulting Services Ltd, London W2 4UA.

23

New directions: regulations for biotechnology products and medical devices

Andrew Willis

INTRODUCTION

It is intended that this chapter should serve as a supplement to the concise overview of medicinal product regulations provided in *Chapter 2*. The two areas defined as biotechnology and medical devices are often considered to be distinct industries within the overall pharmaceutical sector. This chapter will discuss the regulatory aspects pertinent to these two areas.

THE BIOTECHNOLOGY INDUSTRY

The clinical requirements and marketing authorisation requirements for the biotechnology industry are similar to those already defined in *Chapter 2*. However, there are regulatory concerns that are unique to the biotechnology industry, and these are two-fold. First, there are concerns over the environmental risk of exposure or release of genetically modified materials and the consequences of such exposure to the individual and society as a whole. Secondly, the regulators are required to consider specific issues relating to the quality and reproducibility of materials manufactured by such means. This short review of biotechnology products is divided into two sections – environmental control and quality control.

Environmental control

Biotechnology involves the use of modern genetic engineering and, as such, potentially affects many different products and processes. The regulatory

Table 1. Biotechnology guidelines – adopted guidelines published in *The Rules Governing Medicinal Products in the European Union. Volume 3A* (EudraLex, 1998).

Title	Date of item (date of effect)	Reference documents
Production and Quality Control of Medicinal Products derived by recombinant DNA Technology.	December 1994 (July 1995)	Volume III Addendum 3 (1995) (III/3477/92) (Updated Volume III (1998) guideline: III/860/86)
Quality of Biotechnological Products: Analysis of the Expression Construct in Cells used for Production of rDNA derived Protein Products. *(ICH topic Q5B, Step 4 adopted November 1995).*	December 1995 (July 1996)	CPMP/ICH/139/95 (III/5828/83)
Production and Quality Control of Cytokine Products derived by Biotechnological Processes.	February 1990 (August 1990)	Volume III Addendum (1990) (III/3791/88)
Production and Quality Control of Monoclonal antibodies.	December 1994 (July 1995)	Volume III Addendum 3 (1995) (III/5271/94) (Updated guidelines given in Volume III (1989): III/859/86 *(murine)* and Volume III Addendum (1990) *(human)* III/3488/89)
Quality of Biotechnological Products: Stability Testing of Biotechnological/Biological Products. *(ICH topic Q5C, Step 4 adopted November 1995).*	December 1995 (July 1996)	CPMP/ICH/138/95 (III/3772/92)
Gene Therapy Product Quality Aspects in the Production of Vectors and Genetically Modified Somatic Cells.	December 1994 (July 1995)	Volume III Addendum 3 (1995) (III/5863/93)
Use of Transgenic Animals in the Manufacture of Biological Medicinal Products for Human Use.	December 1994 (July 1995)	Volume III Addendum 3 (1995) (III/3612/93)

Virus Validation Studies: The Design, Contribution and Interpretation of Studies Validating the Inactivation and Removal of Viruses.	February 1996 (August 1996)	CPMP/BWP/268/95 (Updated Volume III Addendum 2 (1992) guideline: III/8115/89)
Validation of Virus Removal/Inactivation Procedures: Choice of Viruses.	December 1994 (July 1995)	Volume III Addendum 3 (1995) (III/5543/94)
Minimising the Risk of Transmitting Agents causing Spongiform Encephalopathy via Medicinal Products.	December 1991 (May 1992)	Volume III Addendum 2 (1992) (III/3298/91)
Tests on Samples of Biological Origin.	July 1989	Volume III Addendum (1990) (III/844/87)
Plasma derived Medicinal Products.	March 1996 (September 1996)	CPMP/BWP/269/95 (Updated Volume III Addendum 2 (1992) guideline: III/8379/89)
Plasma Pool Testing.	May 1994 (November 1994)	Volume III Addendum 3 (1995) (III/5193/94)
Harmonisation of Requirements for Influenza Vaccines.	October 1991 (January 1992)	Volume III Addendum 2 (1992) (III/3188/91)
Allergen Products.	May 1996 (November 1996)	CPMP/BWP/243/96 (Updated Volume III Addendum 2 (1992) guideline: III/9271/90)
Assessing the Efficacy and Safety of Human Plasma derived Factor VIII:C and Factor IX:C Products in Clinical Trials in Haemophiliacs before and after Authorisation.	February 1996 (February 1996)	CPMP/198/95 (III/5769/94)
Assessing the Efficacy and Safety of Normal Intravenous Immunoglobulin Products for Marketing Authorisations.	February 1996 (August 1996)	CPMP/388/95 (III/5819/94)

framework for biotechnology within the EU was created in the 1980s to establish an internal market for biotechnological products, and has evolved around two basic areas:

- The contained use of genetically modified micro-organisms (GMMs); deliberate release into the environment of genetically modified organisms (GMOs); and the protection of workers from risks related to exposure to biological agents in the workplace.
- Legislation covering the placing on to the market of medicinal products and additives (used in animal nutrition, plant protection products, novel foods, seeds).

The legal framework developed in Europe ensures that the safety requirements are appropriate to the risks for human health and that the environmental controls reflect the associated risk. The regulations have taken account of current advances in scientific knowledge, established international practices, and existing regulatory experience with modern biotechnology from the USA.

The principal instruments of current legislation are:

- Council Directive 90/219/EEC of 23 April 1990: this covers any contained use of GMMs, both for research and commercial purposes.
- Council Directive 90/220/EEC of 23 April 1990: this relates to experimental and marketing-related aspects of GMOs. The Directive covers any research and development (R&D) release of these organisms into the environment and contains a specific environmental risk assessment for the placing on to the market of any product containing or consisting of such organisms.

In addition to these regulations, a number of further proposals are likely to be incorporated into European law in the near future. The key instrument relating to the pharmaceutical industry is the Draft Council Directive on Legal Protection of Biotechnological Inventions.

The European Commission's view is that, in the future, the whole network of interrelated biotechnological regulations needs to ensure that a broad understanding of the pertinent issues is available and that data are presented that are always appropriate in relation to the risks involved. The Commission, while being fully committed to the protection of human health and the environment, is also concerned with the building of a competitive industry.

Quality control

In addition to the environmental restrictions imposed upon biotechnological products, clinical researchers must also take into account requirements concerning the quality of such products. As listed in Table 1, the current guidelines in operation throughout the EU ensure that sponsors/manufacturers of such products adhere to these quality requirements and provide adequate controls to safeguard the reproducibility of biotechnological products.

Researchers should take into consideration the aspects relating to these quality issues and ensure that the development programme is appropriately designed. Marketing authorisations for biotechnological products are required to adopt the centralised procedure (*see Chapter 2*) and review of any such technical documentation will be based upon the guidelines for this procedure.

MEDICAL DEVICES

Currently the US and European requirements for medical devices are not harmonised: they differ with regard to the documentation needed for product submissions in the US and for conformité européenne (CE) marking in Europe. In the light of this, it is important to follow a detailed strategy that will:

- be effective for US approvals and European CE marking;
- satisfy applicable US and European regulatory requirements; and
- satisfy the US and European quality system requirements.

In this context the EU guidelines present important definitions in three main categories, as described in the following sections.

Medical devices

Article 1 of Council Directive 93/42/EEC defines a medical device as:

'... any instrument, apparatus, appliance, material or other article, whether used alone or in combination, including the software necessary for its proper application intended by the manufacturer to be used for human beings for the purpose of:

- diagnosis, prevention, monitoring, treatment or alleviation of disease,
- diagnosis, monitoring, treatment, alleviation of or compensation for an injury or handicap,
- investigation, replacement or modification of the anatomy or of a physiological process,
- control of conception,

and which does not achieve its principal intended action in or on the human body by pharmacological, immunological or metabolic means, but which may be assisted in its function by such means.'

Active implantable medical devices

According to Article 1 (c) of Directive 90/385/EEC, an active implantable medical device (AIMD) is defined as:

'... any active medical device which is intended to be totally or partially introduced, surgically or medically, into the human body or by medical intervention into a natural orifice, and which is intended to remain after the procedure.'

In-vitro diagnostic medical devices

Finally, Article 1 (b) of Directive 98/79/EC defines an *in-vitro* diagnostic medical device as:

'... any medical device which is a reagent, reagent product, calibrator, control material, kit, instrument, apparatus, equipment, or system, whether used alone or in combination, intended by the manufacturer to be used *in vitro* for the examination of specimens, including blood and tissue donations, derived from the human body, solely or principally for the purpose of providing information:

- concerning a physiological or pathological state, or
- concerning a congenital abnormality, or
- to determine the safety and compatibility with potential recipients, or
- to monitor therapeutic measures.

Specimen receptacles are considered to be *in-vitro* diagnostic medical devices. "Specimen receptacles" are those devices, whether vacuum-type or not, specifically intended by their manufacturers for the primary containment and preservation of specimens derived from the human body for the purpose of *in-vitro* diagnostic examination.

Products for general laboratory use are not *in-vitro* diagnostic medical devices unless such products, in view of their characteristics, are specifically intended by their manufacturer to be used for *in-vitro* diagnostic examination.'

In all three cases, the devices have to meet essential requirements in order to obtain a CE mark in Europe. The common requirement stated in all the legislation is that the device must be designed and manufactured in such a way that it does not compromise the clinical condition or the safety of the patient or the user.

In order to ensure compliance in this respect, the directives lay down all the essential requirements relevant to each type of device and include data requirements and advice, as follows:

- general requirements;
- design and construction;
- complete quality system;
- EC-type examination and verification by notified bodies; and
- clinical requirements, where appropriate.

European CE marking requirements

All medical devices being placed on the market in Europe must comply with the European Directives for medical devices and carry the CE mark.

In order to obtain CE marking in Europe, a number of points first need to be clarified:

- determination of product classification;
- identification of an appropriate conformity assessment route to CE marking; and
- development of the technical dossier.

In addition, for CE-marked products, the manufacturer must adhere to the EU Medical Devices Vigilance System. As such, upon becoming aware of adverse events concerning its product, the manufacturer must immediately notify the Competent Authority. A European Commission guidance document defines the acceptable time limit for such notification as not later than 10 days after becoming aware of the incident.

It should be noted that medical device manufacturers located outside the European Economic Area (EEA) and without subsidiaries in the EEA must designate an authorised representative to conduct certain regulatory activities under the European Directives for medical devices. Therefore, manufacturers should designate an authorised representative who is qualified to represent the company's regulatory interests.

European clinical trials on medical devices

In order to demonstrate compliance with the essential requirements, it will sometimes be necessary to provide clinical data. These data may be in one of two forms:

- either a compilation of the relevant scientific literature currently available on the intended purpose of the device and the techniques employed, as well as, if appropriate, a written report containing a critical evaluation of this compilation; or
- the results and conclusions of a specific clinical investigation.

Critical analysis and evaluation of the scientific literature are broad concepts that can take into account experience with an established device that is already on the market and used in clinical practice. The evaluation can also be based on relevant scientific literature, including data on the materials, on the type of medical procedures used, and other non-clinical test data, including animal studies.

However, unless safety and performance can be adequately demonstrated by other means, a specifically designed clinical investigation will need to be carried out. Such a trial will need:

- to verify that, under normal conditions of use, the performance characteristics of the device conform to those intended by the manufacturer; and
- to determine any undesirable side-effects, under normal conditions of use, and to allow an informed clinical opinion to assess whether these are acceptable when weighed against the intended performance of the device.

Thus, a clinical investigation of a non-CE-marked device must be designed to establish that the performance claimed by the manufacturer can be adequately demonstrated, and that the device is judged by a clinical expert to be safe to use on a patient, taking into account any risks associated with the use of the device when weighed against the expected benefits.

For a device already authorised to carry the CE marking, clinical investigations are also required where the device is to be used for a new purpose. However, submission of a clinical investigation to the Competent Authority for assessment is not required where a device is CE-marked for the purpose intended or in the case of a comparative study of two devices, where each has obtained prior CE marking and each is used for its original purpose.

It is recognised that a manufacturer may wish to subject a small number of 'prototype models' of a device to clinical investigation, in order to assess safety and/or performance, and that such prototypes may need to undergo a number of changes prior to large-scale production. These changes may be regarded as variations included within one application unless, in the view of the Competent Authority, the risk to patients or users is increased by the proposed changes.

Most medical devices about to be placed on the market are likely to fall into one of three categories. The first concerns devices for which previous clinical experience exists. The second relates to a modification of a device where the safety and performance of the modification can be demonstrated without the need for investigation in human subjects, e.g. by means of laboratory testing. For the third category, a specifically designed clinical investigation will be necessary in order to demonstrate device safety and performance.

A clinical investigation of a non-CE-marked medical device will probably be required in the following circumstances:

- when introducing a completely new concept of device into clinical practice where components, features and/or methods of action, are previously unknown;
- where an existing device is modified in such a way that it contains a novel feature if such a feature has an important physiological effect; or where the modification might affect the clinical performance and/or safety of the device;
- where a device incorporates materials previously untested in humans, coming into contact with the human body or where existing materials are applied to a new location in the human body, in which case compatibility and biological safety will need to be considered; or
- where a device is proposed for a new purpose or function.

Discussion with the relevant Notified Body, where applicable, may prove helpful before embarking on the planning of a clinical investigation. Where a clinical investigation is required, the investigation must:

- be performed on the basis of an appropriate plan with well-defined aims and objectives;

- make use of procedures appropriate to the device under examination;
- be performed in circumstances similar to the intended conditions of use;
- include sufficient devices and human subjects to reflect the aims of the investigation, taking into account the potential risk of the device;
- examine appropriate features involving safety and performance and their effects on patients so that the risk/benefit balance can be satisfactorily addressed;
- fully record all adverse incidents and report serious incidents to the Competent Authority. Although this is only a requirement for those devices falling within the scope of the Medical Devices Regulations, manufacturers are encouraged similarly to report for those devices falling within the scope of the Active Implantable Medical Devices Regulations ('Adverse Incidents of Devices Undergoing Clinical Investigation');
- be performed under the responsibility of a medical practitioner or a number of medical practitioners; and
- include a final written report, signed by the medical investigator(s) responsible, which must contain a critical evaluation of all the data collected during the clinical investigation, with appropriate conclusions.

The legal requirements for methodology and ethical considerations relating to clinical investigations are set out in the Active Implantable Medical Devices Regulations: Schedule 3, and in the Medical Devices Regulations: Section 16, which incorporate those parts of the relevant Medical Devices Directives dealing with clinical investigations. Additionally, the principles of clinical investigations with medical devices are set out in the European Standard EN540, Clinical Investigation of Medical Devices for Human Subjects. This is a harmonised standard providing presumption of conformity with Annex X of the Active Implantable Medical Devices Directive and Annex X of the Medical Devices Directive.

Before devices intended for clinical investigation are made available to a medical practitioner for the purposes of clinical investigation, the manufacturer of the device (or the authorised representative in the EU) must give 60 days' prior notice to the Competent Authority. If the Competent Authority has not raised objections within that period of 60 days, the clinical investigation may proceed.

By virtue of the provisions of the Medical Devices Regulations, Member States may authorise manufacturers to commence the clinical investigation prior to the expiry of the 60-day period if the relevant ethics committee has issued a favourable opinion with regard to the investigation in question. The option is, however, left to the discretion of each Member State.

Finally, for all clinical investigations of devices falling within the scope of the Medical Devices Directive, a relevant ethics committee opinion is required (Medical Devices Regulations: Paragraph 16(1)(a) which incorporates Annex VIII, Paragraph 2.2 of the Medical Devices Directive). Although not required under the provisions of the Active Implantable Medical Devices Directive, all clinical investigations of AIMDs should also receive a favourable ethics committee opinion before commencement.

The ethics committee opinion(s), whether approved or qualified, must be sent to the Competent Authority with the other required documentation when notification of a clinical investigation is made.

In the case of a multicentre clinical investigation, the Competent Authority will carry out assessment of that investigation, provided that the opinion from one of the relevant ethics committees is submitted with the original documentation.

The requirements for clinical investigations with medical devices in Europe are presented by country in Table 2.

Table 2. Medical device guidelines – an overview of requirements by country in Europe.

AUSTRIA	
Observations	● Reimbursement of device is regulated in some cases by individual's insurance/health care providers ● Detailed clinical trial requirements defined in law ● Auditing of clinical investigation is mandatory ● It is mandatory to conduct clinical investigations in accordance with GCP
Labelling	● German
Information for subject	● German
Insurance	● Insurance is required by law ● Personal injury insurance applicable ● Austrian law applies in all cases
Ethics committee	● Mandatory for all clinical investigations ● For multicentre trials, one ethics committee approval required although all ethics committees require to receive list of *all* participating investigators ● Hospital ● May charge fees
Notification	● Notification required for all trials ● For trials conducted under the Medical Devices Directive (MDD), a 60-day waiting period obligatory ● No waiting period for trials not conducted under the MDD ● No fees ● No standard form required

Table 2. *Continued.*

BELGIUM

Observations	• No reimbursement for clinical investigation devices
Labelling	• French, Dutch/Flemish, German • English may be possible
Information for subject	• French, Dutch/Flemish, German
Insurance	• Insurance is required by law
Ethics committee	• Hospital • Some may charge fees • Applicable to all clinical investigations
Notification	• Notification for MDD trials but authorities do want to know about all trials in their country • Authorisation may be given prior to 60-day period if ethics committee approval is received for clinical investigations conducted under the MDD • May start immediately after ethics committee approval for all other trials • No Competent Authority fees • No standard form at this time

---

DENMARK

Observation	• No reimbursement for devices
Labelling	• May be Danish or other language • Must be agreed with the ethics committee
Information for subject	• Most likely Danish but must be agreed with ethics committee
Insurance	• The law does not mandate the necessity of insurance although the Competent Authority is considering requiring insurance by law; it is nonetheless recommended to have insurance to ensure full compliance • Competent Authority considering regulation for mandatory insurance
Ethics committee	• Central Scientific Ethical Committee, part of the Danish Ministry of Health (i.e. Competent Authority) • Must submit for approval of all types of clinical investigation • Fees charged
Notification	• Approval by ethics committee does not require notification to Competent Authority • For all clinical investigations, no waiting period once approval given

Table 2. *Continued.*

FINLAND

Observations	• Drafting clinical trial guidelines • Reimbursement dependent on hospital/patient insurer
Labelling	• Finnish or Swedish if intended for patient • English permitted for professional use
Information for subject	• Finnish or Swedish
Insurance	• The law does not mandate the necessity of insurance, although it is recommended to have insurance to ensure full compliance with GCP
Ethics committee	• Hospital • Fees exist • Applicable to all clinical investigations
Notification	• Notification required for all clinical investigations • 60-day waiting period for clinical investigation under MDD • Can start all other trials directly after notification provided there is ethics committee approval • Fees for Competent Authority notification based on level of risk associated with product: the higher the risk, the higher the fee • Standard form may be applicable

---

FRANCE

Observations	• No reimbursement for clinical investigation devices • *Loi Huriet* (i.e. French GCP) applies to clinical investigation • Multicentre clinical investigations require one principal investigator • Devices to be given free-of-charge to clinical investigation sites
Labelling	• French
Information for subject	• French
Insurance	• Insurance (specifically, liability and risk) required by law • Insurance with a French company mandatory • Duration may be set by ethics committee for certain products
Ethics committee	• Regional • Charges fees, approximately FF10 000 • Applicable to all clinical investigations
Notification	• Must notify Ministry of Health for all trials • No delay in starting once ethics committee approval is granted • No standard form to be submitted but should consult with Ministry of Health in advance due to changes within the agency which are taking place • No fees

Table 2. *Continued.*

GERMANY

Observations	• *Länder* authorities supervise the clinical investigation process. Each *Land* could stipulate additional requirements • May be dealing with 16 different sets of requirements at *Land* level • No reimbursement for clinical investigation devices/treatments
Labelling	• German or another Community language according to Law on Medical Products (MPG) • *Länder* authorities could require German only
Information for subject	• German
Insurance	• Insurance required by law on subject insurance (*Probandenversicherung*) • Coverage set for a minimum of DM 1 million
Ethics committee	• Registered with and approved by Competent Authority • Currently 22 ethics committees, appointed and recognised under MPG • Private institutions • Fees applicable • Required for studies involving human subjects
Notification	• Notification for all trials to the *Land/Länder* authority(ies) where clinical investigation site(s) located • Technically a 60-day waiting period for trials done for MDD purposes. *Länder* authorities may regulate differently, e.g. trial could commence directly upon ethics committee approval • Use of standard form may be required – depends on the *Länder* authorities • No fees charged

GREECE

Observations	• No reimbursement for clinical investigation devices/treatments
Labelling	• Greek (including software)
Information for subject	• Greek
Insurance	• Insurance required by law
Ethics committee	• Hospital • Applicable to all clinical investigations • Charging of fees is unknown
Notification	• Notification for all trials involving products that are not conformité européene (CE)-marked • No notification for trials using CE-marked products. Can commence trial on ethics committee approval. • Application may be in English, French or German although English is preferred • Must wait 60 days prior to beginning the clinical investigation for those conducted under the MDD • No fees known

Table 2. *Continued.*

IRELAND

Observations	• No reimbursement for clinical investigation devices/treatments
Labelling	• English
Information for subject	• English
Insurance	• Insurance necessary. Authorities must be satisfied that investigators and clinical investigation sites are indemnified in case of injury
Ethics committee	• Hospital • May charge fees • Required for all clinical investigations
Notification	• Notification on all clinical trials • Class I and all other devices used in trials not conducted under the MDD may commence immediately after notification, provided ethics committee approval has been issued • For Class II-a, II-b and III devices, notification to Department of Health (DoH) at least 60 days prior to making devices available for clinical trial • Within 60 days of giving notice, DoH gives written notice to sponsor if objections to trial or trial can commence if ethics committee approval obtained • No fees • Standard form most likely applicable

ITALY

Observations	• Reimbursement depends on hospital and insurer • Clinical investigation must be done in public hospitals only • Must comply with Italian GCP laws
Labelling	• Italian (including all labelling on or provided with the device as well as software)
Information for subject	• Italian
Insurance	• Required by law
Ethics committee	• Hospital • May charge fees • Required for all clinical investigations
Notification	• Notification required for all clinical investigations • Application may be in Italian, English or French although the Competent Authority prefers either Italian or English • Must wait 60 days for clinical investigations conducted under the MDD • Other trials require notification but can commence directly upon ethics committee approval • No fees at present

Table 2. *Continued.*

LUXEMBOURG	

Observations	• Trial devices could be expected to be free-of-charge to clinical investigation sites
Labelling	• Must be in French, German or Letzeburgish • English may be accepted for professional use
Information for subject	• Must be in French, German or Letzeburgish
Insurance	• Insurance required
Ethics committee	• Hospital • May charge fees • Required for all clinical investigations
Notification	• Notifications for all clinical investigations which are being conducted under the MDD • Applications may be in French, German or Letzeburgish • 60-day waiting period for clinical investigations conducted under the MDD • Other clinical investigation may commence directly after ethics committee approval received • No fee structure determined as yet • No standard form/application

NETHERLANDS	

Observations	• CE-marked devices may be used in clinical investigation if the device is being used in accordance with its intended purpose • Reimbursement depends on the hospital and insurer • GCP compliance is mandatory. Recent changes have far-reaching implications
Labelling	• Dutch, although English may be accepted. Requires approval from Competent Authority • Clinical investigation devices must include a statement that they cannot be CE-marked
Information for subject	• Dutch
Insurance	• General liability and risk insurance required
Ethics committee	• Hospital but also a central ethics committee exists. In some cases a central ethics committee opinion must be obtained in place of hospital ethics committee • May charge fees • Required for all clinical investigations
Notification	• Specific guidance issued by health authority outlining procedure for clinical investigation application and data to be presented to Competent Authority • Applications must be in English • Must wait 60 days for clinical investigations conducted under the MDD • Can commence directly after favourable ethics committee opinion for CE-marked devices used in clinical investigation • No standard form although there is a requirement for specific documentation to be submitted • No fees

Table 2. *Continued.*

PORTUGAL	
Observations	● None
Labelling	● Portuguese
Information for subject	● Portuguese
Insurance	● Insurance is required
Ethics committee	● Hospital ● No fees at present, although this could change
Notification	● Notification for all clinical investigations ● 60-day waiting period for clinical investigations conducted under MDD ● Other clinical investigations may commence directly after ethics committee approval ● Applications may be submitted in Portuguese, English, French or Spanish ● No fees charged by Competent Authority at present, although this could change ● No standard forms at present

SPAIN	
Observations	● A number of additional requirements exist in Spain which do not exist elsewhere ● Clinical investigation covered by a separate decree ● Autonomous regions are entitled to require details of all clinical investigations being conducted in their territories ● Devices to be provided free-of-charge to hospitals
Labelling	● Spanish
Information for subject	● Spanish
Insurance	● Insurance is required by law
Ethics committee	● Mandatory under law ● Hospital ● Fees may be charged
Notification	● Notification for all clinical investigations ● 60-day waiting period for clinical investigations conducted under MDD ● Other clinical investigations may commence 15 days after receipt of acknowledgement from Ministry of Health. Must have ethics committee approval ● Applications to be in Spanish ● Must notify Ministry of Health of all changes to the clinical investigation plan ● Clinical study report to be provided to Competent Authority at the closure of the trial ● No fees at present ● Standard format for application required

Table 2. *Continued.*

SWEDEN	
Observations	• National Board of Health (NBH) regulates the clinical investigations • Medical Product Agency (MPA) is responsible for assessing trial design and performance • Swedish guidelines exist on the performance of clinical investigations to GCP • No reimbursement for non-CE-marked devices • Reimbursement for CE-marked devices used in a clinical investigation
Labelling	• Swedish, although English may be acceptable
Information for subject	• Swedish
Insurance	• Insurance required
Ethics committee	• Hospital • Fees may be charged
Notification	• Notification for all clinical investigations to authorities • 60-day waiting period for clinical investigations using non-CE-marked devices • Applications should be in Swedish although English will be accepted • Applications to be submitted in quadruplicate • Fees charged (Skr 10 000) • Standard format to be used, applications must be signed by investigator, sponsor, monitor and chief of the department at the clinical investigation site

Table 2. *Continued.*

UNITED KINGDOM

Observations	• None
Labelling	• English
Information for subject	• English
Insurance	• No statutory insurance requirements, recommended to have insurance to ensure compliance with GCP • Ethics committees require sponsor to have insurance
Ethics committee	• Regional for each trial site • Fees charged and are variable
Notification	• Notification for clinical investigations being conducted for purposes of the MDD • Must give at least 60 days' prior notice to Medical Devices Agency (MDA) of the trial. MDA gives sponsor (within 60 days) a written notice if any objections to the trial exist, if there are no objections, trial may commence after the 60-day waiting period for clinical investigations conducted under MDD provided there is a favourable ethics committee opinion • May commence other clinical investigations only when there is ethics committee approval • May submit application to Competent Authority for multicentre sites when a favourable ethics committee opinion has been obtained for one of the sites; other ethics committee opinions, however, must be submitted to Competent Authority prior to commencing trial in those hospitals • Applications to be submitted in English • Standard application format mandatory • Fees charged linked to risk classification of device

CONCLUSION

The volume of information relating to the regulatory aspects of biotechnology products and medical devices appears daunting at first sight. In real terms, however, much of this information is given to provide a menu for guidance and the apparent complexity can be overcome by a combination of considered application and experience. Those new to clinical research involving biotechnology products and medical devices should seek local support and advice, paying particular attention to the specific country nuances for clinical trials in these and other evolving areas.

REFERENCE

EudraLex (1998). *The Rules Governing Medicinal Products in the European Union. Volume 3A: Medicinal Products for Human Use. Quality and Biotechnology – Guidelines*, European Commission, Brussels.

24

Fraud and misconduct in clinical research

Frank Wells

INTRODUCTION

Patients are entitled to receive treatment that is based on sound evidence. This is fundamental to the practice of medicine. That there are so many effective treatments available for the cure or control of so many diseases is largely the outcome of decades of successful research. Such research must continue for the indefinite future, however, in order to master diseases including the cancers, psychoses, dementia and many others, which are currently untreatable successfully. This will include genetic and biotechnological research, recognising that the welfare of patient-subjects involved in such research must be safeguarded.

Though rare, one of the greatest pitfalls threatening the welfare of patients is their exploitation by fraud in the context of clinical research. It remains difficult to quantify, but whatever the actual occurrence rate, even one case is one too many. Fraud in any context is deplorable, but if it is primarily prescription, tax or financial fraud, the only party at risk is the victim of the fraud – and this may be the Government or, ultimately, the taxpayer. *Research* fraud is far more heinous: it distorts the database on which many decisions may be made, and possibly has adverse repercussions for thousands of other individuals. *Clinical* research fraud has the potential to be horrifyingly dangerous: if licensing decisions were to be based on efficacy and safety data that are false, the result could be disastrous. Fortunately, there is no strong evidence that such a sequence of events has yet occurred, but the importance of the roles of both the clinical trial monitor and the independent auditor cannot be over-emphasised in this regard. Nevertheless, they are inadequate by themselves when fraudsters are determined to cheat and to cover their tracks so that auditors are hoodwinked into believing that all is well. While fraudsters are confidence tricksters who deceive their victims remarkably convincingly, there is sufficient published evidence to confirm that fraud in clinical research is ever-present (Campbell, 1997).

The conduct of most clinical research is honest and honourable. Occasionally, however, the sponsor of a clinical study may be faced with data that are suspect. Such data might or might not be fraudulent. It is vitally important for society in general, and for the pharmaceutical industry in particular, that all possible attempts are made to eliminate fraudulent research. This chapter is addressed to all those responsible for sponsoring, monitoring and auditing biomedical research projects, including research ethics committees. Its twin aims are to alert them to fraud and to provide guidelines for its detection, investigation, prosecution and prevention. Many companies and institutions already have standard operating procedures (SOPs) in place which outline the steps to be adopted by any staff or colleagues suspecting fraud and which emphasise the philosophy and management commitment of the organisation concerned. This chapter is therefore also intended to stimulate and assist organisations in establishing a relevant SOP where one does not already exist.

The ideal world where fraud does not occur is remote from the real world in which we live. Although high standards are invariably set for clinical research, to which all interested parties are expected to adhere, fraud can still occur. Indeed, it is highly unlikely that anyone working in the field of clinical research will not have met a case of fraud during their professional career. Procedures must therefore be in place for the time when fraud is suspected, despite the existence of these standards. Within the pharmaceutical industry, the standards needed for the conduct of clinical research already exist, and have been adopted by all regulatory bodies licensing medicines, international pharmaceutical companies and contract research organisations. Although predated by the Committee for Proprietary Medicinal Products (CPMP) guidelines on good clinical practice (GCP) in the European Community (CPMP, 1991) and the requirements of the US Food and Drug Administration (FDA), the GCP guideline adopted under the International Conference on Harmonisation (ICH) process now takes global precedence (ICH Guideline, 1996). With ICH at the Step 5 stage, global guidance and therefore global standards now exist which have been adopted by Europe, the USA and Japan. Although the standards referred to above are in place, no such harmonisation exists for dealing with fraud and misconduct in the context of clinical research. Indeed, even within Europe, there is as yet no agreed attitude towards tackling the problem. However, whatever its incidence, this unacceptable aspect of clinical research must be tackled if we are to achieve and maintain confidence in scientific integrity and in the clinical research process.

DEFINITIONS

Distinctions must be drawn between clinical research of poor quality and that which is fraudulent. Data with minor flaws should be detected by the clinical trial monitor of the pharmaceutical company or contract house, and drawn to the attention of the investigator who can check if errors have been made, and can correct them, though without deleting the original flaws. Such flaws result from lack of attention to detail, pressure of work, inadequate or over-complex case record forms or guidelines for their completion, or carelessness, and not from malice aforethought. Corrections can be made without loss of integrity.

Fraud is much less frequent than carelessness: although difficult to quantify, its incidence has been estimated at between 0.1 and 0.4% (Hone, 1993). Based on my current work on cases of fraud, however, I believe that the true incidence may be nearer to 1%. On this basis, in the UK therefore, some 30 studies that may be fraudulent could be in progress at any one time. Extrapolating this to the rest of the world, and there is no evidence that the incidence of fraud in clinical research differs across Europe or North America (although it is dealt with more openly in the UK), there may be between 125 and 150 clinical trials currently in progress where some of the data being generated are fraudulent, where investigators are fabricating some of the data to be submitted to a company and – worst of all – where patients are being exploited in the process.

Fraud can be defined in many ways, but two definitions will prove useful. The first, which was agreed at the Joint Consensus Conference on Misconduct in Biomedical Research convened by the Faculty of Pharmaceutical Medicine and the Royal College of Physicians of Edinburgh in October 1999, defines *research misconduct* as: 'Behaviour by a researcher, intentional or not, that falls short of good ethical and scientific standards' (Royal College of Physicians of Edinburgh, 2000). According to the second definition, *frank fraud* in the context of research is: 'The generation of false data with the intent to deceive'. If we discount carelessness, these definitions cover everything that comes into the category of suspect data.

HISTORICAL ASPECTS OF FRAUD

Most of the earlier documented cases of fraud in the medical research field are from the USA, and many of these refer to published papers, but the phenomenon is global. Five examples will suffice here, although further details of most of them, and several additional case histories, can be found in the definitive book on the subject (Lock and Wells, 1996).

The first example is that of John Darsee, a research cardiologist, first at Emory University, then at Harvard Medical School (LaFollette, 1992). He committed an extensive series of frauds, including non-existent patients or collaborators as well as fabricated data. During his career he published over 100 papers and abstracts, many of which have had to be retracted from the prestigious journals in which they first appeared.

Robert Slutsky was a resident in cardiological radiology at the University of California, San Diego. Between 1978 and 1985, he published 137 articles, either as principal author or co-author, most of which were based on non-existent data (Friedman, 1990). Interestingly, although roundly discredited, only some of his fraudulent articles have subsequently been retracted by the editors of the journals in which they were published.

The story of thalidomide is well-known; less well-known are the attempts by William McBride, one of the first to describe the effects of thalidomide on the developing foetus, to discredit another drug, Debendox (known as Bendectin in the USA) along similar lines (Swan, 1996). McBride had never in fact conducted controlled trials to determine the thalidomide effect, but had at least accurately observed its toxicity. The situation with Debendox/Bendectin was different because McBride was ostensibly responsible for conducting studies on rabbits during the late 1970s which had shown up the product's toxicity. It took a decade to demonstrate publicly that such studies did not exist, and almost another decade before McBride was publicly denounced in 1996 – much too late to save what was possibly a valuable therapeutic product. Here was an example of an eminent public figure whose reputation was such that it was unthinkable that he might be telling lies. Furthermore, this case demonstrates the messianic complex occasionally seen in fraudsters who seem to believe that they have a divine right to state falsehoods as if they were proven facts.

Dr Roger Poisson was a researcher at St Luc Hospital, Montreal, Canada. In 1993 he was investigated by the Office of Research Integrity (ORI) and found to have fabricated and falsified patient data submitted to the National Surgical Adjuvant Breast and Bowel Project regarding a number of multi-centre clinical studies on breast and bowel cancer. As a result of the ORI's investigation, Dr Poisson was debarred for eight years from the receipt of any federal funding. It took until 1996, however, before he appeared before the Discipline Committee of the Quebec College of Doctors. He pleaded guilty to 13 counts of committing 'acts derogatory to the honour and dignity of the medical profession' and he was subsequently reprimanded, fined and permanently restricted from several activities, including serving as a principal investigator in medical research (Anonymous, 1997a).

The first extensively documented British case, in 1988, was that of Dr Uzair Siddiqui, a psychiatrist in the city of Durham (Anonymous, 1988). An astute pharmaceutical company clinical trial monitor found that Dr Siddiqui had fabricated some of the laboratory data for most of the patients purported to have taken part in a clinical trial and had invented one patient altogether. The laboratories used for this study were located in two hospitals inside and outside the city, and the monitor could not find any evidence at either laboratory that specimens had been submitted for analysis. When challenged, Dr Siddiqui claimed that he had not performed the study himself, but had delegated it to his medical registrar (a doctor in training); however, he had forgotten her name and did not know where she now worked. The help of the UK trade association, the Association of the British Pharmaceutical Industry

(ABPI) was sought, and it was not difficult to ascertain the name and location of the junior doctor accused by Dr Siddiqui. She, however, very strongly denied any involvement in the study and her evidence was accepted and subsequently confirmed.

The case was a strong one to take to the General Medical Council (GMC) but, understandably at the time, the pharmaceutical company was very concerned that it might be criticised for making an allegation of fraud. Indeed, it was worried that it would lose the confidence of doctors if it were seen to be taking such an action. With some misgivings, therefore, the case was submitted to the GMC and eventually its Professional Conduct Committee (PCC) found Dr Siddiqui guilty of serious professional misconduct and his name was erased from the medical register.

The reaction of doctors in Durham was exactly as the pharmaceutical company had feared: they were furious that a company, even though it had been supported by the ABPI, had dared to refer an eminent consultant psychiatrist to the GMC. They imposed a sanction against the company by banning it from the local postgraduate medical centre, to which all pharmaceutical companies normally had access for sponsored meetings. Fortunately, within two weeks, it proved possible to hold an independent meeting in Durham, at which the full facts were explained (the case having been conducted in complete confidentiality until the public hearing of the PCC), and the *status quo ante* was restored.

In some respects this event marked a watershed in the UK. It has subsequently come to be expected of the pharmaceutical industry that it *would* take forthright action against any doctor found beyond all shadow of doubt to have committed fraud. Since Dr Siddiqui, 16 further cases have been submitted by companies and the ABPI to the GMC: all have been found guilty of serious professional misconduct and the majority of them have been struck off the medical register. The most recent cases are summarised towards the end of this chapter.

These events manifestly demonstrate that clinical research fraud is a problem against which all possible steps should be taken. Until relatively recently, however, little had been done historically to formalise these steps. Even now, and even within the developed world, little has happened apart from isolated initiatives in the Scandinavian countries and Austria, where there are Committees on Scientific Dishonesty (Andersen *et al.*, 1992), in the UK where the pharmaceutical industry, through the ABPI and a private agency (MedicoLegal Investigations Limited) has been very active (Smith, 1997), and in the USA where both the FDA and the ORI (which also operates in Canada) are active in this regard. Thus, for some time before anything was done about it, there was an impression amongst pharmaceutical physicians, clinical trial monitors and quality assurance professionals, that a small but significant amount of data supplied by clinical investigators was fraudulent. Eventually, this view came to be shared by the Royal College of Physicians

(RCP), which set up its own working party on fraud and misconduct in clinical research in 1990, following the publication of a leading article in the *British Medical Journal* (Lock, 1988). This RCP initiative was important, lending voice to the suspicion that several serious instances of fraud and misconduct had occurred which had not been investigated or reported. Sadly, no action followed the publication of its report (Royal College of Physicians of London, 1991), and it was consequently left to the ABPI to set up its own working party to produce its own report, on which action *was* taken (Wells, 1994). Clear agreed guidelines for the UK industry thus exist from which many actions have followed.

Before this forthright UK industry policy was adopted, UK pharmaceutical companies suspecting fraud seemed greatly concerned about the risk of recrimination, adverse publicity, and loss of favour, support and indeed prescriptions if they were seen to be critical of the medical profession. These concerns had some justification at the time, but not now. Indeed, in the UK at least, were a pharmaceutical company or contract research organisation *not* to take action to investigate any case of suspected fraud, it would be very vulnerable indeed, and likely to be pilloried by the media if its lack of action were to be discovered. Regrettably, as already mentioned, other than in Scandinavia, the situation is far less robust in continental Europe where there is still considerable reluctance to take action against an errant investigator, seemingly for the very reasons that prevailed in the UK a decade ago. Nevertheless, there is now evidence of some movement towards adopting clear courses of action in cases of suspected fraud in France, Germany and certain other European countries, and the author of this chapter has already obtained some experience in the forensic investigation of such cases outside the UK.

SUSPICION

The ABPI working party began its deliberations against a background of increasing confidence on the part of UK pharmaceutical companies to take action against doctors found to have submitted fraudulent data, but uncertain how best to investigate or to handle suspicions that such data might be fraudulent. The working party recognised that a facilitating mechanism was needed to enable member companies to pursue such suspicions without prejudice.

The RCP report had suggested the appointment of a 'screener' who would decide whether or not an allegation of fraud should be investigated (Royal College of Physicians of London, 1991). To enable that decision to be made, the screener would first receive and consider a detailed confidential statement in support of the allegation. If it were clear that the suspicion was justified, then an investigation should be conducted to enable a case, if proved, to be presented to a court of law, or to the GMC. However, if it were found that the allegation was not substantiated, then an informal enquiry would be conducted, subject to the utmost degree of confidentiality, by a panel of three 'appropriate' persons. The enquiry would either lead to the allegation being withdrawn or to it proceeding to an investigation, as above. The ABPI has adopted a considerably modified version of this procedure, vesting responsibility for advising on the methods of enquiry in its Medical Director. In practice, this responsibility has been shared with the author of this chapter in his capacity as consultant medical advisor to both the ABPI and to MedicoLegal Investigations Limited.

PREVENTION

Outside the discipline of clinical research, few individuals are aware of, or understand, the principles of Good Clinical (Research) Practice (GCP). Those within the discipline, though, tend to take it for granted that everyone is aware of what they are doing and why. It is therefore essential to spend some time and effort in explaining the principles of good clinical research practice not only to individual investigators but also to their colleagues, their peers and, indeed, the leaders of the medical profession. There are several reasons for doing this, not least of which is the prevention of fraud. Fraud is most likely to be prevented if investigators, and their colleagues, are fully aware of GCP standards, of the requirement for the pharmaceutical industry to operate to them, and of the commitment of companies to act vigorously against any irregularities. The ICH GCP guideline emphasises the importance of monitoring, and of audit procedures (ICH Guideline, 1996). The need for this information to be promulgated, and for investigators to be trained in the principles of GCP continues. Outside the context of industry sponsorship, clinical research is not subject to any agreed standards, though organisations such as the Medical Research Council (MRC) in the UK have set out their own commendable guidelines (Medical Research Council, 1998). It is therefore appropriate to suggest that the equivalent of GCP standards should apply equally to non-industry-sponsored scientific studies.

Despite GCP, there is always a possibility that investigators will deliver unsatisfactory clinical data. This can be for a number of reasons, including pressure of work or fatigue. Frequently, it can be because of carelessness. Careful, meticulous, clinical investigators who are trustworthy are essential. It is the responsibility of the pharmaceutical physician, in co-operation with the clinical trial monitor, to ensure that only reliable investigators are recruited.

Local research ethics committees (LRECs) have an important role to play in ensuring that investigators are approved as rigorously as protocols. Indeed, section 3 of the ICH GCP guideline clearly sets out these two quite different but equally important responsibilities (ICH Guideline, 1996). Thus, although it would be inappropriate to suggest that LRECs should adopt a 'policing' role with regard to investigators, they must satisfy themselves that local investigators – about whom only they will possess relevant local knowledge – are competent in all respects. LRECs also have a responsibility to assist if or when fraud is suspected (see below).

THE REASONS FOR FRAUD

There are many reasons why doctors may volunteer inappropriately to become investigators. These are well recognised in the report of the Royal College of Physicians on fraud and misconduct in medical research (Royal College of Physicians of London, 1991). For some, it may be pressure to publish, and recent industry experience confirms this. However, it is well-known that doctors in training, ultimately hoping to obtain consultant appointments, seek to enhance their list of published papers, which will be closely scrutinised when they come to apply for a career post. Also, doctors in academic departments require a list of up-to-date references of their recent publications when, in the UK for example, submitting their bids under the Higher Education Funding Council's quadrennial assessment scheme or when applying for extra staff or for scarce additional research grants. There is, of course, nothing inherently wrong in undertaking research with a view to publish, but the pressure to fabricate, duplicate, slice-up or plagiarise must be vigorously resisted.

Some doctors might wish to take part in a clinical trial because of their perception of the excessively routine nature of day-to-day clinical practice. Involvement in a research project injects a break into that routine, and such doctors may produce very good data because they have been stimulated by their involvement in research. However, it is also recognised that a doctor who has become bored may well have difficulty in maintaining standards, and the involvement of such a doctor in a research project must be monitored with care.

Some doctors will admit that they offer to take part in clinical trials primarily because of the money they will earn for doing so. As far as this aspect is concerned, there should be two safeguards. The first is the approval of the LREC that the amount to be paid to the investigator is acceptable. The second is to have an agreed figure suggested by a body whose influence is largely accepted by doctors throughout the country concerned. For the UK, until recently, the British Medical Association, through its Professional Fees Committee, suggested an hourly figure for payment by pharmaceutical companies to investigators taking part in clinical trials: this was generally accepted by pharmaceutical companies as the benchmark level throughout the UK. Unfortunately, fair trading laws have prevented this service continuing, but the historical figure, established in 1992, was GBP 100 per hour and *pro rata*.

Doctors undertaking research work mainly for money are particularly likely to take short-cuts, or to produce fraudulent data. In the light of recent experience they undertake too many clinical trials with the patient population or the time at their disposal, and they are tempted to invent patients or to invent data attributed to genuine patients. As the RCP report has stated (Royal College of Physicians of London, 1991), some doctors may be emotionally disturbed (an excuse for fraudulent data used on more than one occasion recently) or frankly mentally ill; bizarre aberrations of data may be supplied by a doctor who is suffering from a psychotic illness.

Again, as the RCP mentioned in its report, some doctors are motivated by the incentive of vanity. They need their partners or their colleagues or the world at large to see how busy or how clever they are, without having any real commitment to undertaking clinical research in accordance with the principles of GCP.

Companies are therefore advised to take the utmost care in recruiting, remunerating and retaining appropriate investigators. They should reject any potential investigator about whom doubts have arisen as a result of past involvement in a research project. A mechanism now exists for sharing doubts outside the company where those doubts were originally generated. This is the 'grey list', for which the ABPI Medical Director has a 'possibly suspect doctor name-holding' responsibility. Companies may ask whether the name of a possibly suspect doctor has already been given to the ABPI by another company, a question that receives a Yes/No answer. No list of names is promulgated although the information is held on computer.

THE DETECTION OF FRAUD

Most investigators conduct research projects entirely satisfactorily. However, despite careful selection of investigators, standards occasionally slip, and if this process is insidious, fraudulent investigators can be exceedingly difficult to detect. The general principles for the detection of fraud are all commonsense, but it is often the complexity of clinical trials that makes the application of commonsense difficult and fraud hard to detect.

Methods for detecting fraud

A clinical trial monitor must remember that fraud can occur anywhere and at any time. The biggest case of fraudulent research in the USA was first investigated after the research team at a pharmaceutical company became suspicious when the data submitted by a specialist physician were found to be 'too perfect'. The data were indeed just that – too good to be true. On the other hand, a very few investigators *are* obsessional and have a fanatical attitude towards neatness and tidiness, and these blameless few must, of course, be recognised.

It used to be felt that the precise methods used by companies for the detection of fraud should be kept secret; detection may indeed often depend on a particular way of selecting numbers or on patterns within written text. However, while it was once thought that potential fraudsters would be helped to avoid making easily detected mistakes if they were forewarned, this is now felt to be fallacious. This attitude therefore no longer applies, as it is clearly in the public interest that the chances of fraud occurring should be minimised. This chapter is therefore intended to help pharmaceutical companies to set up their own internal procedures and methods to avoid fraud being perpetrated against them.

Although they do not appear in the published literature and are fortunately few and far between, it should be mentioned that cases are known where there has been suspected collusion on the part of the company employee or department with the person perpetrating the fraud. Usually this happens when the company employee involved – sometimes a very senior executive – is simply not prepared to think the unthinkable. This situation is exemplified by a recent case in which the head of research, who had held this post for many years, resisted any attempt to investigate a clear case of patient exploitation in the research context, solely because he could not accept that someone whom he held in the highest regard had exploited him as well as patients in the conduct of a pivotal research project. Such occurrences can be minimised by having an SOP in place which clearly requires any company employee who believes that their concerns are not being taken seriously to report such concerns to management at the most senior level or to a relevant outside body. Such a body could be the Committee on Scientific Dishonesty in Denmark, Finland, Norway or Sweden, the FDA or the ORI in the USA, or ABPI/MedicoLegal Investigations Limited in the UK.

Fraud is often detected by the clinical trial monitor working in the field. These monitors may well be junior staff entering their first professional post after obtaining a degree. They need to be trained so that if they have the slightest concern that something is not right with the centre or investigator, this should be discussed immediately with their project manager or other responsible person within the company. Many new graduates find this very difficult to put into practice, particularly if dealing with well-known investigators or centres. Strong reassurance on the importance of discussing this type of concern must be given.

It is therefore critical that methods for communicating doubts about the integrity of any data should take this into account. All such doubts, even if based on only the most circumstantial evidence, should be communicated by the project manager to the Medical Director or other independent person. If the person expressing concern does not think that the matter has been followed up appropriately, company procedures should also provide appeal, without prejudice, to the next level of management or to the Quality Assurance Manager.

If the basic and refresher training programmes for clinical trial monitors discuss fraud case studies, all staff will learn to pick up signs which should prompt them to be suspicious of an investigator or centre. With encouragement, clinical trial monitors may rapidly build up a 'library' of quotes or attitudes that may indicate fraud. Examples include:

- 'I won't actually be doing the work myself, my registrar will, but you can't meet her today because she is off somewhere else.'
- 'I will be getting the patients from several other clinics/outpatients, but I am not quite sure which ones I will be using yet.'
- 'I don't have the patients' records here – but if you let me know what the questions are, I will follow them up and send the answers on to you.'

Monitoring for patterns and trends in documentation

Primary and secondary research monitors, either field- or office-based, often become suspicious because of patterns or trends in the appearance of case record forms (CRFs). Initially, their concerns may be nothing more than a 'gut feeling'. Monitoring visits are often spaced out over many weeks or months and the CRFs concerned will have moved on to the next level within the data processing organisation. It is useful to reacquire all the CRFs relating to a particular doctor or centre and to review them all together. This may highlight suspicious similarities that were missed when the CRFs were dealt with individually as they moved through the data processing system. With experience, clinical trial monitors may become astute in detecting tell-tale signs, e.g. the use of one pen for a study involving 30 patients from three different centres over a six–month period.

Patient diary cards, particularly those involving visual analogue scales for rating disease parameters, can be especially revealing. The way that the 'patient' has marked the visual analogue lines often gives the first clue. The consistent use of a cross, tick, vertical line, idiosyncrasies such as the use of dots, or connecting strokes between figures, or any other device to mark the scale across many individual subjects over time, should be viewed with suspicion. Consent forms are a relatively frequent source of forgery. Because the original consent forms are not retained with the CRFs, nor are they held by the company (in accordance with the requirement to maintain complete patient confidentiality), fraud in this area is more difficult to detect than elsewhere. The original patient notes (where the consent forms will be filed) need to be seen alongside other patients' notes and the consent forms compared side by side. If there are any suspicious circumstances arising from such a comparison, e.g. similarity of handwriting, a signature that does not flow, or different signatures ostensibly from the same witness, then it is legitimate to make copies of such discrepancies. Authorisation for such an action may be needed from the Medical Director or equivalent within the company, but it is wise to record in a lasting format, without delay, any evidence of irregularity.

Check the dates

Many cases of fraud are perpetrated in a great hurry. The fraudster is more concerned with checking that the 10- or 14-day or 1-month follow-up visits actually occur 10, 14 or 28 days after the first visit than with ensuring that the resultant dates make any sense. There are numerous examples where public holidays, notably Bank Holiday Mondays, tend to be forgotten.

Examine returned clinical trial materials and drug usage

The regular examination of returned clinical trial materials can be very worthwhile. Both subjective and objective parameters may give a clue that the materials have not been used correctly. A good example of the subjective clue is that of a particular study involving a topical non-steroidal anti-inflammatory drug. The clinical trial monitor noticed that the first two 'used tubes' returned to her looked odd. On further investigation, they seemed to have been grasped in the middle of the tube and squeezed. In fact, the indentations on the first and second tubes were identical, despite the fact that they were meant to have been used by different patients. Subsequent follow-up revealed that the 10 remaining tubes returned from this particular investigator had been squeezed in an identical manner. This is obviously a most unlikely occurrence because all individuals seem to have their own unique way of squeezing tubes. This example also illustrates how objective data can be useful. When the returned tubes from this centre were weighed, the mean weight was 20.4 g, whereas the tubes returned from the other centres had a mean weight of 12.1 g.

Further examples include the objective observation that all patients taking a particular treatment distributed in calendar packs had seemingly started on exactly the same day of the week; and that trial materials which should have been in patients' homes for two months or more were returned in pristine condition. Also of interest, and worthy of investigation on a routine basis, is the consumption of other supportive medication during double-blind or placebo-controlled studies. Good examples come from research based on the investigation of non-steroidal anti-inflammatory drugs. Such studies often involve either a placebo control group or a wash-out period in which placebo is administered. To allow the ethical use of placebo, an analgesic, such as paracetamol, is often provided, and counts of analgesic consumption are used as an index of efficacy of an active drug. In one specific case, suspicion was aroused when the apparent consumption of 'escape' analgesics remained the same during administration of the active agent as during the placebo-controlled/wash-out period. This showed up particularly when the pattern from other centres, which had received clinical trial materials from the same batch, showed a significant reduction of analgesic consumption during active treatment. A whole range of methods of looking at data derived from medication consumption can be developed, aimed at detecting patterns that do not make sense.

Sometimes electrocardiograms (ECGs) are falsified. A number of cases are on file where a single tracing has been divided up and used for the same patient as if recorded on different dates, or as if obtained from different patients. Other cases involving ECGs include speeding up or slowing down the recording, or switching leads so that the tracings differ – again, as if obtained from more than one patient.

One case was detected when source document verification revealed that the forms used for apparent magnetic resonance and echocardiography readings were six months out-of-date, confirming that the data that they showed were clearly generated fraudulently with intent to deceive.

Routine examination of the data

Once numerical data have been loaded into a database, their comprehensive analysis becomes possible. However, although this is sometimes useful, it can be very time-consuming and very seldom leads to the primary detection of fraud. The fundamental question being posed is a well-known statistical conundrum: are there any groups of patients whose data are atypical compared with other patients within the same centre or from the other centres within the same study? The methods for carrying out these analyses require the expertise of statisticians and include:

- estimated probability distribution function plots,
- stem and leaf plots,
- ordinary data plots,
- 'contour' plots,
- Mahalanobis distance calculations,
- kurtosis.

Routine and graphic systems can readily be established to allow such comparisons to be run on a regular basis as part of a quality control audit check. The interpretation of these routine tests also requires the application of straightforward commonsense. For example, doubts raised about the authenticity of the data created at one so-called 'atypical centre' were based on the observation that the patients recruited there showed a different age distribution (i.e. they were much older) compared with the age distribution at the other centres in the study. However, the medical adviser responsible pointed out that this practice was situated in a town on the south coast of England with a large retired population. It was then easy to confirm that the age/sex distribution at this centre was skewed towards elderly females, and any doubts were allayed.

A far greater difficulty is posed by the detection of a single fraudulent entry, or a series of entries relating to a particular visit. This situation may arise if a patient misses a follow-up appointment for any reason and the data for that visit are invented. The detection of this type of fraud is very difficult if the investigator has inserted clinically sensible values and has taken account of previous and subsequent results. However, the audit procedures and requirements for source document verification inherent in good clinical (research) practice may reveal discrepancies that require further investigation.

Another example in this context relates to a study with a non-steroidal anti-inflammatory drug involving measurement of the erythrocyte sedimentation rate (ESR). During active treatment, the ESR of patients with rheumatoid arthritis fell progressively in the majority of cases; trend lines were plotted for each patient and an outlier far above the trend line led to an investigation for fraud. Although these techniques may help the pharmaceutical industry, it cannot be emphasised too strongly that requirements for source document verification inherent in GCP, and all the associated audit procedures, are essential components of the processes of both the detection and investigation of suspected fraud. Furthermore, it requires the utmost vigilance from clinical trial monitors and the consistent application of quality control checks to minimise the risk of fraud going undetected.

THE PROSECUTION OF FRAUD

Once an investigator has been shown beyond all reasonable doubt to have submitted fraudulent data to a pharmaceutical company or contract house, it is essential in the interests of the public, the medical profession and the industry for that doctor to be dealt with in a forthright manner, either by appropriate disciplinary process or by prosecution. In the UK, referral to the GMC is considered appropriate, for consideration by the PCC. Alternatively, the doctor may be referred to the police, the likely outcome being prosecution for the criminal offence of deception. In the UK, the former alternative is preferable as it is a more rapid procedure than the courts of law.

The General Medical Council

Disciplinary powers were first conferred on the GMC by the Medical Act 1858, which established the Council and the Medical Register (Lock, 1990). The Council's jurisdiction in relation to professional misconduct and criminal offences is now regulated by sections 36 and 38 to 45 of, and Schedule 4 to, the Medical Act 1983. This Act provides that if any medical practitioner registered with the GMC:

● is found by the PCC to have been convicted in the British Isles of a criminal offence, or
● is judged by the PCC to have been guilty of serious professional misconduct,

the Committee may, if it thinks fit, direct that his/her name shall be erased from the medical register, or that his/her registration be suspended for a period not exceeding 12 months, or that his/her registration shall be conditional on his/her compliance, during a period not exceeding 3 years, with such requirements as the Committee sees fit to impose for the protection of members of the public or in his/her interests.

Cases submitted to the GMC must be presented in the form of a statutory declaration, a model for which appears in Figure 1. The majority of cases

---

The President
General Medical Council
44 Hallam Street
LONDON W1M 6AE

Sir

We, the undersigned, Dr......... (position occupied) .... of the Association of the British Pharmaceutical Industry, of 12 Whitehall, London SW1A 2DY, and Dr............ (position occupied) .... of (company) .... Limited, of (company address) .... do solemnly and sincerely declare as follows:

That Dr (name) .... general practitioner (or professional status), of (address of doctor) .... has acted in a manner which has brought the medical profession into disrepute. Having considered details of the case which are summarised in the report, a copy of which is attached to this formal declaration and forms part of it, we allege that a question of serious professional misconduct is raised by (brief statement of the irregularities) ....

We make this Declaration conscientiously believing the same to be true by virtue of the Statutory Declaration Act 1835.

Signed   (a) ....
             (b) ....

Declared at: (address where declared) ....
On: (date of declaration) ....
Before me: ....
(Justice of the Peace or Solicitor)

Figure 1. Model statutory declaration.

submitted to the GMC by pharmaceutical companies recently have been mediated through the ABPI and, most recently, facilitated by MedicoLegal Investigations Limited. The simple statutory declaration must be accompanied by a report setting out the details of the case, including a description of the clinical study, the method of recruitment of the doctor to whom the report refers, the monitoring process, how suspicions were first raised, how they were investigated, and how the conclusion was reached that led to the case being presented to the GMC. Supporting documents are required, although these best follow the declaration and the report. These supporting documents include the clinical study protocol, the recruitment letter(s) to the doctor concerned, the formal agreement with the doctor, including details of the financial arrangement, and copies of all the CRFs, laboratory or other reports and/or diary cards which may be suspect.

The GMC secretariat will acknowledge receipt of the statutory declaration, and will subsequently request any additional documents considered necessary to process the case before or after it has been considered by the Preliminary Screener. Every complaint is scrutinised meticulously, and if it appears that the evidence submitted is insufficient, the Council's solicitors may be asked to make enquiries to establish additional facts. Cases recently submitted by the industry have nearly all provided sufficient evidence for this stage to be unnecessary. Nevertheless, it may not be possible for a pharmaceutical company to obtain access to patients themselves – for example, to verify whether the patients had completed diary cards submitted by the doctor concerned – before deciding to refer a matter to the GMC. If the GMC considers such verification necessary, it will advise the pharmaceutical company accordingly, and do what it can to assist.

A decision whether action shall be taken over an allegation of serious professional misconduct is then taken by the President or by another member of the Council appointed for the purpose (the Preliminary Screener). If it appears to the President that the matter is trivial, or irrelevant to the question of serious professional misconduct, he will normally decide that it shall proceed no further. To date, none of the cases referred by or in conjunction with the ABPI and MedicoLegal Investigations Limited has come into this category. If it is decided to make allegations of serious professional misconduct, the doctor is informed of the allegations against him/her and is invited to submit a written explanation. If the doctor responds to this invitation, the explanation offered, which may include evidence in answer to the allegations, is placed before the Preliminary Proceedings Committee which next considers the case.

After considering a case of alleged serious professional misconduct, the Preliminary Proceedings Committee may decide:

1. to refer the case to the Professional Conduct Committee for inquiry;
2. to send the doctor a letter; or
3. to take no further action.

The letter referred to under 2. above may be a warning letter or a letter of advice, in cases where it appears that the conduct of the doctor has fallen below the proper standard but not to have been so serious as to necessitate a public enquiry. A small number of cases referred by the pharmaceutical industry has been dealt with in this way. The names of the doctors concerned have remained confidential.

Additionally, if it appears to the Preliminary Proceedings Committee that the doctor may be suffering from a physical or mental illness that seriously impairs his/her fitness to practise, the Committee may refer the case to the Health Committee instead of to the PCC. This safeguard for the doctor concerned is important, and has been used in at least one case referred to the GMC by the industry.

The rules governing the operation of the PCC require that any allegation of serious professional misconduct, unless admitted by the doctor, must be strictly proved by evidence, and the doctor is free to dispute and rebut the evidence called. It is therefore essential that cases referred by pharmaceutical companies to the GMC must be supported by the strongest possible evidence. The doctor is entitled to submit evidence and witnesses to rebut the allegations, and to call attention to any mitigating circumstances and to produce testimonials or other evidence as to character. Pharmaceutical companies may be required to provide witnesses for cross-examination, but the case may be so strong that such witnesses are not needed. This is what has happened in the majority of cases referred by pharmaceutical companies in conjunction with the ABPI that have been considered to date by the PCC (Anonymous, 1991; Anonymous, 1995; Dillner, 1991). If the facts alleged are found by the PCC to have been proved, then it is incumbent upon the committee to determine whether, in relation to those facts, the doctor has indeed been guilty of serious professional misconduct.

At the conclusion of any inquiry in which a doctor is found guilty of serious professional misconduct, the PCC must decide on one of the following courses of action:

- to conclude the case without affecting the doctor's registration, but with provision for admonishing the doctor;
- to postpone its determination;
- to direct that the doctor's registration be conditional on his/her compliance, for a period not exceeding 3 years, with such requirements as the PCC may think to impose for the protection of members of the public, or in the doctor's own interests;
- to direct that the doctor's registration shall be suspended for a period not exceeding 12 months; or
- to direct the erasure of the doctor's name from the medical register.

Doctors whose registration is suspended or erased have 28 days in which to give notice of appeal against the direction to the Judicial Committee of the Privy Council.

In the 16 cases referred to the PCC by the pharmaceutical industry (ABPI and MedicoLegal Investigations Limited), all 16 doctors were found guilty of serious professional misconduct: three were admonished, two were suspended for 6 months and 11 were erased from the medical register. There was one appeal, but the Privy Council, while reducing the penalty, confirmed that the doctor was indeed guilty of serious professional misconduct.

Other legal routes

If a pharmaceutical company decides, for whatever reason, that it does not wish to use the GMC procedure, or if, in another European country, for example, a company wishes to prosecute a doctor who is not registered with the GMC, it is always open to that company to use a legal process. The GMC has made it clear that it would not seek to usurp the proper authority of the police or of the Crown Prosecution Service where a criminal offence may have been committed. Alternatively, a company that considers itself fraudulently exploited by a doctor may take out a civil prosecution. A prosecution, however, would take considerably longer to process through to conviction than the GMC procedure and, if successful, would automatically (in the UK) lead to the GMC disciplinary procedure being invoked. It is therefore strongly recommended that companies should consider it most appropriate that offending doctors in the UK should be submitted to the professional disciplinary proceedings laid down by law for the GMC.

SOME RECENT CASES

Malcolm Pearce, at the time an eminent obstetrician and gynaecologist at St George's Hospital in London, claimed during 1995 to have performed a pioneering operation, when a subsequent enquiry found that he had not done so (Lock, 1995). He claimed to have successfully transplanted an ectopic pregnancy, a procedure leading to a normal full-term vaginal delivery. Had this really happened, it would have been the first time such an operation had been successfully performed. The subsequent history of this case is interesting on several counts. First, the enquiry into the fabricated operation revealed that Pearce had previously reported on a study on 191 patients with polycystic ovary disease: this was also found to be fraudulent. Secondly, both reports were published in the *British Journal of Obstetrics and Gynaecology*: the article on relocation of the ectopic pregnancy was co-authored by two others, one of whom was Professor Geoffrey Chamberlain who was also Pearce's head of department. Furthermore, Chamberlain was editor of the journal in question and President of the Royal College of Obstetricians and Gynaecologists. Obviously, Chamberlain could have had no part in the non-existent operation, and his co-authorship was thus untenable. He subsequently resigned both his editorship and his presidency. Thirdly, there is no question of Pearce conducting these false activities for financial gain: his case demonstrates the objective of some fraudsters, who are usually very vain, of wishing to be seen to be a pioneer. His case was referred to the GMC and his name was erased from the medical register.

Animal research can also be fraudulent, although it may be much more difficult to detect. Mr Yi Li was reported in the *ORI Newsletter* early in 1997 for having fabricated an experimental study on the behaviour of rats during his candidature for a PhD degree in the neuroscience programme at The University of Illinois, Urbana-Champaign. His fraud came to light following a review by the ORI, and he subsequently entered into a Voluntary Exclusion Agreement in which he agreed to exclude himself from publicly funded research activity for a period of 3 years (Anonymous 1997b).

Dr Geoffrey Fairhurst was an eminent general practitioner in St Helens, Lancashire – a town in the northwest of England (Dyer, 1996). On this occasion it was the doctor's partner who acted as 'whistle-blower' and who alerted the authorities to activities which Fairhurst was clearly doing his best to conceal. The partner discovered a number of consent forms that were not signed by the patients in question, who were therefore not aware of their involvement in a clinical trial. Furthermore, on pain of losing her job, the practice nurse had been required to alter the dates printed by the electrocardiograph on tracings taken for clinical trial purposes, sometimes by as much as 9 months. After extensive further enquiries, Fairhurst's case was referred to the GMC and his name was ultimately also erased from the medical register.

The final example concerns Dr John Anderton, a distinguished academic consultant renal physician in Edinburgh who in his time had been Secretary of the Royal College of Physicians of Edinburgh (Dyer, 1997). An astute clinical trial monitor discovered that, some 6 months prior to the commencement of the particular study, the laboratories concerned had discontinued the forms on which Dr Anderton had submitted magnetic resonance and echocardiography data. This led to the involvement of an investigational agency which conducted further enquiries, including questioning a number of patients, whose consent to be so questioned had first been obtained by the local hospital authorities. These enquiries revealed that Dr Anderton had not obtained consent from a number of patients for their involvement in a clinical trial and, worse, that he had required his personal assistant to sign that she had witnessed non-existent signatures from patients from whom Dr Anderton had purportedly obtained consent. His case went before the GMC during the summer of 1997: he too was found guilty of serious professional misconduct and his name was erased from the medical register.

Two further cases will never be fully documented because they involved doctors who died prematurely – in one case the coroner recorded that death was due to suicide, and in the other the coroner reached an open verdict. In both cases, the fraud discovered was multiple and very extensive. The doctors involved had gone to extreme lengths to disguise the nature of their fraudulent activities and had thus hoodwinked clinical trial monitors and auditors who had not detected anything amiss. Original patient records were themselves fabricated in one case, and a vast 'library' of spare ECGs, presumably performed on a small number of patients over periods of hours and then divided up, were drawn upon in the other. Hundreds of consent forms were forged, with signatures varying considerably, but none of them being the signatures of patients purported to be involved in the various studies.

Other cases are known where independent ethics committee (IEC) approval has been forged (Anonymous, 1996), patients have been put into several studies at once without the sponsors' knowledge, nurses have been required to recruit patients with disregard to inclusion or exclusion criteria, and investigators have sampled blinded material themselves in an attempt to unblind it.

THE SHARING OF INFORMATION

One of the most frequently reported problems arising from the detection of suspected fraud is deciding what to do with the information that has been gathered. Might there be other cases of suspected fraud that other companies have detected from the same investigator, but is it right and proper to contact other companies at random to raise such queries? And would company pharmaceutical physicians be laying themselves open to the laws of libel or defamation if they suggested to others that a doctor might be acting fraudulently?

The ABPI working party referred to above considered these questions at length, and concluded that it would be in the public interest for pharmaceutical physicians to report to an independent third party any serious concerns which they may have, in good faith, regarding a specific investigator. This third party was appropriately considered to be the Medical Director of the ABPI, who has subsequently received most of the information from individual companies leading to action by the GMC. The current ABPI Medical Director, who shares this information in total confidence with his predecessor, the author of this chapter, is in a position to answer a query from another pharmaceutical physician who has doubts about an investigator on whether or not any information has already been submitted, regarding a suspect investigator. No active dissemination of information by the ABPI Medical Director or his predecessor ever occurs, but he is in a position to answer 'Yes' or 'No', when asked. He is also in a position to advise companies when, in his opinion, the accumulated evidence reported from more than one company creates a strong enough case to submit to the GMC, even if the evidence from one company alone does not.

CONCLUSIONS

In a climate that is increasingly critical of research processes, particularly those involving the biosciences, the possibility of fraud occurring must be clearly recognised by those whose responsibility it is to maintain standards. Furthermore, it is essential that those responsible for sponsoring research, at whatever level, and wherever located, should take forthright action not only to prevent fraud from occurring wherever possible, but also to detect and investigate it if it does occur, and to prosecute anyone who is guilty of fraud.

Every organisation responsible for sponsoring clinical research should therefore be reminded of its obligations under the principles of GCP, and should be required to state its commitment to reporting all cases of fraud and to taking appropriate action. Every such organisation should introduce SOPs for handling suspected fraud, and these should cover the following items at least:

- A clear statement of the organisation's policy towards the handling of suspected fraud.
- A stated policy that any cause for concern regarding suspected fraud must be referred to the medical director or other appropriate senior or independent person at the earliest possible stage.
- Clear guidelines defining the path to be followed if fraud is suspected, culminating in the appropriate prosecution of the investigator if the suspicions are proved to be justified.
- Clear guidelines as to the right of appeal if a complainant feels that his/her concern is being inappropriately addressed within the organisation, so that the 'whistle-blower' is appropriately protected.

Every person involved in clinical research, be they a monitor, an auditor, a statistician, a medical adviser, a medical director, a head of department, a co-investigator, a company or health service chief executive or a university vice-chancellor, should be committed to such a policy and to its publicity, not least to act as a deterrent, in a determination to stamp out fraud in clinical research, as far as is humanly possible. Every international company, every regulatory authority and every individual pharmaceutical physician should strive to ensure that there is an effective mechanism in place, in every country, by which anyone who commits fraud can be summarily dealt with. Only the utmost vigour in applying this policy will be successful; but it is in the ultimate interests of patient safety that this must happen.

REFERENCES

Andersen, D, Attrup, L, Axelsen, N and Riis, P (1992). *Scientific Honesty and Good Scientific Practice*, Danish Medical Research Council, Copenhagen.
Anonymous (1988). GMC professional conduct committee. *Br Med J* **296**, 306.

Anonymous (1991). Doctor struck off register for drug test misconduct. *The Scotsman*, 11 December.

Anonymous (1995). Consultant struck off for fraudulent claims. *Br Med J* **310**, 1554.

Anonymous (1996). Bias doctor who forged key letter keeps his job. *Manchester Evening News*, 14 September.

Anonymous (1997a). Medical discipline committee takes actions. *ORI Newsletter* **5**, 7.

Anonymous (1997b). Case summary. *ORI Newsletter* **5**, 4.

Campbell, D (1997). Medicine needs its MI5. *Br Med J* **315**, 1677–1680.

Committee for Proprietary Medicinal Products (CPMP) Working Party on Efficacy of Medicinal Products (1991). *Good Clinical Practice for Trials on Medicinal Products in the European Community* (111/3976/88–EN Final), European Commission, Brussels.

Dillner, L (1991). GMC gets tough with fraudulent doctors. *Br Med J* **303**, 1493.

Dyer, O (1996). GP struck off for fraud in drug trials. *Br Med J* **312**, 798.

Dyer, C (1997). Consultant struck off over research fraud. *Br Med J* **315**, 205.

Friedman, PJ (1990). Correcting the literature following fraudulent publication. *JAMA* **263**, 1416–1419.

Hone, J (1993). Combatting fraud and misconduct in medical research. *Scrip Magazine* (Mar), 14–15.

ICH Guideline (1996). *Topic E6: Good Clinical Practice – Consolidated Guideline*, International Federation of Pharmaceutical Manufacturers Associations, Geneva (Issued as CPMP/ICH/135/95).

LaFollette, MC (1992). *Stealing into Print: Fraud, Plagiarism, and Misconduct in Scientific Publishing*, University of California Press, Los Angeles.

Lock, SP (1988). Misconduct in medical research: does it exist in Britain? *Br Med J* **297**, 1531–1535.

Lock, SP (1990). Research fraud: discouraging the others. *Br Med J* **301**, 1348.

Lock, SP (1995). Lessons from the Pearce affair. *Br Med J* **310**, 1547–1548.

Lock, S and Wells, F (1996). *Fraud and Misconduct in Medical Research, 2nd edn*, BMJ Publishing Group, London.

Medical Research Council (1998). *Guidelines on Fraud and Misconduct in Research*, Medical Research Council, London.

Royal College of Physicians of Edinburgh (2000). Joint Consensus Conference on Misconduct in Biomedical Research. *Proc R Coll Physic Edinb* **30** (Suppl. 7), 1–26.

Royal College of Physicians of London (1991). *Report on Fraud and Misconduct in Medical Research*, Royal College of Physicians, London.

Smith, R (1997). Misconduct in research: editors respond. *Br Med J* **315**, 201–202.

Swan, N (1996). Baron Munchausen at the lab bench? In: Lock, S and Wells, F (Eds), *Fraud and Misconduct in Medical Research, 2nd edn*, BMJ Publishing Group, London, pp. 128–143.

Wells, FO (1994). Fraud and misconduct in clinical research. In: Griffin, JP, O'Grady, J and Wells, FO (Eds), *The Textbook of Pharmaceutical Medicine*, Queens University, Belfast, pp. 341–355.

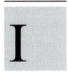

I

World Medical Association Declaration of Helsinki

Ethical Principles for Medical Research Involving Human Subjects

Adopted by the 18th WMA General Assembly Helsinki, Finland, June 1964 and amended by the 29th WMA General Assembly, Tokyo, Japan, October 1975, 35th WMA General Assembly, Venice, Italy, October 1983, 41st WMA General Assembly, Hong Kong, September 1989, 48th WMA General Assembly, Somerset West, Republic of South Africa, October 1996, and the 52nd WMA General Assembly, Edinburgh, Scotland, October 2000

A. INTRODUCTION

1. The World Medical Association has developed the Declaration of Helsinki as a statement of ethical principles to provide guidance to physicians and other participants in medical research involving human subjects. Medical research involving human subjects includes research on identifiable human material or identifiable data.

2. It is the duty of the physician to promote and safeguard the health of the people. The physician's knowledge and conscience are dedicated to the fulfillment of this duty.

3. The Declaration of Geneva of the World Medical Association binds the physician with the words, 'The health of my patient will be my first consideration', and the International Code of Medical Ethics declares that, 'A physician shall act only in the patient's interest when providing medical care which might have the effect of weakening the physical and mental condition of the patient'.

4. Medical progress is based on research which ultimately must rest in part on experimentation involving human subjects.

5. In medical research on human subjects, considerations related to the well-being of the human subject should take precedence over the interests of science and society.

6. The primary purpose of medical research involving human subjects is to improve prophylactic, diagnostic and therapeutic procedures and the understanding of the aetiology and pathogenesis of disease. Even the best proven prophylactic, diagnostic, and therapeutic methods must continuously be challenged through research for their effectiveness, efficiency, accessibility and quality.

7. In current medical practice and in medical research, most prophylactic, diagnostic and therapeutic procedures involve risks and burdens.

8. Medical research is subject to ethical standards that promote respect for all human beings and protect their health and rights. Some research populations are vulnerable and need special protection. The particular needs of the economically and medically disadvantaged must be recognized. Special attention is also required for those who cannot give or refuse consent for themselves, for those who may be subject to giving consent under duress, for those who will not benefit personally from the research and for those for whom the research is combined with care.

9. Research Investigators should be aware of the ethical, legal and regulatory requirements for research on human subjects in their own countries as well as applicable international requirements. No national ethical, legal or regulatory requirement should be allowed to reduce or eliminate any of the protections for human subjects set forth in this Declaration.

B. BASIC PRINCIPLES FOR ALL MEDICAL RESEARCH

10. It is the duty of the physician in medical research to protect the life, health, privacy, and dignity of the human subject.

11. Medical research involving human subjects must conform to generally accepted scientific principles, be based on a thorough knowledge of the scientific literature, other relevant sources of information, and on adequate laboratory and, where appropriate, animal experimentation.

12. Appropriate caution must be exercised in the conduct of research which may affect the environment, and the welfare of animals used for research must be respected.

13. The design and performance of each experimental procedure involving human subjects should be clearly formulated in an experimental protocol. This protocol should be submitted for consideration, comment, guidance, and where appropriate, approval to a specially appointed ethical review committee, which must be independent of the investigator, the sponsor or any other kind of undue influence. This independent committee should be in conformity with the laws and regulations of the country in which the research experiment is performed. The committee has the right to monitor ongoing trials. The researcher has the obligation to provide monitoring information to the committee, especially any serious adverse events. The researcher should also submit to the committee, for review, information regarding funding, sponsors, institutional affiliations, other potential conflicts of interest and incentives for subjects.

14. The research protocol should always contain a statement of the ethical considerations involved and should indicate that there is compliance with the principles enunciated in this Declaration.

15. Medical research involving human subjects should be conducted only by scientifically qualified persons and under the supervision of a clinically competent medical person. The responsibility for the human subject must always rest with a medically qualified person and never rest on the subject of the research, even though the subject has given consent.

16. Every medical research project involving human subjects should be preceded by careful assessment of predictable risks and burdens in comparison with foreseeable benefits to the subject or to others. This does not preclude the participation of healthy volunteers in medical research. The design of all studies should be publicly available.

17. Physicians should abstain from engaging in research projects involving human subjects unless they are confident that the risks involved have been adequately assessed and can be satisfactorily managed. Physicians should cease any investigation if the risks are found to outweigh the potential benefits or if there is conclusive proof of positive and beneficial results.

18. Medical research involving human subjects should only be conducted if the importance of the objective outweighs the inherent risks and burdens to the subject. This is especially important when the human subjects are healthy volunteers.

19. Medical research is only justified if there is a reasonable likelihood that the populations in which the research is carried out stand to benefit from the results of the research.

20. The subjects must be volunteers and informed participants in the research project.

21. The right of research subjects to safeguard their integrity must always be respected. Every precaution should be taken to respect the privacy of the subject, the confidentiality of the patient's information and to minimize the impact of the study on the subject's physical and mental integrity and on the personality of the subject.

22. In any research on human beings, each potential subject must be adequately informed of the aims, methods, sources of funding, any possible conflicts of interest, institutional affiliations of the researcher, the anticipated benefits and potential risks of the study and the discomfort it may entail. The subject should be informed of the right to abstain from participation in the study or to withdraw consent to participate at any time without reprisal. After ensuring that the subject has understood the information, the physician should then obtain the subject's freely-given informed consent, preferably in writing. If the consent cannot be obtained in writing, the non-written consent must be formally documented and witnessed.

23. When obtaining informed consent for the research project the physician should be particularly cautious if the subject is in a dependent relationship with the physician or may consent under duress. In that case the informed consent should be obtained by a well-informed physician who is not engaged in the investigation and who is completely independent of this relationship.

24. For a research subject who is legally incompetent, physically or mentally incapable of giving consent or is a legally incompetent minor, the investigator must obtain informed consent from the legally authorized representative in accordance with applicable law. These groups should not be included in research unless the research is necessary to promote the health of the population represented and this research cannot instead be performed on legally competent persons.

25. When a subject deemed legally incompetent, such as a minor child, is able to give assent to decisions about participation in research, the investigator must obtain that assent in addition to the consent of the legally authorized representative.

26. Research on individuals from whom it is not possible to obtain consent, including proxy or advance consent, should be done only if the physical/mental condition that prevents obtaining informed consent is a necessary characteristic of the research population. The specific reasons for involving research subjects with a condition that renders them unable to give informed consent should be stated in the experimental protocol for consideration and approval of the review committee. The protocol should state that consent to remain in the research should be obtained as soon as possible from the individual or a legally authorized surrogate.

27. Both authors and publishers have ethical obligations. In publication of the results of research, the investigators are obliged to preserve the accuracy of the results. Negative as well as positive results should be published or otherwise publicly available. Sources of funding, institutional affiliations and any possible conflicts of interest should be declared in the publication. Reports of experimentation not in accordance with the principles laid down in this Declaration should not be accepted for publication.

C. ADDITIONAL PRINCIPLES FOR MEDICAL RESEARCH COMBINED WITH MEDICAL CARE

28. The physician may combine medical research with medical care, only to the extent that the research is justified by its potential prophylactic, diagnostic or therapeutic value. When medical research is combined with medical care, additional standards apply to protect the patients who are research subjects.

29. The benefits, risks, burdens and effectiveness of a new method should be tested against those of the best current prophylactic, diagnostic, and therapeutic methods. This does not exclude the use of placebo, or no treatment, in studies where no proven prophylactic, diagnostic or therapeutic method exists.

30. At the conclusion of the study, every patient entered into the study should be assured of access to the best proven prophylactic, diagnostic and therapeutic methods identified by the study.

31. The physician should fully inform the patient which aspects of the care are related to the research. The refusal of a patient to participate in a study must never interfere with the patient–physician relationship.

32. In the treatment of a patient, where proven prophylactic, diagnostic and therapeutic methods do not exist or have been ineffective, the physician, with informed consent from the patient, must be free to use unproven or new prophylactic, diagnostic and therapeutic measures, if in the physician's judgement it offers hope of saving life, re-establishing health or alleviating suffering. Where possible, these measures should be made the object of research, designed to evaluate their safety and efficacy. In all cases, new information should be recorded and, where appropriate, published. The other relevant guidelines of this Declaration should be followed.

Index